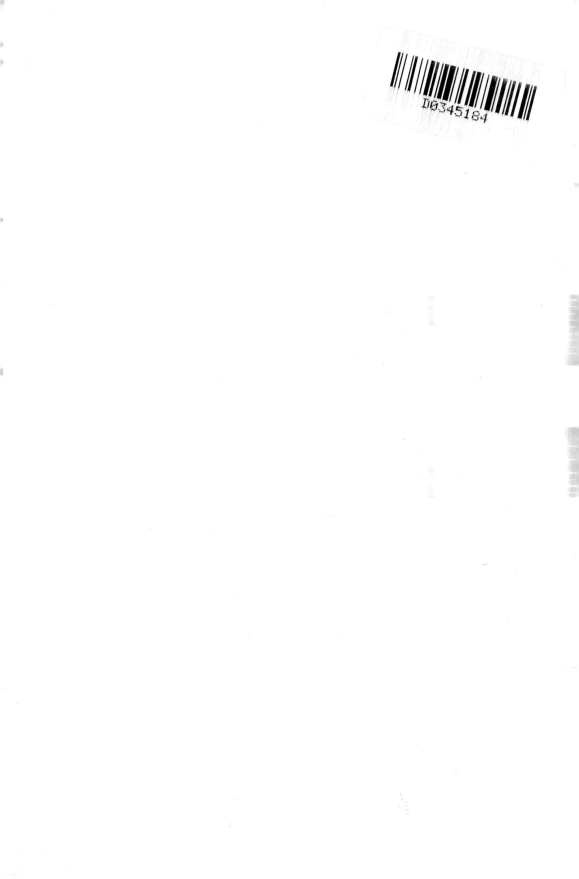

DRUG MUGGERS®

Which Medications Are Robbing

Your Body of Essential Nutrients—

and Natural Ways to Restore Them

SUZY COHEN, RPh

Author of *Diabetes without Drugs* and *The 24-Hour Pharmacist*

RODALE.

Direct online and trade editions published in January 2011.
Direct mail exclusive edition published in July 2011.

All recipes on pages 384–447 (except page 446) © Rodale Inc.

Book design by Christina Gaugler

Library of Congress Cataloging-in-Publication Data
Cohen, Suzy, R. Ph.
    Drug muggers : which medications are robbing your body of essential nutrients—and natural
ways to restore them
        p.   cm.
    Includes bibliographical references and index.
    ISBN 978-1-60529-415-5   direct online hardcover
    ISBN 978-1-60529-416-2   trade paperback
    ISBN 978-1-60961-056-2   direct mail hardcover
    1. Dietary Supplements–Popular works.   2. Nutrition–Popular works.   3. Vitamins–
Popular works.   I. Cohen, Samuel M., 1946-   II. Title.
RM258.5C65   2011
615'.1–dc22   2010040375

    4   6   8   10   9   7   5   3   direct mail hardcover

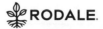

We inspire and enable people to improve their lives and the world around them.
For more of our products visit **rodalestore.com** or call **800-848-4735**.

This book is lovingly dedicated to those who continue to endure each day and know that better times are ahead.

And with great affection and love, this is also for my children, Samara, Michael, and Rachel. You make the sun shine every day!

Contents

Part I: Protect Yourself from Drug Muggers

Part II: Vital Nutrients

Part III: Getting the Most from Your Supplement

Part IV: Where Do I Begin?

Introduction

I emptied my brain into this book. I hope it answers every question you have, even the ones you haven't thought of yet. I'd like to think this book is priceless because I wrote it with the intention of fostering your good health and maybe even saving your life.

In pharmacy school 20-something years ago, I learned about the value of medicine. Through the years I've personally seen the benefits of certain medications that save lives. So I know that when your doctor prescribes medication or when you purchase over-the-counter medications, you take those meds in the sincere hope that they'll help you feel better. Yet, despite that miniature pharmacy in your medicine cabinet, it is entirely possible that you still feel awful. Why is that?

The fact is, you can't cure disease with drugs made of synthetic chemicals, especially when they often suppress your body's ability to produce or use natural, healthy nutrients.

Drugs have an intended effect on the body, but in the process of helping you, they can sometimes put your body in a dangerous state by slowly depleting you of the very nutrients you need to maintain your health and to help you heal. This slow depletion can make you feel miserable. It can even hasten your death. I know we all have to face death one day, but why do something that might make that happen sooner rather than later?

Since I became a pharmacist 22 years ago, I've seen an exponential rise in the use of medications, many of them helpful and necessary, but some of them dangerous and dubious. And I know that when drugs deplete the body of essential nutrients, it's easy to replace them by taking the right kinds of supplements. But most people never hear about what they need to take in order to protect themselves from what I call the drug muggers—medications that rob you of the very nutrients you need in order to produce energy, fend off infections, and live in good health. All this is lunacy!

The vast majority of people take a lot of drugs. It's possible that you are among that number and that you feel okay taking these drugs . . . for now at least. It's also quite possible that you feel just horrible, worse than you did back when you went to the doctor with your original complaint! There's a good chance that the information you receive in this book will fix that problem and help you feel good again. This *Drug Muggers* book is really your solution to side effects.

As a newspaper columnist with many millions of readers, I get a lot of mail. I can't count how many e-mails and letters have just broken my heart. I read so many of them thinking, "This pain and suffering is so needless and is so avoidable!" Because of all those letters, I've written this book, which is intended to protect you and help you find solutions to uncomfortable problems caused by common medications that you take every day. You see, it's essential to replenish what drugs steal from your body, otherwise you could experience side effects and possibly catastrophic health consequences.

If you have to take medicine, then you should know how to stay safer on it. I want to give you and your physician(s) some insight into why you may not be feeling well and why you are plagued with uncomfortable or bizarre side effects, and I hope to provide some clues about the state of your health along with a major "Aha!" Armed with the information in this book, you'll be able to make changes to your drug regimen or reduce symptoms by installing a nutrient security system so you won't be robbed blind by drug muggers. In fact, if you turn to the Punch List, which begins on page 92, it will take you only a moment to look up your medications and find out what nutrients you need to be paying special attention to.

I've always wanted to help people understand their bodies and feel their best, and, with all my heart, I present this book to you. It was really hard getting people to understand the concept at first, and getting it recognized by a publisher so that it could be sold to you in bookstores nationwide. Thankfully, Rodale has seen the value of this information, for which I am most grateful. This book could be a lifesaver for you or someone you love. It allows you to remain compliant with your medication regimen while offering side-effect solutions.

I am known as America's Most Trusted Pharmacist, and I am serious about helping you. I put my heart and soul into this book, and I sincerely hope it is of service to you.

A Word of Caution

Drug Muggers is intended to help you regain health and vitality. However, it's just a book, and there are limitations with any book. First off, not every single drug is listed in it, as there are thousands. Finding a clinical study that discusses the depletion impact of every single drug is not humanly possible, and even if it were, I'm not the human for that job.

What I have done is fill these pages with the most popular medications in use today—a thorough listing of the leading drug muggers in the marketplace. In a few cases, I've included all of the drugs that fit into a particular class, even if there was evidence of depletion impact in only a few of the drug muggers in that class. For example, I may include four different acid blockers because they are in the same drug category, although it's possible that only three of those four drugs actually have studies that demonstrate their depletion impact. Basically, I have applied the commonsense principle, "If it walks like a duck and quacks like a duck, it's a duck!" I believe that if a drug hangs with the drug muggers, then it probably is one. Perhaps some might say that I'm painting with too broad a brush, but where your health and well-being are concerned, I think that the best approach is to err on the cautious side.

As with any book that addresses health, individual safety must be the top priority. So please be advised that my nutrient dosages are only general guidelines, not gospel. If a suggested dosage doesn't seem like the right one for you, then you should determine which one is. If your doctor suggests taking a lower (or higher) dosage, then follow his instruction because he knows your medical history. A few of the dosages I suggest are extremely high by some standards (like the USDA's Recommended Daily Allowance), and they aren't right for everyone. Excessive nutritional supplementation can be harmful to certain people, and I can't tell from here if you're one of them, so follow your instincts and comply with your doctor's advice.

I did not include chemotherapy on the drug mugger lists even though these medications can deplete many nutrients. They are not here because some oncologists ask you to avoid dietary supplements totally during treatment. So if you are receiving chemo or have used it in the past, ask your oncologist and other practitioners exactly what they would like you to take (if anything).

One more thing: I am not suggesting that the depletion impact of a drug mugger is the cause of your illness. You must discuss every aspect of your personal health with your team of practitioners. I am not a doctor; I am just a nerdy pharmacist who likes to write and eat chocolate. I have my heart in the right place, but I cannot assume the burden of treating you, nor can I be responsible for what happens to you if you take my advice. It is not my intention to diagnose, treat, cure, or prevent any disease. I just want to share information. Finally, my statements have not been evaluated by the US Food and Drug Administration.

How to Use This Book

If you are familiar with my syndicated column "Dear Pharmacist" and my other books, you know that I write in simple terms. Big, complicated words give most people a headache. In this book, I've done my best to keep concepts simple, but I'm aware that many of you may want to bring *Drug Muggers* to your physician's office to get approval for certain nutrients you want to take. Your doctor may scratch his head and say that he's never heard about "drug muggers." This is your cue to hand him my book. The concept is real, but the term was invented by my husband, Sam, who came up with it during a flash of brilliance (which occasionally happens if I bake him banana nut bread). I have offered a few deeper scientific explanations within the book for the benefit of physicians, nurses, chiropractors, acupuncturists, naturopaths, and other practitioners who may be seeking more background.

If you have only a few minutes, then just look up your medication in the Punch List, which begins on page 92. If you have more time to spare, then read this book cover to cover. You can do it in bits and pieces rather than all at once, since there are 512 pages. Let me just tell you now: It's okay with me if *Drug Muggers* becomes your bathroom reading material. Splendid. I understand that this may be the only 5 minutes you have to sit down all by yourself without a kid in tow or a boss breathing down your neck.

The index is comprehensive. Your medications are referenced by both generic and brand name. I've even indexed symptoms of common disorders that you may be dealing with. For example, "Heart disease" and "Depression" are indexed. I wrote a fascinating section on lifestyle drug muggers as well, so don't miss Chapter 3: Lifestyle Drug Muggers.

When my editors reviewed *Drug Muggers*, they said that they felt compelled to take every single nutrient I wrote about. I don't recommend that you do that. Rather, read Chapter 27: Where Do I Start to Stop a Drug Mugger?, to help you identify the health concerns you should address first.

Chapter 28 explains how to jump-start your healing with a 7-day body tune-up. I'm sure you'll be hungry after reading so much helpful advice, so browse Chapter 29 to find 100 or so nutrient-dense recipes you'll want to add to your diet this week.

To help you digest all of this information, I've divided the book into parts. Part I gives you some helpful general information about drug muggers, what they are and how to protect yourself. Part II provides information on the vital nutrients that drugs can steal from your body and why it's so important for you to replace them. Part III gives you some general information on how to purchase and use top-quality supplements. Part IV tells you how to get started and how to stay well with good nutrition.

This is also a good place to tell you not to stop taking your medications, although I'm sure you are tempted to do so every time you find your medication on a drug mugger list. My purpose in writing this book is to help you stay safe on your medications if you must take them. It's your side-effect solution. It's not to make you stop taking them. Now, if you seriously want to try natural remedies or use integrative medicine, which combines both natural and holistic options, refer to my other books, visit my Web site, and be sure to sign up for my free e-newsletter, which will update you each month. Speak to your physician about your intentions and any changes to your health regimen.

www.SuzyCohen.com

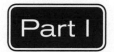

Part I

Protect Yourself from Drug Muggers

What Is a Drug Mugger?
And Why Should You Care?

As a licensed pharmacist for 22 years, I have a confession to make: Some medications scare me! Don't get me wrong. As someone who has been dispensing prescription and over-the-counter (OTC) drugs for many years, I have a deep respect for what they can do. Pharmaceuticals can ease your pain, help you breathe better, keep you from having a seizure, and alleviate allergy symptoms that make your life miserable. The list of life-enhancing benefits goes on and on and on.

But—and, oh boy, is this a big but—while fixing the one problem that you take the pharmaceutical to fix, that drug is likely robbing you of life-sustaining nutrients in the process. Many, in fact most, of the medicines you're taking have the potential to steal the life out of you slowly. How does that grab you? The ultimate effects of this nutrient depletion explain everything from nagging aches to life-threatening diseases.

Millions of people are slipping through these drug-caused nutrient deficiency cracks as they get sicker and sicker each year. The system is so out of whack that people think it's normal to see eight or nine different physicians for an ailment that eludes diagnosis. And there's a good chance that the ailment can be traced back to a single nutritional deficiency!

While drugs often do provide blessed symptom relief, in most cases they don't actually cure the disease. By virtue of the fact that they steal nutrients from your system or prevent their absorption, they could even be causing more diseases. As you will soon see, if you run low on even one vital nutrient, you can experience a veritable cascade of uncomfortable side effects. Then these will likely be diagnosed as a new disease, for which you will be handed yet another pricey prescription.

Sad to say, you'll get on a medication merry-go-round, and it's a hard ride to get off of. That's why I wrote this book. I want to empower you to learn what is causing your problems and to help you feel better. Also, knowing what nutrients to replenish will help you to stay compliant with your medications, and this will please your physician, too.

Let's talk about nutrients and their dosages, because you will soon find out while supplement shopping that dosages vary widely from brand to brand. You may be afraid to take more than the US Recommended Dietary Allowance, which I sometimes suggest you do, so allow me to give you a primer on the RDA and dosages in general.

The RDI Is Not the Be-All and End-All

In my professional opinion, the Reference Dietary Intake (RDI) is just a starting place. It's not the be-all and end-all of good nutrition. The suggested amounts for each nutrient are definitely not enough to provide optimal health or offset the drug mugging effects of your medicines and lifestyle. To tell you the truth, I don't pay much attention to the RDIs on labels because I don't eat a lot of foods that come with labels. That's because I lean toward vegetarianism. (If you do, too, then please eat intelligently, because many vegetarians do not know how to eat properly. They quickly run out of important vitamins, amino acids, and minerals, among them vitamin B_{12}, L-carnitine, and iron.)

Fruits and veggies don't come with a food label stating the RDI. I assure you that these foods are highly nutritious even if they don't have a label to prove it. Not only are plant foods good for you, but they also do away with the compulsive need to read the RDI and make sure you're getting it.

I am bent on keeping a nutritious kitchen, so you won't find many canned foods in my pantry. I keep a can of ravioli for my dad because he loves it and has stayed alive for 80-something years despite eating it. It would take you an hour to find this can. I realize that I'll be in serious trouble if another hurricane barrels through Florida, where I live, but canned, boxed, or highly processed foods are simply not part of my family's diet. This does not mean that you won't find chocolate-covered macadamias if you search hard enough. Okay, fine, there are some in the top drawer of my desk in case of an unlikely emergency, like if my computer freezes or umm, I umm . . . develop writer's block . . . or misspell a werd :-).

I do not normally buy, eat, or store foods that have lengthy nutrition labels on them. We as humans are at the top of the food chain, so we have the most highly developed brains and impressive cognitive function. This enables us to make a choice to eat consciously, or not. If we all ate organic fruits and vegetables, we could get by with fewer drugs. There would be no stress about whether or not we met the RDI for a nutrient. We would be getting enough of each nutrient naturally.

This whole rant isn't to nag you. I do it because I care. I've read thousands of readers' e-mails and letters over the years. I know that many people are concerned about improving their diets, losing weight, and avoiding a heart attack or diabetes. Many of my readers must take medications that are drug muggers, sometimes multiple drug muggers. Perhaps you are among this number. I can imagine how you feel, taking so much medicine and feeling worse and not knowing what else to do or who else to ask.

This is like being stuck in the middle of a giant whirlpool and not being able to get out. As a pharmacist, I want to get as many people as possible on the right track of taking fewer prescribed drugs. My point is that if you're eating really well—and I know you can—then it won't matter much what the fine print on your food labels says. The same goes with your vitamin or dietary supplement. It may have the RDI listed on it, but if you are being mugged by a drug, you are going to need much more than the RDI suggests. Let me tell you a good story.

A woman came to the pharmacy 1 month after I had suggested that she take additional vitamin B_6 to help her with her carpal tunnel syndrome. She had been taking birth control pills, which I knew to be a drug mugger of vitamin B_6. She told me she wasn't doing any better on the B_6 she had picked up and showed me the bottle. It was a popular multivitamin that contained 2 mg of B_6. I told her it was abysmally low for her needs, but she insisted that it met 100 percent of the DV and pointed out the ingredient label to prove it. We went round and round for a few minutes until I walked her over to the vitamin aisle and showed her a bottle of B_6 that contained 50 mg and suggested she try that for another month. She happily returned a month later to tell me she was totally relieved of her pain.

I'm one of the health-care professionals who happens to think that the RDI is just a minimum requirement that should keep you from developing a deficiency of a nutrient and perhaps dying of that deficiency. For example, the RDI for vitamin C will keep you from developing and dying of scurvy. The recommended amount of vitamin B_1 will prevent you from dying of beriberi. The suggested amount of vitamin D will keep you from developing rickets, and the list goes on. This leaves me deflated and thinking, "That's it? I'm meeting 100 percent of the DV and all this means is that I won't die from a deficiency?" Sheesh! There is a huge gap between suffering from a deficiency and being healthy, isn't there? I choose health. That's why I want more than what the DV recommends. For more on Daily Values, see Chapter 26.

Science Looks at Pharmaceuticals

The idea of helping people replenish lost nutrients didn't just suddenly dawn on me; *Drug Muggers* was years in the making. Many other scientists studied this topic before I did. As a pharmacist, I have made it my business to pay attention to every medication on the market and all the interactions that may occur with them. I also watch for news about medications and food or herb interactions. Because I specialize in medication and herbal interactions, I keep files on certain drugs and on all those black box warnings that the FDA comes out with every now and then. A black box warning is basically a warning to physicians stating the possibility of a particularly dangerous side effect. Keeping files and computer documents about such things is part of my professional life. I haven't included every single clinical research study or trial in this book because it would make it very long indeed. When it is most interesting, however, I have included certain citations in each chapter, but most of my references are in the back of this book so you can see them for yourself at your leisure. The fact is that drugs cause side effects, and many do so by stealing vital nutrients from our bodies. I'm proud to share all this information with you in the coming pages.

My information doesn't come only from studies, however. It also comes from my heart. I want you to know that I used to work in nursing homes, where I saw firsthand the horror of living under the shadow of disease and the negative side effects of multiple medications. I so wanted to have a positive impact on people's lives, and I was saddened that many of the medications that came from my pharmacy did more harm than good. Before I teach you how to restore balance to your own life, I need you to master the basic definition of a drug mugger.

Drug mugger: *noun* An over-the-counter or prescribed medication, food, herb, medical condition, or lifestyle choice that is capable of robbing your body's natural stores of an important vitamin, mineral, or hormone.

Usage: Acid blockers are drug muggers of zinc. Smoking is a drug mugger of vitamin C.

Drug mugging: *adjective* Of or relating to a drug mugger.

Usage: My legs are cramping; I could be suffering from the drug mugging effects of my cholesterol medication.

The Nutrient Depletion Effect of Drugs Is Well Known

The drug mugging effect is real. It's not debatable or something that scientists are still trying to figure out. Even though there are hundreds of published articles and studies regarding nutrient depletion by drugs, millions of people continue to suffer. This is because the information has not been widely disseminated. Most physicians have not studied it, and many of them do not even know that depletion occurs.

All those drug commercials on TV bother me. They paint miraculous pictures of medicine, but if you don't let yourself get distracted by the playful images, you might hear the litany of side effects of each new drug. The term *side effect* sounds like it's incidental to the main, desired effect. But I think a side effect, especially if it's a really serious one, is really another main effect that happens to be uncomfortable. Every drug has them. It's important to compare the risks to the benefits before beginning drug therapy or any treatment plan, for that matter.

Drugs are advertised to fix one problem, but in reality (as opposed to what's on TV) they often manage to disrupt other aspects of cellular function. That's common knowledge in my circle of health-care practitioners. Unfortunately, it's not common knowledge to most people. So I need you to fully understand that the information in this book will help to reduce your risk of developing uncomfortable side effects from the medication you take.

Side effects (drug mugging symptoms) may not show up right away. Some can occur months to years after taking a drug. For example, you can take a particular medicine for years and then suddenly have a heart attack. Was your heart diseased to begin with? Maybe. But it's also possible that it was weakened by a nutritional deficiency that went overlooked for too long, a nutrient deficiency caused by a drug you were taking to protect your heart. (I'm referring here to drugs that deplete your body of coenzyme Q10 [CoQ10], a nutrient that helps your heart do its job. You'll learn about this in detail further along in this chapter and in Chapter 8.) This kind of tragedy is completely avoidable as far as I'm concerned. All you have to do is take CoQ10 if you take a drug listed in that chapter.

As you turn the pages, I'd love for you to say, "Aha! I just figured out why I feel so bad. Now I know exactly what to take to feel better!" For pennies a day, you can get your life back! As you read this book, you'll be able to recognize whether you are deficient in a particular nutrient; you can then start to put the right foods on your plate or take absurdly inexpensive vitamins to feel better. Okay, some of the supplements I recommend may cost a little more than you're used to paying for vitamins. But if you compare their cost to the bills for medical care that you won't have to pay down the line, they are, indeed, absurdly inexpensive. Let's take a brief look at some so-called diseases that may be related to the drug mugging effect.

Depression, osteoporosis, and irregular heartbeat: These can all be caused by a deficiency of the mineral magnesium. Common drug muggers of magnesium include female hormones, diuretics, raloxifene (Evista), anti-inflammatories, and aspirin.

Bald patches, loss of taste or smell, erectile dysfunction, and chronic diarrhea: All these conditions may result from zinc deficiency. Common drug muggers for zinc include anti-inflammatories, antibiotics, antacids, ulcer and heartburn medications, diuretics, and estrogen drugs used for birth control and menopause.

Leg cramps, muscle spasms, memory loss, and fatigue: Any of these conditions may develop from a deficiency of CoQ10 (ubiquinone). This life-sustaining antioxidant gets demolished by hundreds of medications, including statin cholesterol drugs, metformin, antidepressants, beta-blockers, and diuretics.

Cataracts, macular degeneration, liver problems, and high levels of the heart-attack-promoting substance homocysteine: Any of these conditions could be tied to low glutathione, a powerful antioxidant needed to get rid of poisons in your body. Acetaminophen is a possible drug mugger of glutathione. (Did you know that taking acetaminophen every day could contribute to vision loss later in life?)

Weight gain, depression, fatigue, anemia, nerve pain, and a sensation of pins and needles: Any of these could be related to a deficiency of one or more B vitamins. Your stash gets depleted by female hormones (used for birth control and to relieve the symptoms of menopause), alcohol, antacids, ulcer medications, diuretics, raloxifene (Evista), cholestyramine, and diabetes drugs.

Delving Deeper: The Statin Dilemma

I'd like to give you a couple of good examples of how the drug mugging effect develops. So I'm going to start with one of the most prescribed classes of pills on the planet, the statins. These drugs are used to lower cholesterol and to reduce the risk of heart attack. Many people have to take them, physician's orders. But because I am a pharmacist, I'm aware that often people secretly stop taking these drugs because they feel bad when they take them. The statin class of drugs is very effective at reducing cholesterol. They do their work in the liver by suppressing an enzyme called HMG-CoA reductase. When you block that enzyme, you also block the production of CoQ10, a nutrient involved in energy production in every single cell in your body. So statins are drug muggers of CoQ10. It's important to note that dozens of other medications also suppress CoQ10.

Why is that important? A deficiency of CoQ10 can cause you to feel very uncomfortable. It can even be deadly for some people. Here's what can happen when you run too low on CoQ10.

- Leg cramps and heavy, achy legs (The doctors may diagnose this as restless leg syndrome and give you another medication for it.)

- High blood sugar (You may get a diagnosis of diabetes.)

- Impotence (The doctor may tell you that you have erectile dysfunction.)

- Shortness of breath or fatigue (You may be prescribed Provigil or another stimulating drug, or assumed to be hypothyroid and started on the thyroid medication Synthroid.)

- Depression and memory loss (You could be told that you have major depressive disorder, dementia, or the beginnings of Alzheimer's disease.)

- Liver enzyme abnormalities (Your liver may be slowly shutting down. For real.)

- Cardiac arrhythmias or palpitations (You will be given medications to treat coronary artery disease or heart failure and offered ablation and a pacemaker, too!)

Are you scared? If you see yourself in that list, do you realize that you may simply be deficient in just one important nutrient? Are you scared that your physician hasn't recognized the fact that your declining health may be because you are a victim of the drug mugging effect? Are you scared because your doctor may not be receptive to your request to look into the situation and give you her blessings to buy an affordable OTC nutrient supplement and see what happens? Are you aggravated because you've been bounced around from clinic to clinic and churned through the system like a cash cow?

In today's pill-happy society, most physicians look to the prescription pad for answers instead of delving deeper into why their patients have particular symptoms. I'm happy to report that an increasing number of physicians and other health-care providers are becoming aware of this problem. And many are willing to work with you, monitoring and supervising your progress as you try supplements that could make all the difference in your health.

Fortunately, you have *Drug Muggers* in your hands, so now you know that all you have to do is replenish your cells with what they are starving for. In our example of statins and CoQ10 depletion, all you have to do to better protect yourself is take this relatively inexpensive nutrient sold over the counter. That beats having to take four different medications for all the new diseases that could develop as a result of not replenishing your CoQ10.

Naturally, I want you to ask your doctor for her blessing, because if you have any of the symptoms or diseases listed above, you need to get approval to take any new supplements. I am not a doctor. I am just shining a flashlight for you to illuminate a brighter path of health. Are you with me? Great!

Delving Deeper: The Hormone Replacement Therapy Dilemma

Now let's talk about something that hits close to home for many women. All those top-selling prescription drugs for hormone replacement therapy (HRT) or contraception are among the most dangerous drug muggers I can think of because their nutrient depletion effects on your body range from fatigue and weight gain all the way to stroke and heart attack. But many women suffer so much from low hormone levels after menopause that they have to take these drugs.

The information I provide in the coming pages should help you over-come some (if not all) of the damage these types of hormones have caused you, whether you've just started taking them or you've been on them for many years. I'll teach you about the nutrients you need to replenish what the drug mugger stole.

If you are taking a prescribed hormone for hot flashes, what I call a menopausal mugger, or contraception, you are getting a synthetic form of estrogen, usually estradiol, or ethinyl estradiol; however, there are other types of hormones used in these drugs. Now let's take a look at some of the nutrients that get mugged and what can happen to you as a result.

Iodine Deficiency

Too little iodine can be catastrophic to the breasts, thyroid gland, and immune system. (For men, drug muggers of iodine impact the prostate gland.) Iodine is also needed for fertility, so it is essential in pregnancy. Does it shock you to learn that estradiol decreases your cells' ability to take up iodine? You need iodine to make thyroid hormone. So it makes sense that iodine deficiency has been implicated in Hashimoto's disease (a con-dition of low thyroid hormone), fibrocystic breast disease, breast cancer (and prostate cancer), uterine fibroids, ovarian cysts, brain fog, diabetes, heart arrhythmias, and the inability to detoxify the body following expo-sure to mercury, fluoride, and bromide.

Magnesium Deficiency

Oral contraceptives can also wipe out your stash of magnesium, making you very sick because it's involved in about 300 metabolic pathways in the body. Of all the "diseases" you might be labeled with (and that really relate to magnesium deficiency), the most debilitating ones are depression and/or anxiety, high blood pressure, and a chronic pain condition.

Let's start with depression. You need magnesium to make the happy brain hormones serotonin, norepinephrine, and dopamine. If you run low on these hormones, life looks gloomier and you become susceptible to anxiety and panic attacks. In a misguided effort to remedy the situa-tion, your brain releases chemicals that cause you to crave sweets and carbohydrates (candy bars, cookies, chocolate), because carbohydrates increase serotonin levels.

Your blood pressure can rise, causing your doctor to diagnose essential hypertension, and this terrible condition increases your risk for heart attack and stroke. It works like this: Magnesium relaxes your blood vessels, allowing for easier blood flow. When you're magnesium deficient, your blood vessels constrict. As you experience the squeeze, your blood pressure rises.

Running low on magnesium can also cause widespread aches, pain, spasms, and tenderness in the body. You may be told you have fibromyalgia or arthritis. Another type of pain related to magnesium deficiency comes in the form of migraines and chronic headaches. Are you starting to understand how taking one drug (like HRT or birth control pills) can cause you to develop all kinds of new "diseases"?

Zinc Deficiency

When you run out of zinc, you may gain weight, develop hypothyroidism (too little thyroid hormone), experience chronic diarrhea, or lose interest in sex. You may also get sick more frequently. That's because zinc plays an important role in immune function, and without enough of it, you lose your defense system, most notably some of your T-helper cells and natural killer cells. Ultimately this means that you are less able to defend yourself from pathogens in your environment.

Zinc is involved in the creation of thyroid hormone. You need it to activate your hormone T_4, which is a precursor to the active, useful form called T_3; and you need this T_3 to enter the cell, where it wakes you up. With low zinc, you may develop hypothyroidism, which brings with it hair loss, weight gain, feeling cold all the time, depression, thinning eyebrows, irritability, heart palpitations, weakness, insomnia, fatigue, chronic pain, brittle nails, and dull, dry hair and skin.

Lowered zinc levels cause women to stop producing testosterone, the "manly" hormone. You may not realize this, but women need testosterone, too, for sex drive, just in smaller amounts. So low zinc means lowered testosterone, and low T means less interest in sex. It's ironic to me that oral contraceptives, sometimes taken to promote sexual freedom, can cause a woman to lose interest in sex altogether! It's like a cruel twist of fate. The pills make you able to have sex whenever you want to, but you no longer want to!

B Vitamin Deficiency

HRT drugs and contraception can cause your Bs to crash. I'm referring to all of the B vitamins here (think B complex). There is a more complete discussion of each individual B vitamin later in the book, but for now, know that B vitamins are involved in a gazillion biochemical reactions throughout the body, from head to toe. Generally speaking, when you run low on B vitamins, you can start to feel really bad, and very quickly, too, within a matter of weeks. You may notice feelings of depression, poor memory, muscle pain, spasms, and weakness or stiffness in your muscles and joints. You may feel nerve tingling, burning sensations, and numbness. You may get more frequent headaches, fatigue, and nausea. These are just a few of dozens of symptoms that can happen as a result of B vitamin deficiency.

You may also hold on to weight. Thiamine (B_1) works in tandem with the other B vitamins to break down proteins, carbohydrates, and fats and turn them into energy. All the Bs play some role in turning food into energy, so when you take a drug mugger of the B vitamins, you may find it harder to lose a few pounds because your metabolism has slowed down.

B vitamins nourish the nerves and help you form myelin, the protective coating around your nerve cells. When you run low on B vitamins, your nerves get touchy, meaning you may feel pins and needles, numbness, and shock sensations, and you may have a higher propensity to develop conditions like carpal tunnel syndrome or peripheral neuropathy. For more on neuropathy, as well as on natural ways to relieve the pain, refer to my book *Diabetes without Drugs* (Rodale, 2010).

Instead of considering replenishing what the drug mugger stole from you, doctors often prescribe painkillers, anti-inflammatories, and anti-seizure drugs, which dampen these maddening and painful sensations.

Estrogen-containing drugs also have the potential to increase your odds of developing heart attack and stroke by depleting your body's B vitamin stash. Essentially, the lower your B vitamin status, the higher your levels of inflammation-causing chemicals such as homocysteine, C-reactive protein, and interleukins. When these substances get too high, your risk for heart attack and stroke increases dramatically.

Without enough B vitamins, especially folate (vitamin B_9), problems such as abnormal cells in the cervix may occur. In fact, it's possible that cervical dysplasia and cervical cancer may be tied to folate deficiency. The deficiency may occur because of the drug mugging effect or because a woman is unable to utilize folate and convert it to 5-MTHF in the cells. (5-MTHF is also sold as a supplement that can be purchased OTC.)

As far back as 1973, a study in the *Lancet* found that low vitamin B status increases the risk of depression because Bs are needed to make the feel-good brain hormones dopamine, norepinephrine, and serotonin. B vitamins are often referred to as stress vitamins because they help a person cope by making coping chemicals and happy hormones. Along that line, low B status could very well be driving your anxiety, irritability, tearfulness, full-blown depression, adrenal exhaustion, and panic attacks.

Vitamin C Deficiency

This nutrient is needed to make happy hormones in the brain and to keep us looking youthful. Vitamin C is a water-soluble antioxidant that sweeps away toxins that might otherwise damage your cells. It helps your body form collagen in your bones, cartilage, skin, muscles, and blood vessels. Vitamin C helps your body take up and use iron, too, so when you run low on C, you run low on iron, which can lead to anemia and extreme tiredness. A severe deficiency of vitamin C is rare, but the low-grade drug mugging effect of medications can cause your body to become deficient in this important vitamin. Numerous studies suggest that vitamin C's antioxidant effects (how it protects our cells) are important in preventing cancer and diabetes. Vitamin C also powers up the immune system.

The Drug–Disease Connection

If you're still skeptical—even after reading about some of the nutrients that are depleted and what can happen to a woman who takes drugs containing synthetic female hormones without replenishing the nutrients they deplete—read on. Medical research has established there's a definite connection between the drugs and the diseases. Just a few short years ago, one part of the famous Women's Health Initiative (WHI) study was halted in July 2002, earlier than expected, because of problems—namely fatalities—associated with synthetic hormone replacement therapy. The study followed 161,808 generally healthy postmenopausal women for about 15 years. Although not all aspects of the Women's Health Initiative were negative, many researchers did conclude that HRT could increase the risk of breast cancer, heart disease, and stroke. The medications used in the study contained equine estrogen and synthetic progestins. This type of synthetic HRT was abandoned by many doctors after these WHI results were published, except as a way to relieve the most debilitating and stressful symptoms of menopause. (Today, more and more doctors are learning about bioidentical forms of estrogen, since those match a woman's body exactly and may be less harmful.)

One study published in the *Journal of the American Medical Association (JAMA)* reported that once women stopped taking horse-derived estrogens, their risks for heart attack and blood clots went down, although the risk for cancer still remained slightly higher than in women who never took these drugs. A horse has 34 different estrogens; we have 4, none of which matches those of a horse.

Let's focus on one of the diseases found to be more frequent in the WHI research—breast cancer. Breast cancer takes a long time to develop, and its formation is associated with many factors, among them iodine deficiency, progesterone deficiency, insufficient B vitamins, organic pollutants, and a woman's inability to produce protective estrogen by-products versus those associated with cancer. Obviously, the development of cancer depends on many, many other things, too—your genes, your weight, how long you took these drugs, your liver and kidney function, whether you exercise, and what you eat.

Since it takes breast cancer so long to develop, it makes sense that tumors will be fueled when the environment supports their growth. For example, HRT can cause candida overgrowth, and this yeast may fuel cancer growth.

HRT mugs folate, which is needed to protect DNA. So it comes as no surprise that a deficiency of folate contributes to the development of cancer. HRT can steal immune-supportive minerals, such as zinc, iodine, and magnesium. When immunity goes down, cancer growth increases. So the drug mugging effect is a risk factor for developing cancer by virtue of the fact that it robs the body of cancer protective nutrients. Let's just look at facts.

In 2001, the number of hormone prescriptions using equine estrogen (Premarin, Prempro) was 22.8 million from January to March. The incidence of breast cancer was 141 cases per 100,000 women. In 2002, the WHI study results were published and showed unfavorable results (deaths!) associated with some synthetic hormones. At that point doctors stopped prescribing these drugs to many of their patients. Guess what? In 2003, the number of hormone prescriptions dropped to 15.3 million from January to March. And the incidence of breast cancer went down to 124 cases per 100,000 women. Until that time, the incidence of breast cancer had risen for the prior 2 decades. This was the steepest decline in breast cancer incidence I had seen in my career. This 7.2 percent decline was a startling turnaround.

When a woman is no longer exposed to a drug mugger that is stealing the life out of her, then the odds of her contracting a dreadful disease naturally go down. There are other factors, too. The point I am making is that we did something right in 2003, and it stands to reason that this has something to do with removing a drug mugger that steals numerous vitamins and minerals. Unfortunately, there is no study to prove me right. But to me it's just common sense. Think about it: If you need folate to have healthy cells and healthy DNA strands and a drug is stealing your folate, then your DNA isn't normal, opening up the possibility of tumor formation. I wish someone would do a study showing that this is so. But do we really need to spend millions of dollars on a study to prove common sense?

When the harmful by-products of estrogen linger rather than clear your body, your risk of cancer increases. So I always tell my clients that if they must take (or have taken) estrogen-containing hormones of any sort, it pays to focus on ways to unglue the harmful estrogen by-products that are wedged in the body's cells just waiting for the right set of circumstances to start multiplying. What you eat matters, too. It's so simple. Foods rich in a compound called I3C (indole-3-carbinol) turn aggressive estrogens into meek ones that leave the body easily. These foods include cruciferous veggies. Here's yet another reason to eat your broccoli!

Are You Shocked Yet?

Why aren't physicians telling women that these possibilities exist? Why are millions of women still getting these medications without a warning that they may become deficient in life-sustaining nutrients? And worse, how come when new problems and symptoms pop up, people are not given nutritional testing as part of a standard routine to find the underlying cause?

It's so upsetting to me that millions of women pick up their monthly prescriptions for birth control pills, along with their antidepressants, thyroid medications, and pain pills. So many young, happy women in their twenties get their monthly birth control pill packs, and by the time they are 30 or 35, they are already on four or five other medications. Plus, they are overweight, tired, depressed, and anxious. Some become severely riddled with excessive estrogen, a condition called estrogen dominance. This excess estrogen then causes even more symptoms, such as fibroids, endometriosis, and heavy periods. Similar problems happen in older women who are taking prescribed synthetic HRT for hot flashes and other menopausal symptoms.

I realize that this is a pretty glum picture. But does it mean that you must stop taking these drugs? Not at all. I assure you, there is hope and there is help. You are holding it in your hands right now.

Solutions for Nutrient Losses from Synthetic Hormones

You can reduce your disease risks from nutrient deficiency very easily. In fact, you have several choices.

1. You can discontinue the medication you are on. Don't do this on your own, because some meds require weaning. Discuss alternatives with your doctor.

2. You can have yourself tested for micronutrients, find out what you are deficient in, and take nutritional supplements to put the deficiency behind you.

3. You can supplement with nutrients and replenish what the drug mugger steals. You'll find detailed information in this book on specific drugs, which nutrients they steal from the body, and how much of those nutrients you need to take to replenish your cells' warehouses.

4. You can consider taking any or all of the following nutrients to install a tighter security system from the drug mugging effects of synthetic hormones. Some of them should be no problem for you to take, such as probiotics (everyone should take these daily on an empty stomach; see Chapter 17). But for others, you may want approval from your doctor before you begin taking them.

   Magnesium chelate: 250 mg daily, taken at night

   Iodine: 12.5 mg once daily, in the form of the supplement Iodoral

   5-MTHF: 1 capsule 3 times a week or **Folic acid:** 800 mcg daily

   Probiotics: follow label instructions to replenish intestinal flora that protects your immune system

   Calcium D-glucarate: 200–500 mg twice a day to remove used-up estrogen

   Hemp protein: once daily following label instructions, a vegetarian source of healthy amino acids. Whey is fine, too, as long as you handle dairy well.

   Spirulina: daily for energy and detoxification. This restores minerals and B vitamins with each tablet.

   DIM: 100–150 mg twice a day

When Meals and Medicine Don't Mix

As a pharmacist, I am accustomed to answering questions about drug–drug interactions. Most pharmacists are. We know this language inside and out. Since pharmacists are specialists in drug information and the inner workings of medicines, these questions are easy for us to answer. If we don't know the answers off the top of our heads, we have 4-inch-thick books to look in and detailed computer software to consult.

Dangerous Drug–Food Interactions

By and large, people don't think of food as having any impact on their medicine. But it's very true that certain foods do interact with medications. In some cases, the interaction can be deadly. Most of the time, however, it is not. One way that food can affect your medication intake is by giving your body less of the benefit your medication has to offer you. In the case of certain antibiotics, this could be fatal. For example, if you are fighting a staph infection or pneumonia, you need the full effect of your antibiotic to regain your health.

In the case of pain relievers, it's a catch-22. Pain relievers cause so much stomach upset that they are usually taken with meals to minimize this problem. However, if you take the medicine with food, it may mean that you have to wait a while longer before the benefit of pain relief kicks in.

Your medication's effect can be exaggerated if you combine the drug with food or beverages that have the same effect. Take the example of sleeping pills, which slow respiration and heart rate. When combined with a glass of wine, the effect can be so severe that you just stop breathing and die. It's happened many times. Another example of this enhanced effect is with selective serotonin reuptake inhibitor (SSRI) antidepressants (like Paxil, Zoloft, or Prozac). If you take these along with that morning cup of joe, the caffeine in the coffee reacts with your medicine and the two together wire you so much that it can cause tremors, panic attacks, and insomnia.

Let's take a look at amlodipine (Norvasc, and the newest Exforge) for another example of potentially deadly interactions. This blockbuster blood pressure pill interacts with grapefruit juice. Grapefruit isn't bad; in fact, the citrus fruit offers tremendous health benefits. But compounds in it can interact with dozens of meds. The untoward effect may be a serious drop in blood pressure or a dangerous rise in heart rate (tachycardia). In fact, consuming grapefruit (and especially its juice) can spike the levels of many drugs. The effect of grapefruit on the body is long lasting, up to 24 hours in some people, depending on how well their liver works, so even separating administration of your medication from the grapefruit doesn't help. See pages 88–89 for a list of interactions with grapefruit.

Take the case of some other antidepressants, such as the monoamine oxidase (MAO) inhibitor Nardil (phenelzine). It can interact with cheese, specifically the tyramine in cheese, and in some cases, the interaction can be fatal because it causes a dangerous rise in blood pressure.

In 2008, 64 percent of Americans took three or more drugs and 36.7 percent took five or more. This creates a tremendous potential for interactions between medication and food. The degree of the interaction varies, depending on your age, your sex, your liver function, your genetic blueprint (SNPs, or single nucleotide polymorphisms), your overall health, and your weight. Elderly people and those who are chronically ill or have a poorly functioning immune system should pay especially close attention here. This chapter may even save your life. I've worked hard to create a comprehensive list of drug and food interactions to keep you safe. This type of information is hard to find, and I'm proud to be the one to give it to you.

Some people take medications with a narrow therapeutic index, which means that there is a very thin line between what is an effective dose and what's dangerous. These patients are always more likely to experience toxic effects from eating the wrong food because the line between toxicity and safety is so thin. In addition, there are differences in the way individuals metabolize (or process) their food and medicine. Let's face it, we all have our own genetic footprints.

Here are some important questions you should ask both your doctor and your pharmacist. They apply to every medicine, prescribed or OTC. Don't be shy. Getting this information is vital for your safety.

- Is a glass of wine (or beer) with dinner safe while taking this medication?

- Will this medication make me sleepy? If so, is it okay for me to have a drink with it?

- Should this medicine be taken in the morning or at night?

- Is it okay to drink caffeine-containing beverages while on this medication?

- Can I have a glass of milk or eat ice cream or yogurt with my medicine?

- Can I eat grapefruit or drink grapefuit juice while on this medicine?

- I spice my foods with ginger, which is a natural blood thinner. Is this okay to do while I'm taking this medicine?

- I take fish oil and/or ginkgo, which are natural blood thinners. Is it okay to take these while on this medicine?

The bottom line is that many commonly prescribed drugs have the potential to interact with everyday foods and beverages. Rather than playing a deadly game of Russian roulette, you need to educate yourself about the medications that you're taking. Talk to your pharmacist, ask questions, and read the informational inserts that come with your medicines. What follows is a list of common drugs and the food and beverage interactions you need to be aware of.

Common but Rarely Discussed Drug–Food Interactions

Acetaminophen or Paracetamol

Examples: Dristan, Excedrin QuickTabs, Midol, Sine-Off, Sinutab, Sominex, Tylenol, and certain Benadryl or St. Joseph Cough Suppressant formulas. Prescription drugs that contain acetaminophen (known as paracetamol overseas) include Lorcet, Lortab, Percocet, Roxicet, Vicodin, and multiple strengths of generic pain relievers labeled hydrocodone-APAP or hydrocodone/acetaminophen.

Acetaminophen, sold primarily under the brand name of Tylenol, is used most frequently to control fever, aches, and pains. It is available without prescription and is actually derived from coal tar. Many people use it to control mild arthritic pain. Scientists don't know exactly how it works, but it's clear that it increases the pain threshold. There are hundreds of combination drugs sold OTC that include acetaminophen on their ingredient list. For example, menstrual products often contain it, and many cough and cold preparations and sleep aids also have acetaminophen. You will have to be a sleuth. Break out a magnifying glass and read the fine print. This is especially important if you take prescription medications that also contain acetaminophen. So, for example, read your prescription bottle of Lortab and see that it contains 500 mg of acetaminophen per dose, and then read the label on your cough and cold product to find out if acetaminophen is in the medicine. Be careful not to ingest more than 4 grams (4,000 mg) per day. The following foods may interact with this medicine:

Alcohol: It can damage the liver, and so can acetaminophen. The combination of these two can be dangerous even if you don't take high doses of the drug or drink an abundant amount of alcohol. Separating the drink from the medicine in time won't matter. To avoid this problem, don't drink at all.

Citrus fruits and vitamin C: These can increase the side effects and toxicity of acetaminophen. Don't take dosages greater than 500 mg of vitamin C per day with acetaminophen.

Oatmeal and high-fiber cereal: These slow down the absorption of acetaminophen; therefore, you won't get as rapid an effect. This isn't a big deal if you're taking it for minor joint pain, but if you're counting the minutes before it relieves your stubbed toe, you'll be waiting longer. Oatmeal is good for you, so just separate the administration of your drug from your food by 2 or more hours.

Echinacea: This herb, which boosts the immune system, comes in supplements and teas. Combining acetaminophen and echinacea can inflame the liver in sensitive people.

Acid Blockers and Antacids

Examples: There are hundreds of brands and different blends. It's impossible for me to include them all; however, I'll list the most common ones found at health food stores and pharmacies. These can be broken down into three types of medications.

Antacids: Aluminum and magnesium hydroxide (Gaviscon, Maalox, Mylanta), aluminum carbonate gel (Basajel), aluminum hydroxide (Amphojel, AlternaGEL), calcium carbonate (Tums, Titralac, Rolaids), magnesium hydroxide (Phillips' Milk of Magnesia), sodium bicarbonate (Alka-Seltzer, baking soda).

H₂ blockers: Cimetidine (Tagamet, Tagamet HB), famotidine (Pepcid, Pepcid AC, Pepcid Complete), nizatidine (Axid), ranitidine (Zantac, Taladine).

Proton pump inhibitors (PPI drugs): Esomeprazole (Nexium), lansoprazole (Prevacid), omeprazole (Prilosec and Zegarid, a rapid-release form), pantoprazole (Protonix), rabeprazole (Aciphex).

Acid blockers and antacids are used to prevent damage to the stomach lining by neutralizing stomach acid. The proton pump inhibitors are often used for gastroesophageal reflux disease (GERD or reflux), ulcers, and Zollinger-Ellison syndrome. PPIs can block acid production pretty much 24/7 in an effort to temporarily curb heartburn, coughing, difficulty swallowing, and other painful symptoms associated with these conditions. When you suppress the natural acid that your body uses to break down food, medication, and supplements, you could develop more serious problems, such as food allergies, heart arrhythmias, tingling in fingers and toes, depression, dizziness, and headache. Therefore, these drugs should be reserved for peptic or duodenal ulcers, or for people who secrete an abnormally high level of acid. Did you know that heartburn is a common symptom of gluten intolerance and low acid in the gut? Acid blockers are drug muggers of most nutrients, even though they don't appear in every chapter of this book. But think about it. Acid blockers suppress acid-alkaline balance and thereby alter pH (acidity) throughout the gut, so the absorption of every single nutrient is suppressed. Here are some other things you need to know about acid blockers.

Alcohol: It can irritate your stomach, erode the delicate lining, and literally poke a hole in it. You shouldn't drink if you have heartburn, reflux, perforations, or ulcers.

Cranberry juice: The combination of cranberry juice with these drugs is actually a good and positive interaction. The juice offsets the drug mugging effect of acid blockers. Without the juice, it appears that you are more susceptible to the drug mugging of B vitamins, particularly B_{12} (methylcobalamin). So cheers! Bring on the juice.

St. John's wort: Teas and supplements of this herb interact with acid-blocking drugs and might make you more sensitive to sunlight, so it's easier to burn or develop skin blotches.

Spicy food, garlic, and onions: These foods tend to upset the stomach and may necessitate more medication. Avoid them altogether, or eat in moderation according to how you feel.

Fast food, greasy food, and sugary desserts: These foods strip the gut of healthy enzymes and beneficial flora. This will cause you to run out of every nutrient in the book!

Feverfew: This herbal supplement is prized for its ability to ward off migraines and allergies, but it is a mild blood thinner. It's reasonable to suspect that it can exacerbate your condition and increase your risk for a gastrointestinal (GI) bleed.

Coffee and nicotine: Coffee (both caffeinated and decaffeinated) reduces pressure on the esophageal sphincter, so there's more reflux. Nicotine irritates the delicate stomach lining and can lead to reflux, heartburn, or an ulcer. You are tempting fate with these.

ADHD Drugs (Psychostimulants)

Examples: Adderall (amphetamine), Concerta, Dexedrine, DextroStat, Metadate CD and ER, Methylin, Ritalin (methylphenidate), and Vyvanse.

These medications are classified as psychostimulants because they drive up the amounts of stimulating natural substances in the brain. Ironically, all this "speed" calms anyone who happens to have attention-deficit/hyperactivity disorder. They're prescribed for children (and adults) with attention deficit disorder, behavioral issues, or hyperactivity to control behavioral outbursts and improve focus, concentration, and learning. The medications are sometimes prescribed for narcolepsy, a disorder in which one drops off to sleep without a moment's notice. Many of these drugs must be swallowed whole, without crushing or chewing, because they are extended-release formulations. Breaking them is very dangerous and has led to death. (Always ask your pharmacist if you can crush your medicine before doing so.) Here are the dangerous drug–food interactions.

Fruit juice: This creates more acid in the stomach and may alter the absorption of medication, by increasing or decreasing it. To avoid this, separate the juice from the medicine by an hour or two.

Alcohol: Methylphenidate can cause poor physical coordination along with dizziness or drowsiness in some people. Alcohol may intensify these effects, so don't combine the two. Also, alcohol is a bit of a "downer" on the nervous system, whereas psychostimulants are "uppers"—another reason not to combine them.

Vitamin C: Supplements have similar interactions as fruit juice, either increasing or decreasing the drug effect.

Coffee, tea, soda, and chocolate: Anything with caffeine can speed the heart just like ADHD drugs. Avoid stimulating foods and drinks altogether while taking this medicine. The reaction can cause nervousness, irritability, insomnia, and heart rhythm abnormalities. If you are one of those people who consider soda a staple in your house and will not give it up, let your doctor know so that your drug dosage can be adjusted. (You can read about soda substitutes on page 76.)

Ma huang: Found in many OTC diet pills, energy drinks, and supplements, this herb speeds up your heart and raises blood pressure. Taken with stimulants, the combo is dangerous.

Bitter orange: Found in many OTC diet pills. (Same as ma huang, but to a lesser extent.)

Allergy Medicine

Examples: Alavert, Allegra, Benadryl, Chlor-Trimeton, Clarinex, Claritin, Comtrex, Dimetane, loratadine, Tavist, Zyrtec, and other generics. Allergy pills are also sold by prescription as Allegra (fexofenadine), Atarax or Vistaril (hydroxyzine), Periactin, Trinalin, and dozens of combination products that contain an antihistamine ingredient. Additionally, nasal sprays are now available, including Astelin and Nasonex.

Allergic reactions lead to the release of histamine, which causes a cascade of other chemicals, all of which are responsible for a variety of miserable symptoms. These drugs help people with annoying allergy symptoms, such as sneezing, runny nose, itchy throat and eyes, and cough associated with postnasal drip. They work by blocking the histamine produced when we are faced with the allergic trigger. That's why allergy medicine is referred to as an antihistamine. When you block histamine, you cut down on the misery. Unfortunately, these drugs do nothing to boost the immune system, although they are fantastic at drying up mucous membranes. They are best used in advance of meeting a known allergen. For example, if you know your sister's cat triggers your allergy, take the medicine several hours before you go to her house. You can also begin antihistamine therapy 2 months before the season hits you, and this seems to head it off better. This is not always practical, nor is it foolproof. Antihistamines can also be taken during or after an allergic event. Here's what you need to look out for while taking these types of drugs.

Alcohol: This combo can increase the sedation caused by your medicine. The result is excessive sleepiness and slowed heart rate and breathing. There's also the spacey factor. Many antihistamines (especially Benadryl, Chlor-Trimeton, and hydroxyzine) can make you feel spacey, and combining them with alcohol makes it even worse.

Grapefruit and its juice: The combination of grapefruit with antihistamines may increase or decrease the blood levels of the allergy medicine, resulting in serious heart problems. Take allergy medicine with water, not juice of any kind, until more data trickle in about potential effects.

Bitter orange: Found as a stand-alone supplement and also as part of a synergistic blend in many OTC diet pills, energy drinks, and supplements, this herb has the potential (though fairly mild) to speed up your heart. I recommend that you not combine it with amphetamine-like medications.

Antianxiety Medicines

Examples: Ativan (lorazepam), Klonopin (clonazepam), Valium (diazepam), and Xanax (alprazolam).

Doctors prescribe these medications for people who are feeling anxious or dealing with grief. They are a form of tranquilizer and work within an hour. These medications are called benzodiazepines, or benzos for short, and they may cause physical or psychological dependence or both.

You should take these meds only for a few weeks, and then you are supposed to wean off them slowly. As a pharmacist, I've seen people rely on these drugs for their anxiety for years, making no attempt to ever get off them. If you are relying on these drugs to get through your day or to help you deal with your life or your spouse, then consider some natural options that are safer, more effective, and not addictive. Some choices are described in Chapter 6, Frazzled, Frustrated, and Freaked Out, in my book *The 24-Hour Pharmacist*. Benzos can cause morning hangovers as well as daytime sleepiness and make it dangerous for you to drive.

When you are anxious or stressed, your brain is in overdrive. Benzos come along and spark the release of GABA (gamma-aminobutyric acid), a calming chemical. In fact, you make a lot of GABA when you are sleeping. The medications are helpful to people prone to insomnia, anxiety, panic attacks, and overactive thinking. They're not my choice for a long-term fix because they do not repair the underlying imbalance of brain chemicals. But in certain situations, these drugs are extremely helpful. They bring a feeling of relaxation to the body very quickly. I've seen them used for people who have to undergo dental procedures, surgery, MRIs, and other intimidating medical procedures. They are sometimes prescribed to people who receive news of a terminal illness or the loss of a loved one. Here is what you need to know.

Alcohol: Drinking increases both the sedative and the intoxicating effects of alprazolam. The use of alcohol should be avoided.

Coffee, tea, and soda: Beverages containing caffeine will work against your tranquilizer.

Kava: You can buy this as a natural tranquilizing supplement or tea. It enhances the effect of prescribed sedatives. The combination is usually dangerous, and there have been fatalities. Completely avoid!

Hops, valerian root, and passionflower: Like kava, these herbs are sold as supplements and teas, and they enhance the effect of sedating drugs.

St. John's wort: This may increase side effects, particularly sedation.

Nicotine products: These can speed up the elimination of your drug, making it less effective.

GABA supplements: These natural tranquilizers can be purchased at any health food store. They increase amounts of GABA in the brain, so combining them with tranquilizers or antianxiety drugs is not recommended.

L-glutamine supplements: I've recommended this dietary supplement (a natural amino acid) quite often in my syndicated columns and books. It promotes regularity, excellent immune system function, better brain health, good blood sugar control, and increased muscle mass, and overall, it's good for digestive health, too. The problem is that it's a precursor to GABA, so the more of this goody you take, the more GABA you will make. I think it's okay to combine an antianxiety drug and GABA, as long as you stick to a lower dosage of GABA, like 1,000 mg per day (total) or less. If you get too drowsy, you'll know to back off the drug (or the glutamine), but talk to your doctor, who will alter your drug dosages as necessary.

Lemon balm (*Melissa officinalis*): I frequently recommend this herb to help people sleep and relieve minor digestive troubles. You can buy it dried, and make tea out of it, or you can buy commercial supplements in capsule or tablet form. Lemon balm has several different mechanisms of action, however. One of its effects is to increase levels of GABA. This means that the combination of lemon balm with antianxiety medications will cause an additive effect (and more side effects or excess sedation).

Marijuana: Marijuana users should not take anything that has a sedative effect. The enhancements caused by the combination could slow breathing and heart rate excessively.

Anticoagulants (Blood Thinners)

Examples: Aggrenox, aspirin (called acetylsalicylic acid in some countries), Coumadin (warfarin), heparin, Lovenox, Plavix (clopidogrel), and Ticlid (ticlopidine).

These medications are used to prevent blood clots, pulmonary embolisms, and strokes. But clotting itself isn't a bad thing. If we didn't have the ability to clot, we would bleed to death from a paper cut. Whenever we hurt ourselves and bleed, specific cells called platelets clog up the hole in the blood vessel by clumping together to form a plug in a process called platelet aggregation. The plug gets stronger when other clotting factors in the bloodstream huddle around it and form a stronger meshwork.

Vitamin K is involved in this process because it helps you make clotting substances. In people with impaired blood flow due to hardening of the arteries, excess cholesterol, or plaque in the arteries, the platelets just stick to the artery wall and impede blood flow to the brain (causing a stroke) or to the heart (heart attack). This is why medications are used to prevent platelet aggregation or thin the blood. Each anticoagulant works in its own way to prevent the formation or sticking of blood clots.

Coumadin (warfarin) works by blocking the actions of vitamin K and preventing the production of clotting factors in the liver. It's used to prevent clots that occur deep in the veins. Sometimes, the blood just gets too thick, and that's where aspirin seems to help the most by keeping the blood thin and keeping the platelets from sticking together.

Here is what you need to know about anticoagulants and food.

Salads, seaweed, and leafy greens: These foods contain a lot of vitamin K, which helps blood-clotting substances thicken your blood, so it works against Coumadin. This means that if you eat a lot of salads, you will require higher dosages of Coumadin. *Note:* These foods should not be a problem if you take Plavix. I'll never tell you to give up leafy greens because they are healthy for you in so many ways. My opinion is to stay consistent, and this concurs with the opinions of other top-notch experts; eat about the same amount of these foods on a daily basis, say one salad per day and one serving of sautéed kale, chard, spinach, or broccoli, and so forth. Your doctor will adjust your Coumadin dose accordingly. Once your dosage has been firmly established, if you change your regular eating habits, your drug levels may spike or plunge. Therein lies the problem, and it can be dangerous.

Feverfew: This herbal supplement is prized for its ability to ward off migraines and allergies. It can thin the blood, as do many herbs, and therefore the combination of feverfew with blood-thinning drugs causes too much blood thinning, possibly leading to easy bruising, nosebleeds, or GI bleeds.

Garlic, ginger, turmeric, and ginkgo biloba: These may increase bleeding because they are so fantastic at keeping your blood thin all by themselves.

Saw palmetto: It may increase bleeding, so use with caution.

Onions: More than a few ounces seem to increase blood warfarin levels.

Excess vitamin supplements: Vitamin E (greater than 400 IU per day) and vitamin A (greater than 10,000 IU per day) can thin the blood excessively when combined with blood thinners.

Citrus juice and vitamin C: They might reduce the absorption of certain blood thinners, including warfarin.

Green tea and matcha tea: These teas have powerful effects on the arteries, helping to unclog them and thinning the blood slightly. This is a good thing, but after a few days or weeks of regular consumption, you will need to ask your doctor to lower your medication dose.

Grapefruit and its juice, and pomegranate and orange juices: Grapefruit can increase levels of certain blood thinners to a dangerous extent. For a complete list of medications that interact with grapefruit, see page 88. Pomegranate juice and orange juice appear to act in a similar way, so they may cause the same complications.

Soy milk: This may counteract your blood thinner.

Avocado: This nutrient-rich food seems to reduce the effect of warfarin. Many practitioners warn against eating it. However, I think it's fine because it's packed with the antioxidant glutathione. Simply have your doctor adjust your medication dose to accommodate your dietary preferences, and stay consistent with avocado consumption.

Coenzyme Q10: This may slightly reduce the effect of your blood thinner. I would not give this nutrient up, though. It's a powerful antioxidant, and it protects the heart. I think it's worth having your doctor make a slight adjustment to your drug dosage if needed.

St. John's wort: This reduces the effect of blood thinners, most notably warfarin, so you'll need a higher dose.

Ginseng: May counteract your medicine.

Anticonvulsants

Examples: Depakene and Depakote (valproic acid); Dilantin and Phenytek (phenytoin); Gabitril, Keppra, and Klonopin (clonazepam); Lamictal and Lyrica (pregabalin); Mysoline (primidone); Neurontin (gabapentin); Nootropil, Phenobarbital, and Tegretol (carbamazepine); Topamax and Trileptal (oxcarbazepine); Valium (diazepam); Zarontin (ethosuximide); and Zonegran (zonisamide).

There are a lot of drugs in this class, and they are usually taken long-term or for a lifetime. These drugs are taken every day and are most often used to control seizures in patients with epileptic disorders. These are not prn (*pro re nata*) drugs; prn drugs are used once in a while when needed. Anticonvulsants can also be used to manage nerve pain, trigeminal neuralgia, headaches, migraines, chronic pain, and complications from other medical conditions. Neurologists use these drugs very carefully because they have dangerous side effects. Adjusting and perfecting the dosage for these medications requires careful analysis of your kidney and liver function. Your doctor will routinely test your blood if you take any of these medications to determine whether your body is capable of processing the dosage you take. This is important because anticonvulsant drugs have a small window of effectiveness before they become toxic. The meds do not cure epilepsy. The goal of treatment is to cut down on the number of seizures experienced. Here is what you need to know to keep yourself safer on anticonvulsant medication.

Alcohol: Drinking interferes with your medicine, so you don't have full protection from the drug. You could have a seizure more easily. Alcohol also adds to the sleepiness and slow heart rate induced by anticonvulsants. This additive effect is dangerous.

Antacids: They will suppress your ability to absorb these important medications. Separate their administration by 4 hours.

Borage oil and evening primrose oil (EPO): These essential fatty acids are wonderful dietary supplements, but they seem to increase the risk of seizures, according to some research. Why this happens is not clear, but avoid this combination if you have poor seizure control or take anticonvulsants.

Rice, bananas, and other constipating foods: Anticonvulsants can be constipating, and these foods may worsen the problem.

Valerian root: This herb is often used for relaxation, sleep, and seizure management. Combining it with anticonvulsant meds can add to the sedative properties, slowing heart rate and breathing.

Ginkgo biloba: This supplement is often used to improve memory, sex drive, and circulation. A very small study that appeared in the American Chemical Society's *Journal of Natural Products* suggests that it can increase the risk for seizure, so this herb may work against your medication.

Grapefruit and its juice: Definitely avoid this if you take Tegretol or Trileptal and probably most of the other drugs on the list.

Fiber supplements: Metamucil and other psyllium-based products can reduce the effectiveness of your anticonvulsant medication.

Folic acid: These meds are drug muggers of folic acid, and you should separate taking the vitamin and the drug by at least 4 hours. If you take the folic acid at the same time as the medication, you might weaken the drug's action.

Antidepressants and Mood Modifiers

Examples: SSRI antidepressants include drugs such as Celexa (citalopram), Lexapro (escitalopram), Paxil (paroxetine), Prozac (fluoxetine), and Zoloft (sertraline). Tricyclic antidepressants include amitriptyline, desipramine, doxepin, imipramine, and nortriptyline. Other antidepressants include Cymbalta (duloxetine), Effexor (venlafaxine), Pristiq (desvenlafaxine, the active metabolite of venlafaxine), Remeron (mirtazepine), and Wellbutrin (bupropion).

As a class, these medications are prescribed to ease symptoms of depression, pain, panic attacks, social anxiety disorder (severe and debilitating shyness), and obsessive-compulsive disorder. Nonlabeled uses for some of these drugs include bed-wetting, fibromyalgia, and migraine management. Some of the drug–food interactions of the numerous drugs in this class are listed here.

Coffee, tea, soda, and chocolate: SSRI antidepressants (Celexa, Prozac, Paxil, Zoloft, and Lexapro) can cause the jitters, tremors, anxiety, and insomnia as side effects. Including caffeinated coffee, tea, or soda in your diet can increase the severity of these effects. Note that chocolate also contains a small amount of caffeine.

Alcohol: It suppresses brain chemicals and may work against your medication. With some antidepressants, particularly those in the class of the tricyclics such as nortriptyline and amitriptyline, drinking alcohol can increase sedation and slow breathing. This is also a dangerous interaction with Remeron (mirtazepine), which causes a great degree of sedation all by itself.

Food: Some antidepressants can cause weight gain as a side effect. Monitor meals and try to include healthy foods rather than just empty comfort foods that will only add to your weight gain.

5-HTP: This supplement is a direct precursor to serotonin, and you can buy it at any pharmacy or health food store. People take it to fall asleep, to reduce carb cravings, to improve mood, and to reduce pain in the body. It works by increasing serotonin levels in the body. A lot of people take 5-HTP with their mood drugs, but I never recommend it. It could cause a problem for people who have poor liver function, take excessive amounts of 5-HTP, or take high dosages of prescribed medication. The problem is that the medications do the same thing 5-HTP does—build up your serotonin levels. Too much of this lovely hormone can result in a dangerous condition called serotonin syndrome. In some cases, the excessive serotonin can cause life-threatening symptoms.

St. John's wort: I wouldn't feel comfortable combining this with prescribed antidepressants for the same reason I don't recommend 5-HTP. It also builds up serotonin levels.

Tyrosine: Some people take this natural amino acid when they have tremors, Parkinson's disease, or hypothyroidism. Tyrosine undergoes a chemical reaction in the body and helps make both dopamine and thyroid hormone. When combined with certain antidepressants that also make dopamine, you could end up with too much dopamine in your body. Heart palpitations are just one quick way to know if you are getting too much tyrosine. I'd stay away from it altogether if you take antidepressants (or a prescribed thyroid hormone).

Arthritis Medicines

Examples: Acetaminophen (Tylenol); aspirin (plain or enteric-coated); celecoxib (Celebrex) and its infamous sister rofecoxib (Vioxx), which is no longer on the market; ibuprofen (Motrin, Advil); ketoprofen (Orudis); nabumetone (Relafen); and naproxen (Aleve, or by prescription, Naposyn and Anaprox).

When you hurt yourself or suffer from a sports injury or arthritis, your body creates all sorts of inflammatory chemicals. One of these classes of chemicals is prostaglandins, or PGs. Even though the PGs are incredibly important and have useful functions (like protecting your stomach lining from the surrounding acid), excessive PG chemicals are not good and can promote inflammation, pain, or fever. That's where the drugs come in. By suppressing your body's production of certain PGs, they can reduce pain, inflammation, and fever.

This is why many cold formulas and premenstrual syndrome (PMS) products contain ibuprofen, the most common one of the bunch. Most anti-inflammatories are classified as nonsteroidal anti-inflammatory drugs or NSAIDs (pronounced *N-sedz*). They bring relief within a few hours. A very popular pain reliever, Celebrex is available by prescription. It works very selectively and has less impact on the stomach, meaning it is less likely to cause stomach bleeding or ulceration like NSAIDs can. On the other hand, Celebrex has a higher likelihood of causing high blood pressure, heart attack, or stroke, especially in sensitive, predisposed people. A study reported in March 2006 in the *Journal of the Society of Medicine* found that celecoxib increases the risk of a heart attack more than twofold. Here's what you need to know.

Alcohol: This combination can increase the risk of a GI bleed or liver damage.

Garlic and ginger: These can thin the blood and slightly increase the risk of bleeding when combined with NSAIDs.

Panax ginseng, red clover, white willow, ginger, and ginkgo biloba: The combination of any of these with arthritis medication may cause an additive blood-thinning effect.

Salt substitutes: These contain potassium. NSAIDs sometimes cause potassium retention in the body. The combination can cause potassium overload (hyperkalemia), with symptoms including nausea, fatigue, and muscle weakness.

Aspirin (Acetylsalicylic Acid)

Examples: Alka-Seltzer products, Ascriptin, Aspergum, Bayer, Bufferin, Ecotrin, Goody's, Halfprin, Norwich, St. Joseph, and certain Anacin products. In prescription formulas, you find aspirin in Darvon Compound, Endodan, Fiorinal, Percodan, and Soma Compound.

Aspirin has many uses and appears in hundreds of OTC products. Today it's primarily used as a blood thinner to help prevent stroke and heart attack. Doctors often tell their patients to take it once a day. The substance is derived from the bark of the white willow tree. The use of aspirin (and its predecessors) is centuries old. It can reduce fever, but it's even better at reducing pain and inflammation. That's why you find it in so many prescription pain relievers. Here's what you need to know in order to be safe while taking aspirin products.

Alcohol: Aspirin and alcohol have some ability to poke teeny tiny holes in your gut, so the combination could increase your risk for a gastrointestinal bleed.

Garlic and ginger: These are excellent at thinning your blood, and I always recommend that people eat them. But combined with aspirin, the blood-thinning effect can become too pronounced and result in easy bruising, nosebleeds, or GI bleeds.

White willow tea: Taking aspirin and drinking this tea can also thin your blood to an extreme.

Green tea and matcha tea: I think these beverages can thin the blood just as well as aspirin. If you drink a lot of green tea, ask your doctor about stopping the drug. (Some say that too much green tea may contribute to kidney stones. The jury's out on this, so drink it in moderation.)

Iron supplements: These are hard on the GI tract, as is aspirin. The combination of both could increase risk of gut problems, particularly bleeding.

Bone-building drugs: These are notorious for their ability to damage the delicate mucosal lining of the esophagus. These are supposed to be taken first thing in the morning on an empty stomach, and you are not to lie down for at least 30 minutes after taking the drug. My advice is to *not* combine this class of medication with aspirin-containing products.

Beta-Blockers (Blood Pressure Medicines)

Examples: Acebutolol (Sectral), atenolol (Tenormin), bisoprolol (Zebeta, Ziac, Cardicor), carteolol (Teoptic eyedrops), carvedilol (Coreg), carvedilol betaxolol (Kerlone tablets and Betoptic eyedrops), celiprolol (Cardem, Celectol, Celipro, Celipress, Dilanorm, Selectol), esmolol (Brevibloc), labetalol (Normodyne, Trandate), levobunolol (Betagan eyedrops), metoprolol (Lopressor, Toprol XL), nadolol (Corgard), oxprenolol (Slow-Trasicor, Captol), pindolol (Visken), propranolol (Inderal), sotalol (Betapace), and timolol (Blocadren tablets, Timoptic eyedrops).

This class of drugs is enormous. There are many types and subtypes of beta-blockers. They are known as beta-blockers because there are beta receptors on your cells and these drugs sit at the doorway like a Rottweiler, preventing other chemicals from latching onto the cell. By blocking the beta doorways (receptors), the drugs block nerve impulses that would otherwise make your heart beat too fast or your blood pressure rise. So beta-blockers slow down the heart.

When you stress out, exercise strenuously, or have great sex, you release a lot of adrenaline (which, by the way, is also your fight-or-flight hormone).

This can cause your heart to beat like crazy and make your blood pressure rise.

Beta-blockers are especially useful in these instances because they block the effect of adrenaline on your heart rate. Sometimes they are prescribed for people who have to do public speaking or other events where their heart rate and blood pressure increase from anxiety.

Beta-blockers reduce blood pressure, prevent angina (chest pain), treat heart failure, and attempt to normalize heart rhythm. Some beta-blockers work in the eye to reduce pressure there, which is why glaucoma eyedrops appear on my list. Certain meds in this class decrease the frequency of migraine headaches. Here are some drug–food interactions that you need to know about if you take a beta-blocker.

Potassium supplements: Your doctor should routinely measure your potassium level. You want them to remain in the normal range. If your potassium level gets too high or too low, then your beta-blocker will cause more complications. If you are taking diuretics that cause potassium loss (like hydrochlorothiazide or furosemide), make sure to get enough potassium each day so you don't run low, especially if you also take a beta-blocker.

Alcohol: Beta-blockers slow the heart rate down. Alcohol does that, too, so it has an additive effect. Beta-blockers can be dangerous in some people because they slow breathing and heart rate. The combination of beta-blockers and alcohol can be so severe that it actually stops the heart. If your health-care provider tells you to drink a glass of red wine with dinner, make sure your medication dose is lowered to accommodate the alcohol intake.

Orange juice: Don't drink this with atenolol (Tenormin) or celiprolol (Cardem). Wait at least several hours because orange juice reduces the availability of the drugs. There isn't enough data to extrapolate whether this effect applies to all beta-blockers, but to be safe, just separate administration of the two.

Animal products: Protein (meats) may increase drug levels. In one study, the combination of propranolol with a protein-rich meal increased the bioavailability of the drug by 53 percent! This boost is dangerous because it can cause light-headedness, dizziness, fainting, and slowed heartbeat.

Salt substitutes: These can increase your potassium levels because that's what's in the salt substitute—potassium chloride. Some blood pressure pills, especially the ACE inhibitors (angiotensin converting enzyme inhibitors) and related ARBs (angiotensin II receptor blockers), when combined with the salt substitute, can cause hyperkalemia, or excess potassium in the blood. ACE inhibitors include captopril, enalapril, lisinopril, quinapril, and moexipril; ARBs include Atacand, Cozaar, Diovan, Micardis, and Avapro. Symptoms include nausea, fatigue, and muscle weakness.

Licorice: Natural licorice, found in some candies, can cause salt and water retention, which increases your blood pressure and acts against your medication.

Bone-Building Drugs: Bisphosphonates

Examples: Aclasta, Actonel, Boniva, Didronel, Fosamax, and Fosavance.

These extremely popular medications belong to a class of drugs known collectively as bisphosphonates. They are approved for use in the United States, Canada, and more than 60 other countries to prevent or treat osteoporosis—the loss of bone density, or simply put, the crumbling of bones that leads to kyphosis, fractures of the spine, broken bones, and hip fractures. You see these medications prescribed primarily to postmenopausal women who are at higher risk for bone loss as a result of waning estrogen levels. On occasion, they are given to men. They are also prescribed to people who take steroid medications, which cause bone brittleness. Guess why? Because steroids are drug muggers of your minerals, especially calcium and magnesium. So when bone mass declines, in come the bone-building meds.

Bisphosphonates work by taking up residence on the surface of your bones. They sit in the doorways of your bone cells and slow down the process of bone erosion. The mechanism is complicated, but essentially their presence allows bone-building cells (osteoblasts) to work more effectively.

You must take these drugs on an empty stomach first thing in the morning with plenty of water because they're really hard on the gut and can damage or create an ulcer in the delicate lining of the esophagus in sensitive individuals. Don't even lie down for at least 30 minutes after you take the medicine; sit up or stand so it can go all the way down.

There is some research suggesting that these medications may cause bone death in the jaw (osteonecrosis, or ONJ). In 2009, a study in the *Journal of the American Dental Association* found that "even short-term oral use of [alendronate] led to ONJ" in about 41 percent of patients. However, drugmakers insist that it's too early to conclude that this condition is related to bisphosphonates. Here's what you need to know if you must take these medications.

Calcium supplements: These may affect the absorption of bone drugs. If you take the two together, the calcium and the drug will latch onto one another like reunited lovers. Their binding may significantly reduce the drug level. Conversely, people being treated with bone-building medication often have low calcium blood levels. Check with your physician or pharmacist prior to taking supplements containing calcium or vitamin D and, if you do take them, make sure to take the supplement at least 2 hours before or after taking the medication.

Iron supplements: The combination fosters another type of reaction that grabs hold of your medicine and reduces the drug level, just like calcium. Take it at least 2 hours before or after your medicine.

Antacids: These often contain calcium or magnesium, both of which affect absorption of the bone-building medication. Separate your bone drug and antacid by at least 2 hours.

Spirulina or trace minerals: Take this dietary supplement at least 2 hours before or after your medication.

Breathing Medications (Bronchodilators)

Examples: Albuterol (AccuNeb, ProAir HFA, Proventil HFA, Ventolin HFA), albuterol and ipratropium (Combivent), ipratropium (Atrovent), levalbuterol (Xopenex), montelukast (Singulair), theophylline (Slo-Bid, Theo-Dur, Uniphyl), and zafirlukast (Accolate).

These medications are known as bronchodilators. They increase air flow in your lungs and can relieve shortness of breath and wheezing. They are most often used for bronchial asthma, but many people with restricted airways or emphysema take them. Certain medications in this group are used for chronic bronchitis and respiratory infections.

Breathing medications can be further divided into three subgroups that I will outline shortly. The drugs in these subclassifications may work differently in the body, but they all seek to do the same thing: dilate your airways, or bronchioles, allowing for greater oxygen exchange. They are categorized as bronchodilators as a result. Here are the three basic classes: beta2-agonists (albuterol and levalbuterol); anticholinergic bronchodilators (ipratropium); and methylxanthines (theophylline).

There is a relatively new class of medications to help people with asthma called *leukotriene receptor antagonists* (LTRAs for short). Singulair (montelukast) and Accolate (zafirlukast) are in this category. They are used to prevent asthma smptoms, often in conjunction with the breathing meds above. LTRAs work by blocking the action of certain natural substances in the body (leukotrienes) that tend to cause swelling and tightening of the airways. By blocking these substances, the drugs minimize breathing issues. They are too new to have a long list of drug muggers and interactions associated with them, but, as data trickle in, I will update you in my health newsletter (subscribe on my Web site).

Breathing medications constitute one of the most useful medication classes on the market today. In fact, I've had to quickly dispense some inhalers to people with asthma right at the pharmacy counter to keep them alive or they literally would have collapsed. Make a note to yourself: Never run out of this medicine. Keep it with you at all times. There isn't much room to play with these drugs: Too little and you can't breathe; too much and you could suffer dangerous side effects. Please be vigilant with your medication dosage and study this list of drug–food interactions.

Caffeine: Tea, soda, coffee, and chocolate all contain caffeine. It's dangerous to combine caffeine with breathing meds because the meds contain a stimulant, too (xanthine). Your heart rate could speed to dangerous levels, and you could experience irritability, tremors, anxiety, chest pain, heart pounding, insomnia, shortness of breath, and cardiac arrhythmias.

Ma huang, panax ginseng, ephedra, licorice root, and bitter orange: These are stimulants, so the combination with breathing medications can be overtaxing.

Grilled meat: The combination of grilled meat and theophylline-based breathing meds can cause such a dangerous reaction that emergency intervention may be needed. It occurs because eating barbecued and grilled meat releases chemicals that keep your liver from eliminating the medicine properly. When this happens, your medication blood level soars to new heights. Danger!

High-carb meals: These may decrease the amount of theophylline in your body, suppressing its effect.

Alcohol: Drinking increases the risk of side effects such as nausea, vomiting, headache, and irritability.

Sugary desserts: Specifically avoid these when taking albuterol because the two together raise blood sugar.

Cough and cold medicines: If your medication contains a decongestant such as phenylephrine or pseudoephedrine (or ephedrine, which is available in other countries), it could stimulate the heart too much, behaving like caffeine. Remember, decongestants used in cough and cold medicines are derived from amphetamines.

Smoking: This keeps your breathing medicine from working by reducing its level in the bloodstream. Smoking is dangerous to your lungs, and you already need breathing medicine in the first place. Quit today. You can do it.

Hawthorne and motherwort: Combining either of these herbs with breathing medications may increase cardiac side effects.

Fiber and bran cereals: Separate intake of these from your breathing medications, including Accolate (zafirlukast), by at least 2 hours.

Diabetes Drugs

Examples: Actos (pioglitazone); Amaryl (glimepiride); Avandamet (rosiglitazone and metformin); Avandia (rosiglitazone); Byetta (exenatide); Diabinese (chlorpropramide); Glucophage, Glucophage XR, Glumetza, Fortamet, Riomet Liquid (metformin); Glucovance (glyburide and metformin); Glyset (miglitol); Janumet (metformin and sitagliptin); Januvia (sitagliptin); Metaglip (metformin and glipizide); Micronase (glyburide); Orinase (tolbutamide); Prandin (repaglinide); Precose (acarbose); Starlix (nateglinide); and Volix (voglibose). Injectable forms of insulin include Humalog, Humulin, Lantus (insulin glargine), Novolin, and NovoLog.

There is an arsenal of diabetes drugs available. The various meds that I have listed may work in different ways. It would be too complicated to go through each mechanism of action here, but it should be enough for you to know that these medications all have one thing in common: They seek to lower the amount of blood sugar in your body or improve the way your body uses the insulin it has. Insulin, by the way, is what neutralizes blood sugar. If you can make your body more sensitive to the insulin that is hanging around, your blood sugar will remain within bounds.

As far as I'm concerned, it's the health of your pancreas that matters most. Unfortunately, we are seeing more and more pancreatic problems today, including pancreatitis and pancreatic cancer. Pancreatic problems are becoming more common and are probably the result of eating excessively processed foods, artificial additives, excessive refined white sugar, and/or too much high fructose corn syrup, or of having allergies to gluten or casein.

When blood sugar remains high long-term, problems come on slowly. They include frequent infections, vision problems, and damage to the brain, heart, and kidneys. On the other hand, low blood sugar (hypoglycemia) often brings on an emergency with symptoms of dizziness, shakiness, sweating, headache, confusion, fainting, and convulsions. Pay attention to the foods that might be a problem for you.

Potatoes, candy bars, and starchy foods: If you increase your blood sugar levels with these foods, then you'll need a higher dose of your medicine.

Aloe vera juice: Some people drink this for constipation. It can lower blood sugar very nicely. When combined with medication, however, this effect is enhanced, and your blood sugar may plummet.

Stinging nettle: This incredibly useful herb actually grows like a weed in parts of North America, Europe, and Asia. Can you imagine? It can help men with prostate problems and prostate cancer, according to a German study published in February 2000. It can also help with sex drive issues and urinary tract problems, as well as raise energy levels and reduce bladder problems in women. This herb is often used for allergies, and it can lower blood sugar just like your medication can, so combining nettle with diabetes meds might drop your blood sugar too fast. Monitor your blood sugar closely because your medication dosage may need to be reduced. Stinging nettle also nourishes the thyroid gland and can enhance your medication's effect. It's not a bad thing. Your doctor will just have to lower your drug dosage as the beneficial effects of stinging nettle become evident.

Alcohol: The use of alcohol should be avoided. It lowers your blood sugar, and when combined with insulin, the effect is additive. This will cause blood sugar to drop way below normal limits, causing hypoglycemia, bringing on cold, clammy skin, rapid heart rate, dizziness, weakness, fainting, and possibly seizures or death.

Diuretics: Prescription diuretics and natural herbal ones such as green tea, matcha tea, yarrow, goldenseal, asparagus extract, dandelion, and stinging nettle cause water in the body to be lost. That's the point. But a person who has diabetes already tends to urinate a lot because the increased glucose level in the blood causes water to be lost through urination. So I suspect that diuretics could cause dehydration in some people taking diabetes drugs.

Spirulina or chlorophyll: This supplement may reduce blood sugar after a few weeks or months. Wonderful! Combining it with medications might make glucose drop too low. Just make sure you monitor your glucose level closely and have your doctor reduce your medication appropriately. More about the powerful benefits of these in my book *Diabetes without Drugs* (Rodale 2010). These supplements are the first step to getting well.

Diet pills and appetite suppressants: These reduce appetite. Insulin increases the munchies. Diet pills and appetite suppressants often excite the heart and lower blood sugar. Insulin lowers blood sugar as well. When you mix the two, you don't know what's going to be the end result. It could cause a dangerous drop in blood sugar, sending it so low that it affects the beating of your heart. I would avoid these supplements unless your doctor allows you to lower your drug dosage.

Fiber supplements: Separate these supplements from oral diabetes medication by 2 or more hours.

Vitamin D: This vitamin turns into calcitriol hormone in the body. It's best known for its ability to rev immune function and lower risk for autoimmune disorders and all types of cancer. Most people don't realize it also can greatly improve insulin sensitivity. This means that your body will respond better to circulating (or injected) insulin, and your blood sugar will go down. When combined with medications, your glucose could drop too low. It's a good idea to monitor your blood glucose closely if you are taking vitamin D long-term (more than a month) and have your doctor reduce your medication dosage as needed.

Blood sugar–lowering herbs: The following herbs and nutritional supplements may effectively lower blood sugar, and they should be used very cautiously if you are also taking medicine. Monitor blood sugar frequently when taking the following herbs, and be aware that medications and insulin dosages should be adjusted downward so you don't get hypoglycemic.

Fenugreek	Holy basil
Gymnema sylvestre	Curcumin/turmeric
Bitter melon extract	Alpha-lipoic acid
Stinging nettle	Saffron
Myrrh	Digestive enzymes
Marshmallow	Cinnamon
Alfalfa	Stevia
Aloe vera	Ginseng

Digoxin

Example: Lanoxin.

This drug is a derivative of digitalis, a natural toxin that was once used on arrowheads as a deadly poison. Digoxin is used most frequently for congestive heart failure because it relieves shortness of breath and wheezing experienced while lying down. It may help with swelling in the hands and feet. It works by slowing down the heart, allowing the chambers to fill up with blood and to pump blood more efficiently, which could improve heartbeat rhythm. Side effects may include abdominal pain, nausea, vomiting, loss of appetite, skin rash, blurred vision, mental changes, and heart rhythm problems. People with chronic kidney disease need lower dosages than others. There is a very fine line between what's effective and what's dangerous, so heed the drug–food interactions very carefully. Because the drug has its primary effects on the heart, a drug–food interaction could have harmful consequences for the heart.

Oatmeal and bran cereal: The combination slows down the breakdown of the drug. This means that it lingers for a long time in your bloodstream without being processed and can cause more side effects. High levels of digoxin can lead to overdose and life-threatening arrhythmias.

Calcium: Excess supplementation with this popular bone-building mineral can lead to digoxin overdose.

St. John's wort: This herb reduces digoxin levels, which could mean therapeutic failure. If you want to take the herb, your doctor will have to increase your medication dose.

Erectile Dysfunction Medicines

Examples: Cialis and Adcirca (tadalafil), Levitra (vardenafil), and Viagra and Revatio (sildenafil).

Pills for erectile dysfunction (ED) are big business in the pharmacy, especially every Friday night, when the meds move like hotcakes. For now sex pills are reserved for men, but soon they will be prescribed for women, too. The drugs rank among the most expensive of our recreational drugs, at $15 a pill. That's why Viagra is affectionately dubbed the blue diamond by many pharmacists. It's a blue pill in the shape of a diamond, and it's expensive.

To understand the way these drugs work, you must understand how the body naturally achieves an erection. First, there is some kind of stimulation, visual or physical, that triggers a biochemical reaction in the penis causing the blood vessels and muscles surrounding that organ to relax. This biochemical reaction involves the nitric oxide pathway; the greater the nitric oxide production, the more blood flow to the region. More blood flow to the penis and voila! Passion is possible. Sex pills work by allowing more blood to flow. They are taken 30 minutes to an hour before desired sexual activity, and some meds like Cialis are approved for use every day.

If you have to rely on these medications frequently, get your heart checked out because if the blood isn't flowing properly down south, it isn't flowing well up north either. Not all men with erectile difficulties have heart disease, but erection problems could be your first sign of it. Here is what you need to know about food interactions.

Grapefruit juice and pomegranate juice: These juices seem to be able to increase the blood level of sex pills, leading to dangerous side effects including headache, indigestion, flushing, vision disturbances, and abnormal heart rate. Grapefruit also delays absorption of the medication. It normally takes about an hour for these drugs to begin working, but if taken with grapefruit, it could take longer than an hour, increasing the risk of dangerous side effects (not to mention disappointment).

Over-the-counter sex enhancement pills: These often contain yohimbe and other herbs that affect blood circulation. The combination with prescribed ED drugs is additive and can lead to more side effects. In addition, these supplements may increase your risk of developing a painful, prolonged erection that requires medical attention. Repeat: painful!

Alcohol: Drinking can cause light-headedness and dizziness and so can the prescribed sex pills. The combination could make you dizzy or faint. Also, both alcohol and ED drugs can cause headache or migraine, and the combination can make your head really hurt.

Hawthorne, devil's claw, mistletoe, fenugreek, figwort, shepherd's purse, digitalis leaf, and motherwort: These herbs affect the heart. Since prescribed sex pills may increase the likelihood of cardiovascular side effects, combining them with any of these herbs can be dangerous. In studies of sildenafil (Viagra), the following cardiac changes were noted with the drug alone: angina pectoris, atrioventricular block, tachycardia, palpitations, myocardial ischemia, cerebral thrombosis, cardiac arrest, heart failure, and cardiomyopathy. You certainly don't want to be taking an herb that can increase the likelihood of these effects.

Lithium

Examples: Apo-Lithium, Eskalith, Eskalith CR, Lithobid, and Lithotabs.

Lithium naturally occurs in the human body, and it's very calming. It boosts memory and helps with brain function. Some brands of sea salt contain a little lithium, too. The mineral affects the flow of sodium through nerve and muscle cells all over the body. Sodium affects excitation or mania. You can buy OTC supplements of lithium orotate in low dosages, and it can improve mood dramatically. It's also available in higher dosages with a prescription. Lithium is most commonly prescribed to lessen the intensity or reduce the number of manic episodes in people with manic depression, or bipolar disorder. The symptoms of this condition could include hyperactivity, rushed speech, poor judgment, reduced need for sleep, aggression, and anger. Lithium has a relatively small target range for what's effective as opposed to what is toxic. If it shifts even a little bit, it could become ineffective or toxic.

Table salt (sodium chloride): Too little salt can decrease the lithium level in the blood, while too much can increase it. Either way, the interaction can be dangerous. Ideally, you should drink about six glasses of water a day and stay consistent with your water and salt intake. The dosage of your medication is determined by lab evaluations (blood tests), so it's actually based on your regular daily consumption.

Coffee, tea, soda, energy drinks, and chocolate: Caffeine can reduce serum levels of lithium. The trick is to keep the amount of caffeine-containing beverages you drink consistent from day to day. Less caffeine can cause your lithium level to increase; more caffeine can cause it to decrease. Consistency is key.

Food: Take lithium with food to prevent digestive upset.

MAO Inhibitors (Monoamine Oxidase Inhibitors) and St. John's Wort

Examples: Aurorix and Manerix (moclobemide), Azilect (rasagiline), Eldepryl (selegiline), Marplan (isocarboxazid), Nardil (phenelzine), and Parnate (tranylcypromine).

These medications possess some MAO activity: Furoxone (furazolidone) and Zyvox (linezolid), which are used as antibiotics, and Matulane (procarbazine), used as chemotherapy.

MAO inhibiting medications have been reserved to treat the most resistant forms of depression. In recent years, they have found new use for conditions such as headache, panic disorder, and Parkinson's disease. These medications have been somewhat effective, but they cause dangerous side effects. Like every drug, there is a risk-to-benefit ratio. With MAO drugs, there is a lot of risk for the benefit.

If you are prescribed one of these, be very careful about drug–food interactions. Most health-care practitioners have a list of do's and don'ts for these medications, so don't be shy about asking for any information that they can give you. The drugs work in part by raising levels of serotonin, so any herb or drug (even if it's not listed below) that raises the level of that feel-good hormone could interact dangerously with MAO meds.

MAO inhibitor drugs are among the most dangerous drugs in the world because they interact with so many foods, herbs, and beverages. The danger is in the sudden spike of blood pressure (vasoconstriction) that can happen when there is too much serotonin released in the body. This life-threatening complication is called *serotonin syndrome,* and symptoms include nausea, confusion, sweating, agitation, and unresponsiveness. MAO drugs interact with more than 200 different medications for one reason or another, so prescribing them to people who already take medicine can be tricky. Sadly, there have been some fatalities reported among users who didn't realize they were eating the wrong food. Here's what you need to know if you take an MAO drug.

St. John's wort: This is used for pain and to boost mood in depression. It's found alone or in combination with other herbs, and it acts on the brain in the same manner as MAO drugs, but to a much lesser extent. Don't combine it with MAO drugs, or within 2 weeks of their use. And while I'm talking about St. John's wort, even if you aren't on MAO inhibitors, stop using it 5 days before surgery to be safe because it has some blood-thinning properties and could affect your ability to clot properly while under the knife.

Ginseng: Phenelzine and other MAOs combined with ginseng supplements or drinks can cause insomnia, headache, tremors, and hypomania, which causes excessive energy, insomnia, unusual exhilaration or excitement, agitation, or depression. Avoid ginseng with MAO inhibitors.

Alcohol: It contains the amino acid tyramine, and this can interact with your medication. The interaction is so serious that it can cause a disastrous rise in blood pressure. Avoid beer, red wine, and liqueurs.

Cough and cold syrups: These usually contain dextromethorphan, a cough suppressant that interacts with the classic MAO medications and increases brain levels of serotonin, causing bizarre behavior. There has been at least one reported case of death. Avoid dextromethorphan while using St. John's wort, too. Steer clear of MAO medications for 2 weeks before using any cough or cold syrup.

Cheese: You can experience a problem with any kind of cheese, including Parmesan, mozzarella, Cheddar, blue, brie, Camembert, and so on. The same is true of sour cream. Cheese contains the amino acid tyramine, which reacts with MAO drugs in the same dangerous way as alcohol does. This reaction is extremely rare with St. John's wort.

Other foods: Avoid the following foods because they can interact with MAO drugs and cause a dangerous rise in blood pressure: yogurt, avocados (especially if they are very ripe), bananas, yeast extract, cured meats (such as sausage, salami, and pepperoni) and dried fish, caviar, raisins, sauerkraut, soy sauce, fava beans, and miso soup.

Coffee, tea, and soda: The caffeine in these drinks makes this combination spike blood pressure.

Diet pills and appetite suppressants: These contain ingredients that squeeze your blood vessels and increase your blood pressure. Do not take these products while taking an MAO drug, or within 2 weeks of stopping an MAO drug. If you do, you may suddenly develop extremely high blood pressure.

Nasal sprays: Afrin, Otrivin, and other nasal sprays that contain a similar ingredient can spell trouble for people taking MAOs, including St. John's wort. These drugs squeeze off your tiny vessels, increasing blood pressure just like MAO drugs. Be clear of your medicine for 2 weeks before using any of these nasal decongestants or taking cough and cold medicine. Ocean nasal spray, which contains saline, is a better choice because it is nonmedicated. Neti pot treatments are fine, too.

Eyedrops: Those that contain tetrahydrozoline (Visine) also cause vasoconstriction. Even though it goes into the eye, some of it gets absorbed into the bloodstream, where it could interact with MAO drugs, including St. John's wort, and spike blood pressure.

Metronidazole

Examples: Flagyl and MetroGel.

This antibiotic is effective against certain bacteria and parasites. It is classically used for giardia, an intestinal parasite that causes severe abdominal pain and diarrhea. It's often used to treat *Clostridium difficile,* an infection of the gut that occurs after the use of other strong antibiotics. Take a guess why *C. difficile* might easily overtake the gut after another antibiotic. Yep, drug mugging antibiotics kill normal beneficial flora, allowing other, bad bugs to take over. *C. difficile* is dangerous, and these types of infections are common in hospitals and nursing homes. Read about probiotics in Chapter 17 on page 229 to find out how to replenish what drug mugging antibiotics steal.

Metronidazole can also be used for vaginal infections and for certain sexually transmitted diseases in both men and women. It's used to treat trichomoniasis, a vaginal infection that causes vaginitis. It can also be used for deep lung infections, meningitis, and many other hard-to-treat bugs. Here's what you need to know if you have to take metronidazole.

Alcohol: This combination could kill you, according to a report published in the *American Journal of Forensic Medicine and Pathology* in 1996. The case described a young assault victim who died from cardiac dysrhythmia due to an acetaldehyde (a by-product of alcohol consumption) and metronidazole interaction. Sudden death is possible, but pretty rare. More often, people experience projectile vomiting, dehydration, headaches, stomach cramps, nausea, heart palpitations, shortness of breath, and heat flushing. Those things don't happen to everyone, but when they do, it is not pretty. Some individuals are so highly sensitive to alcohol in combination with their meds—it's called a disulfiram reaction—that they can't even spray perfume or cologne on their skin because the alcohol in it reacts with the metronidazole medication. Cough syrups that contain alcohol are also a no-no. I always recommend steering clear of anything with alcohol while on this medication and for several days after your course of therapy has been completed.

Nitrates

Examples: Isosorbide dinitrate (Isordil, Dilatrate-SR, Coronex, Apo-ISDN), isosorbide mononitrate (Imdur, Monoket, Ismo), nitroglycerin (Nitrostat, Nitrolingual spray), and skin patches like Nitro-Dur and Transderm-Nitro.

Chest pain (angina) is often caused by the buildup of fatty cholesterol plaques that block blood flow to the heart. The insides of the coronary arteries become narrowed with the gunk. When you have chest pain, it's your body's way of telling you that your heart is suffocating and not getting enough oxygen as a result of the reduced blood flow. Nitrates temporarily widen (dilate) your arteries and improve blood flow to the heart. They are most frequently prescribed for people with angina or congestive heart failure. Nitrates don't alter the course of angina, nor do they cure it, but they do relax your blood vessels and allow them to dilate, which takes the strain off the heart because blood flows to it more easily. Side effects include dizziness and headache (because more blood is also flowing to the head), as well as facial flushing, upset stomach, and low blood pressure. Some people experience a change in heart rhythm, fainting, and restlessness. Here is what you need to know in terms of drug–food interactions.

Alcohol: This can relax blood flow by widening arteries, so combining it with nitrate drugs can result in dangerously low blood pressure.

Arginine supplements and sex enhancement vitamins that contain arginine: The amino acid arginine is used to improve erectile dysfunction and also to increase blood flow to the heart in people with coronary artery disease. The problem is that arginine-containing products can cause a dangerous drop in blood pressure when combined with nitrate drugs. (The same interaction is possible for medications such as Levitra, Cialis, and Viagra.)

Nicotine products: These negate the effect of nitrate medication by increasing blood pressure and heart rate.

Oral Contraceptives and Hormone Replacement Therapy (HRT)

Examples of oral contraceptives: Activella, Alesse, Apri, Aviane, Camila, Depo-Provera shot, Estrace, Estraderm, Estring, Estro-Gel, Estrostep, Femring, Levlen, Levlite, Loestrin, Lo/Ovral, Menostar, Micronor, Mircette, Modicon, Necon, Nordette, Norinyl, Nor-QD, NuvaRing, Ogestrel, Ortho-Cept, Ortho Evra patch, Ortho-Novum, Ortho Tri-Cyclen, Ovcon, Ovral, Seasonale, Tri-Levlen, Tri-Norinyl, Triphasil, Yasmin and Yaz, and Zovia.

Examples of hormone replacement therapy: Climara, Combi-Patch, estradiol, femhrt, Ogen, Premarin, Prempro, other estrogens (bioidentical hormones and natural soy isoflavones).

These types of drugs contain a synthetic hormone that is similar to the one produced naturally in your body. There is a lot of hoopla about hormones now as we debate the use of synthetic hormones versus bioidentical ones.

It's the synthetic ones that I want to discuss here, because these drugs are man-made and are not completely recognized by our bodies. They are recognized by our cells just enough to get into the doorway of the cell and do a small amount of work. But then they persistently stick to these cells, and therein lies the problem.

Hormone replacement therapy (HRT) drugs are used primarily to control hot flashes, night sweats, and possibly bone loss associated with declining estrogen. These medications have widespread effects in the body, including numerous side effects and a host of drug–food interactions. Refer to Chapter 1 to learn how to overcome the drug mugging effect of HRT and contraception. Take a look at the most common drug–food interactions.

Vitamin A dietary supplements: A study utilizing a popular oral contraceptive (Ortho-Novum) found that it could increase the blood level of vitamin A, so combining it with high doses (greater than 10,000 IU per day) could cause a buildup of vitamin A. The potential exists for a high level of A to become toxic, causing temporary skin discoloration (yellowing), diarrhea, easy bruising, and arthritis. It is worth noting that problems with vitamin A and hormone medications do not occur if you take beta-carotene, a plant-derived precursor of vitamin A, or if you eat lots of carrots or drink carrot juice.

Coffee, tea, soda, and chocolate: Hormones increase the effect of caffeine. This combination can leave you feeling jittery, irritable, or hyper, and may cause nausea and tremors.

Diet pills, appetite suppressants, and energy drinks: Some of these contain guarana, yerba maté, bitter orange, or ma huang and can be stimulating. Hormones tend to be stimulating as well, so the combination can cause the same problems as caffeinated drinks. See the section above.

Grapefruit juice: This citrus juice can significantly raise estradiol levels in the body. Estradiol is the most common form of estrogen found in oral contraceptives and most HRT drugs such as Estrace, Climara, Estraderm, Estring, Activella, Femring, CombiPatch, EstroGel, Menostar, and many others. One study found that grapefruit juice can also increase the levels of conjugated estrogens (Premarin, Prempro) by up to 30 percent, increasing the risk for harmful side effects.

Herbs such as chasteberry, black cohosh, licorice, motherwort, saw palmetto, and wild yam: These herbs work on the same hormonal systems as the drugs and may interfere with your medicine.

Pain Relievers (Opiate Analgesics)

Examples: Codeine or codeine and acetaminophen (Tylenol 3), fentanyl patches (Duragesic, Actiq), hydrocodone with acetaminophen (Vicodin, Lortab), meperidine (Demerol), morphine sulfate (MS-Contin, Roxanol), oxycodone with acetaminophen (Percocet, Roxicet, Tylox), propoxyphene with acetaminophen (Darvocet-N 100), and tramadol (Ultram, Ultracet).

Opiates and their derivatives are usually prescribed for patients going home after surgery, childbirth, or dental work. They also ease back pain, headaches, arthritis, and pain from broken bones. Opiates are effective at relieving pain, and I'm one of those pharmacists who believe in their use as long as there is a genuine indication, but many clinicians are afraid of these drugs because physical dependence occurs after a few weeks. It's common for people to need more and more medication to confer the same pain-relieving effect as the body grows tolerant to lower doses, but if you have chronic pain, so what? No one should have to suffer as far as I'm concerned.

Opiates were created and intended for short-term use, not forever. I have seen many people who cannot go without the medicine because it provides relief from their chronic and intractable pain. The way they work is not completely understood, but in part they reduce levels of substance P, a chemical in the body that causes the sensation of pain. These medications can cause excessive sleepiness, confusion, slowed breathing, reduced heart rate, and constipation. The nausea and vomiting that is sometimes caused by these drugs can be minimized if they are taken with food.

Alcohol: When combined with painkillers, heart rate and breathing slow down and the heart can stop.

Kava: This natural herb is used as a muscle relaxant, an anticonvulsant, an antianxiety med, and a sleep aid. It acts on the nervous system in the same way as painkillers, and the sedative effect can be additive. Don't combine.

Bananas, rice, and other constipating foods: Painkillers are very constipating, and these types of foods can add to your discomfort. Prunes are good for people who take opiate analgesics.

Sedating herbs: When combined with painkillers, passionflower, hops, lemon balm, and other sedating herbs slow down your heart rate and breathing. They can even stop the heart in sensitive people.

Potatoes and apples: These foods are high in pectin, which slows down the effect of your medicine. Other foods containing a lot of starch or fiber can have the same effect.

Smoking: This can reduce the effectiveness of your painkiller because it speeds the processing and elimination of the drug. The faster the drug goes through your system, the less time your body has to extract any benefit from it.

Potassium-Sparing Diuretics (Water Pills)

Examples: Aldactone (spironolactone); Dyazide, Dyrenium, and Maxzide (triamterene); and Midamor (amiloride).

These drugs are used to treat high blood pressure. They make you urinate more by forcing your kidneys to dump out more sodium, which takes water with it. The water it takes comes from your blood, so the pressure in your blood vessels goes down. Makes sense, right? Although most other diuretics cause you to lose potassium along with the sodium, this class of drugs retains potassium in your body. Sometimes you will see them combined with diuretics that spill potassium, like furosemide.

Potassium-sparing diuretics are often prescribed with different types of blood pressure medications, which control heart rate and pressure in the vessels. What's important here again is the potassium. You have to maintain the proper level, regardless of which diuretic you are using. If your potassium falls too low, you will get hypokalemia, a dangerous condition that can slow or stop your heart and cause nausea, fatigue, and muscle weakness. Here is what you need to know to stay safe while taking potassium-sparing diuretics.

Bananas, asparagus, squash, leafy green vegetables, and orange juice: These foods are rich in potassium. Since the water pill is causing you to hold on to potassium, you may get too much—hyperkalemia—which can affect heart rate and muscle coordination. It's okay to eat them, but do so in moderation.

Salt substitutes: These contain potassium and can cause potassium overload when combined with potassium-sparing diuretics.

Monosodium glutamate: If you are sensitive to monosodium glutamate (MSG), a common food additive, the use of potassium-sparing diuretics can make you even more sensitive.

Stinging nettle supplement and tea: Many people take this dietary supplement for prostate problems or allergies. It removes potassium from the body, so even though it enhances water loss, it may alter potassium levels and work against this type of diuretic.

Dandelion: A popular dietary supplement, dandelion is a mild potassium-sparing diuretic. The combination may produce a dangerous increase in potassium levels.

Quinolone Antibiotics

Examples: Cipro (ciprofloxacin), Floxin (ofloxacin), Levaquin (levofloxacin), Maxaquin (lomefloxacin), and Noroxin (norfloxacin). (Megalone, Omniflox, Raxar, Tequin, and Trovan have been withdrawn from the market.)

These medications are used to treat infections and are particularly good at penetrating hard-to-reach tissue like that in the urinary tract, kidneys, and prostate. They can successfully treat life-threatening cases of Legionnaires' disease and pneumonia. Quinolones are often prescribed long-term (for more than 7 days) because the bad bugs are stubborn about retreating.

However, overprescribing of quinolones has contributed to the sobering problem of resistance. In July 2008, the FDA told makers of quinolone antibiotics to issue a black box warning about the potential for tendon rupture or tendon injuries. The warning didn't surprise me. But for tendon rupture? That was unexpected, given all the other serious side effects these drugs can have, including irreversible nerve pain, burning, tingling, numbness, weakness, and a feeling of vibrations under the skin. Quinolones have been linked to liver failure, irreversible neuropathies, and even toxic psychosis. A warning about quinolones causing tendon rupture is the equivalent of warning smokers that their cigarettes will cause bad breath.

I recommend that you immediately discontinue your medication if you experience the side effects listed above. Other side effects include changes in heart rhythm, depression, anxiety, difficulty concentrating, and a strange dissociation with reality or people. These may be a result of the drug mugging effect of the medication. Here are the drug–food interactions with quinolones.

Dairy products: Milk, cheese, yogurt, and butter all contain calcium. Calcium can bind to your antibiotic and suppress its effect, so you don't heal properly and need a second go-around.

Calcium supplements: As above, the calcium diminishes the effect of your antibiotic.

Multivitamins: These often contain minerals such as iron, magnesium, zinc, and calcium, which could attach to your antibiotic and reduce its effectiveness.

Antacids: Products such as Maalox, Mylanta, and Gaviscon contain aluminum, calcium, and/or magnesium, all of which can latch onto the antibiotic and dramatically diminish its effect in the bloodstream. This happens because the aluminum, magnesium, and calcium grab the fluoroquinolone antibiotic and take it out of the body before it can work on your infection.

Iron supplements: These include Fcosol, Nu-Iron, Niferex, ferrous sulfate, ferrous gluconate, iron bisglycinate, chelated iron, and others. Iron attaches to your antibiotic, reducing the bioavailability of your drug and therefore decreasing its effectiveness.

Zinc: These supplements or lozenges, often used for sore throats, coughs, and colds, can latch onto the antibiotic, making it less effective.

Trace minerals supplement: The minerals attach to your antibiotic, reducing the drug's effectiveness.

Birth control pills: Antibiotics (all of them) make your birth control pills less effective because they strip the gut of beneficial flora. You need flora to absorb the Pill, so you become more susceptible to pregnancy whenever you take an antibiotic. Use a second method of contraception during the course of the antibiotic and for 10 days thereafter.

Coffee, tea, and soda: Quinolone antibiotics tend to be stimulating and cause the jitters, irritability, anxiety, and insomnia, so avoid caffeine-containing beverages that enhance this effect. Beware: Diet pills often contain caffeine and ma huang, which acts just like caffeine. The likelihood of these uncomfortable side effects goes up if you combine the quinolone antibiotic with an OTC pain reliever like ibuprofen or naproxen and caffeine.

Sleeping Medications

Examples: Ambien or Ambien CR (zolpidem), Klonopin (clonazepam), Lunesta (eszopiclone), Restoril (temazepam), Rozerem (ramelteon), Sonata (zaleplon), and Xanax (alprazolam).

Sleeping pills have become fast movers in the pharmacy. We sell so many of these drugs that I think everyone must be up at 2:00 a.m. watching infomercials on how to steam clean grout or get a six-pack of abs. My problem with sleeping pills in general is that the sleep they induce is really not natural, refreshing, or restorative. True, you are in a sleep-type funk, if you will, but it's artificial. All the drugs in the list above (with the exception of ramelteon) trigger the release of one relaxing brain chemical called GABA, and GABA floods your brain and makes you sleepy. It slows everything down, in fact, including heart rate and breathing. Ramelteon increases melatonin, not GABA, and melatonin helps you stay asleep at night.

These medications were designed to be temporary fix-me-ups, but I've seen physicians prescribe them to people for years at a time. They were not intended to treat chronic insomnia. I agree that the thought of having a pill to get you to sleep within a few minutes can be appealing if you are exhausted and simply unable to sleep. But there are many valid concerns about these drugs. For example, many of them cause tolerance, and thus physical dependence as you need higher and higher dosages for them to work. Also, you can't suddenly stop taking them without withdrawal symptoms (with the exception of Rozerem, because this drug does not cause physical dependence since it's a melatonin-derived drug).

Side effects can be bizarre, ranging from forgetfulness and morning hangover to dry mouth and amnesia, and occasionally behaviors that are out of character for an individual, such as driving without remembering the trip or cooking dinner at 4:00 a.m.! There are a slew of drug–food interactions, so be careful if you take this medicine.

Alcohol: Just say no. The combination of alcohol with sleeping pills is incredibly dangerous and can cause a fatal reduction in heart and breathing rates.

Marijuana: You should not be taking anything that has a sedative effect because it can enhance the effect of the medication. With this combination, you might not wake up, especially with cannabis strains high in indica versus sativa.

GABA supplements: These are sold at the health food store because they are an effective natural sleep aid. The combination of sleeping pills with GABA is not safe because of the enhanced levels of GABA the combination causes.

Sedating herbs: The combination of sedating herbs with sleeping pills is unsafe. They include catnip, ginseng, hops, kava, lemon balm, sage, St. John's wort, skullcap, valerian root, yerba mansa, passionflower, and sassafras. Kava is particularly worrisome.

Coffee, tea, and soda: Coffee, black tea, green tea, and matcha tea all contain caffeine. This substance undermines your sleep medication.

Statin Cholesterol Reducers

Examples: Atorvastatin (Lipitor, Avicor), fluvastatin (Lescol), lovastatin (Mevacor, Altocor, Altoprev), pravastatin (Pravachol, Lipostat, Selektine), pitavastatin (Livalo, Pitava), rosuvastatin (Crestor), simvastatin and ezetimibe (Vytorin), and simvastatin and niacin (Simcor).

These are among the most prescribed drugs in the world. They are said to lower your risk of heart disease by reducing the amount of cholesterol your body makes and are often prescribed along with diet and exercise regimens. These meds decrease the amount of cholesterol your liver makes, and your liver makes about 75 percent of your total cholesterol. (The other 25 percent comes from food.) Statins block an enzyme called HMG-CoA reductase, which would otherwise allow the formation of cholesterol as well as of natural coenzyme Q10. (Read more about the drug mugging effect on CoQ10 starting on page 124.)

The cholesterol molecule is fatty, almost waxy, but your blood is water based. Think of oil and water—they won't mix well unless shaken. The cholesterol produced in the liver can't enter your bloodstream unless it is bound to a protein that acts sort of like a taxi. The protein-cholesterol compound, called lipoprotein, gets shuttled all around your bloodstream. There are good lipoproteins like HDL (high-density lipoprotein), which tote cholesterol back to the liver, where it's disposed of.

There is also a protein-cholesterol compound called LDL (low-density lipoprotein), which lugs cholesterol to your blood, where it clogs up arteries and impedes adequate blood flow to your heart and brain. Now you know why doctors are bent on bringing down your LDL. But are statins the answer? That is between you and your doctor. I've not been shy about my dismay over the indiscriminate prescribing of these drugs to people who don't genuinely need them. Here are some helpful drug–food interactions that you should know about if you are taking a statin.

Alcohol: Alcohol damages the liver all by itself, and when you combine it with a statin drug, you get a double whammy. That's because statins work in the liver, too, and they shift liver enzymes out of balance.

Grapefruit and its juice and pomegranate juice: Grapefruit spikes the blood levels of some statins, and this means more side effects. At the time of this writing, there are at least three statins that interact with grapefruit and may cause severe and irreversible liver damage and possibly a condition known as rhabdomyolysis. The three statins are atorvastatin, lovastatin, and simvastatin. Rhabdomyolysis, whose symptoms are dark, red, or cola-colored urine and muscle tenderness, stiffness, aching (myalgia), or weakness, could come on slowly or all of a sudden. If you have these problems, it could be the beginning of rhabdomyolysis. For you science junkies, the interaction between grapefruit juice and statins occurs because the drugs block the action of an enzyme called cytochrome P450 3A4 (CYP3A4).

Other citrus juices (like tangerine and orange) may be a problem as well; this is not clear yet. Additionally, the latest research has found that pomegranate juice acts in a similar manner. This has not been completely settled, however. My advice is to avoid or limit these juices to no more than a sip each day because of their great antioxidant protection. But no guzzling of grapefruit or other citrus juices and pomegranate juice.

Of the three statins I mentioned, atorvastatin seems to be the least affected; however, I would not combine the juice with any of them, just to be safe. For the time being, rosuvastatin, pravastatin, and fluvastatin may be better alternatives if you love grapefruit juice and take a statin. (See page 88 for more grapefruit interactions.)

Grapefruit seed extract: This is a dietary supplement that fights candida yeast infections and can be found at the health food store. It carries the same warnings as grapefruit, even though it's an herbal extract.

Oyster mushrooms: These are thought to have natural statin activity. Though weak in comparison with statin drugs (oyster mushrooms contain approximately 0.4 percent to 2.7 percent statinlike activity on a dry-weight basis). There isn't enough activity to enhance your medication, so don't worry about that.

Red yeast rice: A dietary supplement and Asian food, this is a natural statin that contains the same ingredient as the Rx lovastatin. Combining with statin drugs is a no-no.

Thyroid Medicines

Examples: Armour Thyroid, levothyroxine, Levoxyl, Synthroid, Unithroid, and compounded thyroid formulas.

These medications are used for people who have low levels of circulating thyroid hormone, a condition called hypothyroidism. Some hallmark symptoms of low thyroid include fatigue, difficulty losing weight, and hair thinning or loss. These meds are also used in some autoimmune thyroid disorders (Hashimoto's and Graves' diseases), depending on your thyroid hormone level. These medications are somewhat stimulating. They increase heart rate and energy levels, and for that reason they should be taken in the morning rather than at night. Here is what you need to know.

Iron supplements: According to a study published in the *British Journal of Clinical Pharmacology*, taking iron along with thyroid medication will significantly interfere with the amount of thyroid your body absorbs. The iron binds to thyroxine (the active thyroid hormone in the medication. The problem is that many people take thyroid medication because they are deficient in iron (low ferritin), and so they need both of these items in their daily regimen. Just take the thyroid hormone in the morning, upon arising, on an empty stomach. Take the iron with lunch or with dinner, at least 4 hours after the thyroid medication.

Trace minerals: This is incredibly helpful if you have low thyroid. Like iron, separate this from your thyroid med by 4 hours. If you have to take both iron and trace minerals (along with thyroid medication, and this is quite common), then take the thyroid first thing in the morning and take both the iron and the trace mineral supplement at lunch (or dinner), at least 4 hours later.

Tofu and other soy products: These foods fight against you by crashing your thyroid hormone. You will need higher drug dosages to build it back up.

Broccoli, brussels sprouts, turnips, and cauliflower: These foods can also fight against you, lowering your circulating level of thyroid. Consume no more than 1 cup of these veggies three times a week, but if you love them, stay consistent and ask your doctor to raise your medication dose.

Dairy products and calcium supplements: Calcium can interfere with the absorption of thyroid medicine, which means that your thyroid-stimulating hormone (TSH) may rise and your thyroid hormone levels may be suppressed. Take your medication first thing in the morning, and take your calcium supplement after dinner. Separate the medication from dairy foods by at least 2 hours.

Oatmeal, cereal, and other high-fiber foods and supplements: These speed metabolism and force medicine and vitamins to move through the colon much faster. This interaction will reduce your medication's effect. These foods are healthy, though, so I feel it's best to include them in your diet. Just eat your cereal 2 or 3 hours before or after your medicine.

Other foods: Take thyroid meds on an empty stomach because food in general interferes with it and reduces the amount your body gets.

Urinary Incontinence Medications

Examples: Cymbalta (duloxetine, also an antidepressant), Detrol and Detrol LA (tolterodine tartrate), Ditropan and Oxytrol (oxybutynin), and Tofranil (imipramine). Toviaz (fesoterodine) is new to the market and there are no data regarding this drug yet. I only include it here to make the drug list complete for people seeking medication choices.

The medications listed above are prescribed specifically for people with a weakened bladder or urinary sphincter, which causes stress or urge incontinence—the involuntary loss of urine. These people need to take numerous potty breaks during the day and night. Simply put, these medications can help people who can't hold on to their urine and who pee when they sneeze, walk, or get stressed out, or sometimes when there's no trigger at all. The condition arises for any number of reasons, including shifts in hormones, low estrogen, infection, spinal cord injury, pregnancy, childbirth, and prostate surgery. The medications tend to cause dry mouth, constipation, blurred vision, and drowsiness. Here's what else you need to know.

Grapefruit and its juice: These can spike the levels of medication, causing more side effects. (Read more about grapefruit on page 86.)

Garlic and melatonin: These may be inhibitors of CYP3A4. In English, this means that Detrol levels go up in the bloodstream, sparking more side effects.

Alcohol: Drinking may increase drowsiness and dizziness. Alcohol also makes people urinate more frequently, which undermines the effect of the medicine.

St. John's wort: This herb, which is so helpful for many people with depression, should not be used while taking Detrol.

Potassium supplements: Bladder meds slow down motility in the esophagus and intestinal tract, causing potassium to linger and increasing the likelihood of GI corrosion.

Diuretics: Prescription forms as well as natural herbal ones like green tea, matcha tea, yarrow, goldenseal, asparagus extract, dandelion, and stinging nettle will make you have to go to the bathroom more frequently. That interferes with your medicine, which is treating your overactive bladder.

Coffee, tea, and soda: Excessive amounts can cause urinary incontinence and aggravate bladder symptoms. Drink no more than 1 cup a day.

Horsetail tea: This herbal remedy helps people with bladder issues. Horsetail is the name given to the herb *Equisetum arvense*. I feel confident that this tea can be combined safely with the medications above. I've listed it here because it causes enhanced effects, which I consider beneficial in this case.

FOOD RULES: To Eat or Not to Eat

With all this talk of interactions with foods and herbs, it's important not to lose sight of the fact that many medications need to be taken with food while others should be taken on an empty stomach. The reasons for this sometimes have to do with the fact that a little fat in your meal improves absorption or in some cases inhibits absorption of a drug, affecting its bioavailability. If you absorb less of your medication, the therapeutic benefits are lowered. Sometimes, pharmacists advise that you take your medications with food simply because it will minimize stomach upset. There are many reasons for the food rules on your medication label. I've outlined a list of food rules for medications. These are not hard-and-fast rules, just very basic guidance. If you have a particular concern about a specific medication, or if you do not see your medication (or medication category) listed, please ask your local pharmacist what is right for you. There are also thousands of medications that I have not listed here and that may be taken without regard to meals. Here's what you need to know.

TAKE THESE MEDICATIONS WITH FOOD:

Take these medications a few minutes before you eat, while you're eating, or shortly after you finish your meal.

ACE Inhibitors (Angiotensin-Converting Enzyme Inhibitors)

Benazepril (Lotensin)

Captopril (Capoten)

Enalapril (Vasotec)

Fosinopril (Monopril)

Lisinopril (Prinivil, Zestril)

Moexipril (Univasc)

Perindopril (Aceon)

Quinapril (Accupril)

Ramipril (Altace)

Trandolapril (Mavik)

Analgesics/Pain Relievers

Most pain relievers can be taken without regard to meals; however, they are very irritating to the stomach and often cause nausea or vomiting. I always recommend that you take the following with meals.

Codeine and codeine-containing cough syrup

Hydrocodone and acetaminophen (Lortab, Norco, Vicodin)

Hydrocodone and ibuprofen (Vicoprofen)

Morphine (Avinza)

Oxycodone (Roxicodone)

Oxycodone and acetaminophen (Percocet)

Oxycodone and aspirin (Percodan)

Oxycodone extended-release (Oxycontin)

Tramadol (Ultram, Ultram ER)

Antibiotics

Taking these on an empty stomach will improve absorption, but taking them with food will minimize stomach upset.

Amoxicillin/clavulanate potassium (Augmentin)

Azithromycin (Z-Pak)

Doxycycline (Vibramycin, Vibra-Tabs)

Erythromycin and erythromycin ethylsuccinate (E.E.S.)

Metronidazole (Flagyl)

Minocycline (Minocin)

Nitrofurantoin (Macrobid)

Cephalosporin antibiotics:

Cefaclor (Ceclor)

Cefadroxil (Duricef)

Cefazolin (Ancef, Kefzol)

Cefixime (Suprax)

Cefoxitin (Mefoxin)

Cefprozil (Cefzil)

Ceftazidime (Ceptaz, Fortaz, Tazicef, Tazidime)

(continued)

continued from page 69

TAKE THESE MEDICATIONS WITH FOOD *(continued)*

Cefuroxime (Ceftin)

Cephalexin (Keflex)

Anticonvulsants

Gabapentin (Neurontin)

Phenobarbital (Solfoton)

Phenytoin (Dilantin)

Pregabalin (Lyrica)

Valproic acid (Depakene, Depakote)

Antidepressants

See page 34, "Antidepressants and Mood Modifiers," and page 50, "MAO Inhibitors," for a complete list. All categories of these medications (tricyclics, SSRIs, etc.) should be taken with food to reduce stomach upset, nausea, heartburn, and cramps. All of them can be very irritating, so take them with a snack or with a meal.

Antifungals

Griseofulvin (Fulvicin, Gris-PEG, Grifulvin V)

Itraconazole (Sporanox)

Antigout

Allopurinol (Zyloprim)

Anti-Inflammatories

See "Arthritis Medicines" on page 36 for a complete list.

Celecoxib (Celebrex)

Diclofenac (Voltaren)

Hydrocortisone (Cortef)

Hydroxychloroquine (Plaquenil)

Ibuprofen (Advil, Motrin)

Indomethacin (Indocin)

Ketoprofen (Orudis)

Nabumetone (Relafen)

Naproxen (Aleve, Anaprox, Naprosyn)

Sulfasalazine (Azulfidine)

Benzodiazepines

Alprazolam (Xanax)

Diabetes Medications

Take 5 to 60 minutes after eating, depending on drug. Check with your pharmacist for the correct waiting time for your drug. Please read *Diabetes without Drugs* for more information about safe usage.

Acarbose (Precose)

Albiglutide (Syncria injection, pending FDA approval)

Chlorpropamide (Diabinese)

Exenatide (Byetta)

Glimepiride (Amaryl)

Glipizide (Glucotrol, Glucotrol XL)

Glipizide and metformin (Metaglip)

Glyburide (Diabeta, Micronase)

Glyburide and metformin (Glucovance)

Liraglutide (Victoza)

Metformin (Fortamet, Glucophage, Glucophage XR)

Metformin and pioglitazone (Actoplus)

Metformin and repaglinide (PrandiMet)

Metformin and rosiglitazone (Avandamet)

Metformin and sitagliptin (Janumet)

Micronized glyburide (Glynase)

Pramlintide (Symlin injection)

Repaglinide (Prandin)

Tolazamide (Tolinase)

Tolbutamide (Orinase)

Voglibose (pending US FDA approval; known as Basen in Japan and Volix in India)

Estrogen-Containing Drugs

Hormone replacement therapy

Oral contraceptives

(continued)

continued from page 71

Lipase Inhibitors

Orlistat (Alli, Xenical)

Salicylates

Salicylic acid or aspirin (Bayer, Ecotrin, St. Joseph)

Pain Relievers

These include ibuprofen, acetaminophen, and prescription opiates such as hydrocodone, oxycodone, and morphine.

Steroid Dose Pack

Methylprednisolone (Medrol Dose Pack) and prednisolone (Sterapred Dose Pack)

TAKE THESE MEDICATIONS ON AN EMPTY STOMACH:

Technically, taking drugs on an empty stomach is generally understood to mean 1 hour before you eat a meal or snack or 2 hours after you have finished eating.

Antibiotics

Rifampin (Rifadin)

Tetracycline (Sumycin)

Quinolone antibiotics:

Ciprofloxacin (Cipro)

Levofloxacin (Levaquin)

Ofloxacin (Floxin)

Antihistamines

Desloratadine (Clarinex)

Loratadine (Claritin)

Antiarrhythmics

Digoxin (Lanoxin)

Appetite Suppressants

Phentermine (Adipex-P)

Beta-Blockers

For a complete list, see page 38.

Atenolol (Tenormin)

Labetalol (Normodyne, Trandate)

Metoprolol (Lopressor and Toprol XL)

Propranolol (Inderal)

Bone-Building Drugs

Alendronate (Fosamax)

Alendronic acid and colecalciferol (Fosavance)

Etidronate (Didronel)

Ibandronate (Boniva)

Risedronate (Actonel)

H$_2$ Acid Blockers

Can be taken 15 minutes to 1 hour before eating.

Cimetidine (Tagamet)

Esomeprazole (Nexium)

Famotidine (Pepcid, Pepcid Complete)

Omeprazole (Prilosec)

Pantoprazole (Protonix)

Rabeprazole (Aciphex)

Ranitidine (Zantac)

Sleeping Medications

These may be taken without regard to meals, but will work faster on an empty stomach. For a complete list, see page 61.

Eszopiclone (Lunesta)

Zaleplon (Sonata)

Zolpidem (Ambien)

Thyroid Hormones

Armour Thyroid

Levothyroxine or L-thyroxine (Levothroid, Synthroid, Unithroid)

Liothyronine (Cytomel)

T$_3$/T$_4$ compounded hormone

Lifestyle Drug Muggers

The title of my book may mislead people into thinking that the only way they are going to suffer the effects of nutrient depletion is as a result of a pharmaceutical chemical. Not so. In fact, the impact of nutrient depletion is felt by people who don't even use medications. That's because we can lose our nutrients by making certain lifestyle choices, such as drinking soda or coffee or going on yo-yo diets. We all find ourselves stressing over life's situations, don't we? This, too, can slowly steal the life out of you because stress is a mugger of healthy nutrients and hormones. Malabsorption issues related to poor digestion can also cause you to lose important nutrients. You might be surprised by this information, but as you will soon see, a wide assortment of lifestyle drug muggers might be mugging you of important nutrients. To get a glimpse of just how important it is to pay attention to nutrients that might need replenishing, answer the following questions.

Do You Love Coffee or Tea?

These popular beverages contain a lot of tannins, substances that can grab important minerals from your body. So if you like to drink coffee or tea every day, you may be low on calcium, magnesium, zinc, phosphorus, iron, and other minerals. Also, caffeine has a diuretic effect on the body. I didn't really believe this when I first heard it. I went so far as to have a test done on myself because I love tea and coffee. Sure enough, it showed that I was slightly short on zinc and iron. You can read the chapters on zinc and iron (pages 297 and 160) if you want to learn more about these important minerals and see what symptoms may be caused by these deficiencies. Don't worry, though. You don't have to give up these beverages entirely. You can buy a supplement called trace minerals to keep your minerals replenished. Green drinks and spirulina supplements are other ways to give your body healthy minerals in an easy-to-digest form. Herbal tea does not contain tannins and therefore won't mug your minerals.

Caffeine in black or green tea (and in sensitive folks even matcha tea), coffee, and energy drinks can be so stimulating that you may find yourself needing tranquilizers or sleeping pills at night. A better bet would be to forgo caffeinated beverages after 3:00 p.m. and drink herbal tea. You'll sleep better, plus you'll be saving your precious minerals.

Are You a Soda Pop Junkie?

To put it simply, soda pop is not good for you. It doesn't give your body any form of nutrition, despite all the glamorous advertisements for it. Many health experts feel that cola is a powerful drug mugger of bone-building nutrients because of its high content of phosphoric acid, which is so acidic that your body pulls calcium from your bones to buffer all the acid. It's a little more complicated than that, but you get the gist. Soda is also laden with high fructose corn syrup and sugar, contributing to the development of diabetes and obesity. In the 2006 Framingham Osteoporosis Study published in the *American Journal of Clinical Nutrition*, researchers concluded that "Intake of cola, but not of other carbonated soft drinks, is associated with low BMD [bone mineral density] in women." Then, in a surprising animal study conducted in 2009, scientists also found that soda increased both estrogen and testosterone levels by an unknown mechanism. Excessive amounts of these hormones can be dangerous, and tilt other hormones and nutrients out of balance.

Artificially sweetened soda (diet soda) is not any better. The manufacturers are up-front about it and do let you know what you're getting. But not one of those artificial sweeteners—I don't care what kind they are, they're all basically the same—will help you lose weight. There's also evidence to suggest that they lodge in the nervous system and even kill off brain cells by virtue of the fact that they are *excitotoxins*, meaning that they excite or shake up the body's cells until they die. In another study done in 2009 and published in the *Clinical Journal of Pain*, researchers found that artificial sweeteners apparently spark migraines in some people.

In my opinion, your best bet is to stay away from artificial sweeteners completely, not just in soda. The only exception might be if you go on a weight loss program for a few weeks and your program requires this. But again, this is a short-term process for a few weeks. That's much different than consuming these foods and beverages all day long, every day for years. I wouldn't do that! I prefer that you consume natural sugars instead, just less of them. Try honey, raw agave syrup, blackstrap molasses, coconut nectar, turbinado sugar, or brown rice syrup. For more about safe, healthy sweeteners, see Chapter 15 in my *Diabetes without Drugs* (Rodale, 2010).

Back to the fizzy stuff now. For a healthy soda substitute, try this inexpensive homemade recipe of mine. Mix some grape juice with seltzer water, about a 50/50 mix. It will taste just like soda but doesn't have all the junk! Instead of grape juice, you can also buy pomegranate juice or flavored stevia—I like the root beer—and mix a few drops of that with the seltzer water. Here's one last option: Try Zevia Natural Cola. I found out about this company at a health expo. They make all-natural, sugar-free sodas in delicious flavors. They are sweetened with stevia and other natural ingredients, so they're safe for people with diabetes and better for hard-core soda addicts. They are sold in many health food stores. Big cola makers can't help but get in on the action, too. In 2008, Pepsi launched Pepsi Raw in the United Kingdom and, later, the same drink as Pepsi Natural in the United States. It contains natural ingredients such as cane sugar, coffee leaf, natural caramel coloring, apple extract, grape tartaric acid, natural gum arabic, and sparkling water. To give you an idea of the contrast, the ingredients of regular Pepsi include high fructose corn syrup, sugar, artificial colorings, phosphoric acid, and caffeine.

Do You Need to Take Laxatives?

People who are constipated often take laxatives to promote regularity. If you are using this type of medicine (prescribed or over the counter) more than twice a week, you are going to suffer a drug mugging of every nutrient you need for good health. The reason is that laxatives speed the passage of food through the colon. When that happens, your body doesn't have an opportunity to extract all the healthy nutrients from your food. Laxatives have the greatest impact on minerals and fat-soluble vitamins like vitamins D and A.

If you use laxatives regularly, take a good multivitamin, a trace mineral formula, and vitamin D and/or beta-carotene (for vitamin A). And if constipation is such an issue for you, consider also taking probiotics—supplements that contain beneficial bacteria—and a small amount of aloe vera juice each day. You'll also find a low-sugar diet to be helpful, along with taking enzymes with every meal. Regular oatmeal (not the quick-cooking type) as well as prunes (aka dried plums) would be good, too.

Is Red Wine Your Sixth Food Group?

I know how much people like to drink. In fact, one of my good friends has a wine cellar bigger than my house! You already know that drinking in excess is bad for you. That's because it creates a potent neurotoxin called acetaldehyde that damages the brain, liver, and pancreas. I'll spare you the long lecture because I like chocolate martinis, too. Regular use of alcohol will mug your body of all your B vitamins (particularly thiamine), as well as your glutathione, minerals, vitamin C, beneficial bacteria, and other important nutrients you need to stay healthy. Losing a few nutrients may not sound like a big deal, but over time the drug mugging effect of alcohol can shut down the liver and pancreas. Of course, this extreme scenario usually applies to chronic alcohol abusers, but it can also apply to people with chronic gastrointestinal tract problems. The powerful drug mugging effect occurs even in people who drink one glass of wine with dinner each night. If you drink alcohol on a regular basis, protect yourself with high-quality supplements such as B complex, extra thiamine, probiotics, trace minerals, extra selenium, and vitamins C and E.

Are You Stressed?

Welcome to planet Earth. Who isn't stressed? I think stress is why a relaxing glass of wine may be some people's sixth food group.

Doctors have long known that stress of any sort can tax your immune system and wear you down physically and emotionally. Stress, especially when prolonged, hurts your adrenal glands and your thyroid gland, which causes major imbalances of important hormones in your body. The drug mugging effect of stress is widespread even though it comes on slowly.

You may want to supplement with B vitamins because they are anti-stress nutrients. In particular, pantethine nourishes the adrenal gland. Antioxidants are also important for you because stress translates in the body to free radical damage of cells, which can cause infection, cancer, diabetes, and heart disease. Free radicals are naturally occurring molecules that damage cells. A powerful antioxidant called astaxanthin is a great addition to anyone's health regimen. Minerals such as calcium and magnesium are also critical.

And why not drink a superfoods green supplement each day or take chlorophyll or spirulina tablets (if you don't like the taste of green drinks)? These contain chlorophyll, which helps detoxify an acidic and stressed-out body. You might try a supplement that contains greens from the ocean, such as spirulina, chlorophyll, and phytoplankton, or barley grass or any number of green supplements sold at health food stores. There is a long chapter (Step 1) in my diabetes book *Diabetes without Drugs* that will inform you about the tremendous health benefits of green supplements. Each of these products contains fantastic ingredients that can help you improve your health and increase your vitality and energy reserves regardless of your condition. That's why they call them superfoods.

Do You Smoke? And Not Just Cigarettes . . .

Smokers of cigarettes and marijuana have a tendency to run out of vitamin C, an anticancer compound found in citrus fruits. In fact, each cigarette costs you about 30 mg of vitamin C. You need vitamin C to keep your arteries elastic so that blood flows properly to your heart and everywhere else. Since vitamin C isn't stored in the body, the drug mugging effect of smoking is serious. That's one reason smokers and those exposed to secondhand smoke have much higher risks for cancer.

Cigarette smoking imparts the heavy metal cadmium to your body, and cadmium is a potent neurotoxin. If it is present in your body, it throws off your trace minerals, so you might say it's a drug mugger of healthy minerals (which you need to make bones). Smoking steals thiamine as well, and low thiamine can cause cardiovascular, neurological, and neuromuscular problems and can lead to a condition called beriberi.

If that isn't bad enough, smoking also goes hand in hand with lung cancer. There are hundreds of studies that point to a connection between smoking and lung cancer. It's a no-brainer. Vitamin A can help. One study by the American Cancer Society found that heavy smokers with low vitamin A levels had three times as many cases of cancer as heavy smokers with normal vitamin A levels. So low vitamin A translates into higher cancer, and so does smoking itself! If you smoke and want to add beta-carotene (vitamin A) to your regimen, please refer to Chapter 5, page 101, to make sure you get the natural, healthy sort. Vitamin A protects the lungs and can repair some of the damage done to those delicate tissues. A little added protection with a good antioxidant, vitamin C, N-acetyl-L-cysteine (NAC), and thiamine supplements would be helpful to people who smoke or have a history of smoking.

Do You Sit in an Office All Day?

If you're like me, going out into the sun happens rarely. I don't golf, sunbathe, or play tennis. I just sit here, write cool books, and answer health questions from around the world. If you have a job that keeps you indoors, you may run out of vitamin D. Sunlight stimulates your skin to form vitamin D, but it's blocked by smog, fog, curtains, sunscreen, even window glass.

You need vitamin D for strong bones, to prevent cancer, and to prevent diabetes. I'm not going to recommend supplementation right off, unless you are over the age of 40 or chronically ill. I'm going to tell you to get out of your office and go for a walk outside. We'll do this together, right now. Just go out for 15 minutes. My book will wait. Spending 15 minutes outdoors in the sunlight each day can make a tremendous difference in your health. In a perfect world, the sunlight you get is on your belly and back, not your arms or face. Improving serum levels of vitamin D reduces the incidences of multiple sclerosis, breast cancer, prostate cancer, leukemia, and autoimmune disorders. Read Chapter 23, Vitamin D, to learn more about the benefits of this amazing nutrient.

Do You Feel Like You're Losing Your Mind?

If you are starting to forget little things, are feeling depressed, and are getting confused, your family and doctor may recommend that you start taking a powerful mind-altering drug. Before you do, read on: When I worked in nursing homes and assisted-living facilities years ago, many residents were prescribed psychiatric drugs. When I ordered their vitamin B_{12} levels to be tested, many were shown to be deficient.

Why is this important? Vitamin B_{12} plays a tremendous role in how well your brain functions. And many people have a hard time getting enough of this important nutrient as they age. If you have been diagnosed with senile dementia or Alzheimer's disease or even if you're simply having issues with your memory, get your B_{12} levels checked. (For more information, see page 193.) Because B_{12} is found in meats, strict vegans of any age can run low unless they supplement.

If you have a B_{12} deficiency, you could also develop little sensations of pins and needles in your hands or feet. You might have sores in or around your mouth. When you run out of B_{12}, your other B vitamins may run low, too, and this can be dangerous. For example, you may be short on riboflavin, pyridoxine, or thiamine. This can happen to seniors and to people with *Candida albicans* infection or malabsorption disorders like celiac disease, Crohn's disease, or irritable bowel syndrome. It can happen to folks who have had gastric bypass surgery, too.

I believe that vitamin B_{12} deficiency is so widespread among the elderly that they are often sent to nursing homes when supplementation of B_{12} (in concert with B complex) could have done the trick. That and a fish oil supplement each day (particularly DHA) go a long way toward correcting the problems described here. I know this because many letters from people who read my "Dear Pharmacist" column thank me for this simple solution. I have other simple solutions posted at my Web site, www.dearpharmacist.com, where I have archived my columns for you to learn about your health.

So if you think you're losing your mind, you might be, but it could be easier to fix than you think.

Do You Take Fat Blockers or Follow Fad Diets?

The most popular fat blocker is called Alli and is sold over the counter. It can latch onto fat in your food that would otherwise land on your thighs. Its prescription counterpart, Xenical, comes in a higher dose. If these drugs can grab hold of fat in your foods, what do you think they are doing to the fat-soluble vitamins in your foods? Yes, they are drug mugging those essential nutrients, too. So if you take Alli or Xenical, you may run short on vitamins A, E, K, and D.

This is a huge problem, because if you don't have enough of these nutrients, your risk for heart attack, blood clotting problems, blindness, and cancer go up. I'm not saying that these drugs cause these conditions, because they don't. I'm just saying that they do a number on your stash of nutrients that protect against these problems. You may be at high risk for any of these conditions and not be aware of it, so why not take the right nutrients to replenish your stash and protect yourself?

Now a word about fad diets. Low-fat diets do the same thing as fat blockers. Low-carb diets, such as the Atkins diet, aren't much better. Diets like this rob you blind of vitamin C, beta-carotene, folic acid, B_6, and many minerals. In practical terms, another way to say "low carb" is to say "high fat." Why would you want to be on a diet that clogs your arteries? Why would you even think of following a diet in which bacon and salami are considered better for you than a sweet potato or apples?

If you want to see some nasty pictures of salami and hot dogs up close, get on the computer and visit Health Ranger Mike Adams's Web site, www.naturalnews.com. He's posted highly magnified pictures of what is in these foods, which you will promptly give up.

What about the pizza diet? Are you kidding me? C'mon, this is silliness. I confess that there were very few home-cooked meals at my house while I was locking myself in the office to write this book. My husband, Sam, threatened to buy one of those diet plans featured on TV infomercials so he could get regular meals. I heard him hollering from the living room couch: "Hey, Suzy, did you hear that? We can get some food delivered here every day! Every single day! And I'm *really* hungry!" Wise guy!

So what could possibly be wrong with that? A lot of diet plans on TV sell you the same processed foods that you can get at the grocery store, except in smaller portions. But the boxed foods from diet plans aren't very healthy. They're not grown organically, they're highly processed, and they have way too many funky ingredients in them. I don't believe that they are as good as real food that you can grow in your garden or buy at organic farms or grocery stores, and cook yourself. When you cook your own meals, you know exactly what's on your plate. Natural is always better. It comes from the earth and goes directly to your plate. That has to be better for you than boxed food that gets mailed to you. That said, please know that not all weight clinics make you eat boxed foods. One of the best weight loss centers I've come across is Metabolic Research Center, because you can eat real food and they help you lose weight by balancing your hormones. I'll save the rest of the story on weight loss for my next book.

Do You Have Food Allergies?

People who are allergic to whole groups of food have to be vigilant about avoiding them and finding substitutes for the nutrients they must sacrifice. If you are allergic to the casein or lactose found in dairy products, for example, then you lose a popular source of calcium. The good news is that greens, such as kale, Swiss chard, and broccoli, are all superior sources of calcium anyway. These natural sources are better ways to get calcium than cow's milk or fortified soy milk because the calcium is easier to absorb and digest.

In my opinion, soy is potentially problematic because it behaves much like the female hormone estrogen in the body. Even calcium-fortified soy milk is not your best source of calcium. Get this mineral like the cows do—from eating plants! (There is more on milk and its potential problems at the end of this chapter, as well as on page 113.)

If you are allergic to gluten, on the other hand, you lose a source of folic acid since breads and pastas are often enriched with this B vitamin. It's no biggie, if you make sure to eat other sources of B vitamins such as quinoa. This grain is safe for gluten-sensitive people, including those with celiac disease, and it's loaded with vitamin E, calcium, iron, and B vitamins.

If you're allergic to corn, you lose a good source of fiber, thiamine, folate, and pantethine (the active form of vitamin B_5). Just be sure to eat lots of other veggies to make up for it.

Are You a Drive-Thru Junkie?

If your favorite food comes wrapped in waxed paper or in Styrofoam, we need to talk. They call it fast food for a reason: A regular diet of this kind of food is the fastest way to clog your arteries and develop heart disease. Generally speaking, these foods are laden with artificial colors, preservatives, MSG, high fructose corn syrup, refined white sugar, trans fats, and chemicals that I can't pronounce or find in my medical resource references. Even the healthier choices on the menu often contain chemicals and preservatives that some people are sensitive to such as sulfites and nitrites.

Watch the documentary *Super Size Me* for a fascinating look at one man's experience with fast food. He ate every meal at McDonald's for 30 days straight. After only 2 weeks, his doctor warned him about his increasing risk for dangerous cardiovascular complications. After 30 days, he'd gained 18 pounds, lost his sex drive, and developed mood swings, not to mention mild liver damage.

The drug mugging effect of eating nothing but fast food is huge. I can't even point to just a nutrient or two. You'd have to take hundreds of dollars' worth of supplements each month to offset a daily intake of a cheeseburger, fries, and a shake. Consuming these foods once in a blue moon is fine, but I know people who eat this way or feed their kids this way every day, sometimes twice a day!

I know, it's yummy. Hey, I was young and reckless once upon a time, too. But eating fast food puts you on the fast track to developing type 2 diabetes, heart disease, high blood pressure, brain fog, obesity, arthritis, fatigue, fibroids, osteoporosis, pancreatitis, breast cancer, colon cancer, prostate cancer, and on and on. But don't worry, pharmacies are happy to sell you lots of medications in an attempt to treat these conditions. Why am I telling you this? Because they don't call me America's Most Trusted Pharmacist for nothing. I promise you, it will be far less painful and produce fewer side effects to clean up your diet. Changing to a healthy diet is so much safer (and cheaper) than all those drugs (each with drug mugging effects) that you'll wind up taking if you don't change it.

I realize you can't suddenly stop eating fried chicken (or can you?), but certainly it's possible to ease into a new diet. Just introduce something new and living each week. Try asparagus this week. Sauté it in olive oil with a little goat cheese and sea salt. Next week, try beets. Peel and shred a little bit into your salad. Make your own fresh guacamole. Try cilantro. It's a great heavy metal chelator, which means that it yanks toxic mercury out of your body. Put a little in your salad or sprinkle it into soup at the very end of cooking. See Chapter 29 for recipe ideas that help you restore essential nutrients.

Learn to shop around the perimeter of your supermarket. Buy nutritious foods and salads, which naturally help you feel better and offset the drug mugging effect of medicines. I'll be very blunt here: If you regularly eat fast food and processed boxed or canned meals, your gut is in such bad shape that you won't be able to absorb or incorporate any benefits from the vitamins you take anyway! (Read about probiotics in Chapter 17, page 229, to learn about the importance of healthy bacteria.) Eat more plant foods and fewer foods that are boxed, canned, and processed.

Look at the word D-I-E-T. If you scramble the letters, you get the word E-D-I-T. That's what I want you to do—edit what you eat. Apples instead of apple pie. Brown rice instead of white rice. A baked potato instead of french fries. See, it's not that hard! For more on how to edit what you eat and lose weight, refer to *Diabetes without Drugs*.

Do You Drink More Milk Than Water?

I'm firmly convinced that humans should get their calcium from greens rather than from milk, unless it's raw milk that is not pasteurized so it still has nutrients in it. When I say greens, I mean turnip or mustard greens, Swiss chard, kale, broccoli, cabbage, spinach, and so on.

You'll never catch me wearing one of those milk mustaches you see in popular advertisements. The ads have convinced mothers to feed their babies lots and lots of milk. Maybe this type of advertising programs the minds of Americans to think that milk is a healthy beverage. It's healthy for calves who need it to gain hundreds of pounds within a few months, but I don't think that large amounts of it are healthy for humans. Scientifically speaking, casein, the protein found in milk, causes allergies in many people. Let me make it clear: I'm not suggesting milk is bad. I just think there is a high incidence of allergies to some of its components. You can take an antibody blood test to find out if you're allergic to casein. You have to take the test very early in the morning in order for it to be accurate.

I constantly see people in the pharmacy who are wheezing, sniffling, or dealing with asthma or bronchitis all the time. I see them in Florida getting bagfuls of nebulizing solution, inhalers, breathing pills, and nasal inhalers. I can't help but wonder if some of these people are allergic to milk and other dairy products.

Recently, I suggested a dairy-free diet to two mothers who had toddlers living on multiple breathing medications. Following a dairy-free diet means consuming no milk, butter, cheese, ice cream, yogurt, pudding, milkshakes, or any other food containing dairy products. I suggested they do this for 30 days solid, no cheating. I have to tell you, it's hard to get mothers to agree to this when they think milk is good for you and it's even recommended by their pediatricians as the best source of calcium. But it took me only a few minutes to convince them to try my plan. I guess these two moms were open-minded and motivated to try something new since the medications weren't helping much.

Within a month, both mothers came back to happily report that their children needed fewer treatments and less emergency breathing medication. One of the youngsters was able to stop using his albuterol inhaler altogether as a result of going dairy-free.

If you already avoid milk but miss yogurt, I have a surprise for you. Turtle Mountain makes So Delicious yogurt, which is made with coconuts—coconut milk to be exact, a very healthy ingredient. This brand is so good you'll want some every day. It contains six live and active cultures of probiotics along with natural sweeteners. Their soy-free, dairy-free line also includes frozen desserts. You can learn more by visiting www.sodeliciousdairyfree.com.

Do You Love Grapefruit?

Foods can act like drugs. The interaction of grapefruit with numerous medications can cause the medication level to spike. That's why you see medication labels warning you not to eat grapefruit.

It's a shame, too, because this incredible fruit can help you lower cholesterol, burn fat, and reduce cancer risk. But it does prevent proper breakdown of some medications, causing the blood level to spike. It's because of the seeds, which are the primary source of naringenin, the bitter chemical that causes the pucker. If you take supplements of grapefruit or naringenin you should be aware that interactions may occur. You'll see it listed in various ways, such as naringenin, grapefruit seed extract, or GSE, and sometimes it's part of a comprehensive bioflavonoid formula that also contains hesperidin, rutin, or quercetin. These types of products are widely available at health food stores and are used to eliminate candida (yeast) overgrowth since they have strong antifungal properties. I've recommended them frequently, but it's important for you to know that there could be consequences when you combine this delicious fruit or supplements derived from it with a handful of medications.

Some research suggests that pomegranate juice can do the same thing but to a lesser extent. The same may be true for tangerines and some oranges. Grapefruit is definitely the most important of this fruity bunch, however.

Calcium channel blockers are greatly affected by citrus juices. A 1991 study published in the *Lancet* found that grapefruit juice may dangerously enhance the effectiveness of these medications, including felodipine and nifedipine (note that Norvasc belongs to the same class). In simple terms, if you spike the drug level, you also enhance the effects of the drug. This means the combination of certain juices may possibly cause an excessive lowering of blood pressure. This is why I feel you should avoid combining citrus juices with medications, or, at the very least, be consistent if you choose to combine them. And keep your doctor informed.

One more thing: It doesn't matter what time of day you eat grapefruit or drink grapefruit juice, or if it's been separated from your medication by a few hours. It's still going to have the same effect because it's not as simple as an interaction between the fruit and your drug. Grapefruit actually temporarily changes the way your liver behaves, so your liver and its detoxification pathways are affected all day long.

When you drink grapefruit juice (and possibly pomegranate juice), your body stops breaking down your medicine and the drug level starts to build up in some cases. The most commonly used medications that interact with grapefruit and other juices are sildenafil (Viagra), buspirone (BuSpar), sertraline (Zoloft), triazolam (Halcion), diazepam (Valium), carbamazepine (Tegretol), cyclosporine, tacrolimus, felodipine, nifedipine (Procardia), HIV medications, certain statin cholesterol drugs (simvastatin, atorvastatin, lovastatin), amiodarone, methadone, digoxin (Lanoxin), and losartan (Cozaar).

Please refer to the chart on page 88. If you take medications, just to be safe, no guzzling any of these beverages, okay?

GRAPEFRUIT INTERACTION CHART

I've prepared the following list in case you are wondering whether a medication is safe to combine with grapefruit. Scientific research yields new findings constantly and only one medication in a particular category may be represented (because I found a study for it), but there are numerous drugs in each category and your medication just may not be listed as of yet.

DRUG CLASS	MEDICATION	GRAPEFRUIT INTERACTION RESULTS
Antiarrhythmics	Amiodarone (Cordarone) Propafenone (Rythmol) Quinidine (Quinidex)	Heart rhythm problems
Antibiotics and antifungals	Ciprofloxacin (Cipro) Levafloxacin (Levaquin) Doxycycline (Doryx or Vibra-Tabs) Itraconazole (Sporanox) Ketoconazole (Nizoral)	Elevated drug level in the bloodstream may enhance dangerous side effects associated with these drugs.
Anticoagulants	Warfarin (Coumadin)	Elevated drug level, which may lead to excessive blood thinning. This may or may not be seen, as it may be internal. Nosebleeds sometimes do occur as a first hint, as does easy bruising.
Anticonvulsants	Carbamazepine (Tegretol)	Sedation, slow breathing
Antidepressants	Sertraline (Zoloft) Fluvoxamine (Luvox)	Elevated drug level, so it increases side effects such as anxiety, dizziness, nausea/vomiting, diarrhea.
Anxiety	Amitriptyline (Elavil) Buspirone (BuSpar) Clozapine (Clozaril) Diazepam (Valium) Haloperidol (Haldol) Midazolam (Versed) Trazodone (Desyrel)	Sedation, impaired thinking Breathing problems Slow pulse
Blood pressure medication, including calcium channel blockers	Amlodipine (Norvasc)	Rapid pulse, low blood pressure, fainting
	Diltiazem (Cartia)	This interaction is slight.
	Felodipine (Plendil)	Rapid pulse, low blood pressure, fainting

DRUG CLASS	MEDICATION	GRAPEFRUIT INTERACTION RESULTS
Blood pressure medication, including calcium channel blockers	Losartan (Cozaar)	Elevated drug level, low blood pressure, dizziness, fainting, rapid pulse
	Nifedipine (Procardia)	Rapid pulse, low blood pressure, fainting
	Verapamil (Calan, Isoptin)	This interaction is slight.
Breathing medicine	Theophylline (Theo-Dur, Theo-24)	Might decrease effectiveness.
Cardiac glycoside	Digoxin (Lanoxin)	Either reduces absorption or increases it, depending on the individual and hydration status.
Diabetes	Saxagliptin (Onglyza) [Note: Interaction does not normally occur with sitagliptin (Januvia) or vildagliptin (Galvus).]	Elevated drug level, so it increases side effects such as headache, tremors, dizziness, weakness, fluid retention, and nausea.
Erectile dysfunction drugs	Sildenafil (Viagra) Vardenafil (Levitra)	Headache, flushing, gastrointestinal problems
Estrogen drugs	Birth control and hormone replacement therapy	May produce more estrogen side effects such as dizziness, breast pain, irritability, insomnia, nausea/vomiting, joint pain.
Immunosuppressants	Cyclosporine (Sandimmune, Neoral)	Liver and kidney damage
	Tacrolimus (Prograf)	Increases dangerous side effects.
Insomnia medication	Triazolam (Halcion) Diazepam (Valium) Ramelteon (Rozerem)	Excessive sedation, slowed breathing and pulse
Pain medication	Methadone Oxycodone (OxyContin) Oxycodone and acetaminophen (Percocet)	Increases drug levels, causing excess sedation, slowed breathing, impaired thinking, and bradycardia.
Statin cholesterol reducers and red yeast rice	Atorvastatin (Lipitor, Advicor) Fluvastatin (Lescol) Lovastatin (Mevacor) Pravastatin (Pravachol) Rosuvastatin (Crestor) Simvastatin (Zocor, Vytorin, Lipex, Simcor)	Muscle aches, headache, rhabdomyolysis, liver or kidney damage, leg cramps, and neuropathy

Also, there are a few medications that have been listed for your safety, even though the data is inconclusive or conflicting. Other medications such as the Alzheimer's drug donepezil (Aricept), the breast cancer agent tamoxifen (Nolvadex) and possibly related breast cancer drugs, the prostate medication tamsulosin (Flomax), and the popular nonsedative types of antihistamines like loratadine (Claritin) and fexofenadine (Allegra) seem to also interact with grapefruit juice. However, the significance of these interactions is still unknown.

The Punch List of Drug Muggers

The following pages are designed to make it quick and easy for you to install a nutrient security system. The chart features the most popular categories of medications, providing information about which nutrients are lost when you take a particular medication. Then you will see what could happen to you if you don't replenish what the drug mugger stole. Most drugs deplete the body of many nutrients. I'm not advising that you automatically take every single nutrient on the list. Please ask your doctor which ones are right for you based on your symptoms and medical history.

I want you to be sensible about taking supplements. Micronutrients have broad and powerful effects on the body, so when replenishing these lost compounds, you could experience side effects, especially if you are taking poor-quality products. A sensible approach to integrating new supplements is to begin taking only one supplement at a time and, as far as dosages go, start low and go slow. See how your body reacts to it. Then, if everything goes well, after a week or two bring in the next nutrient. See Chapter 27 for tips on getting started.

It takes only a few weeks or months to replenish depleted nutrients. However, if you must continue to take drug muggers, you may find that you need perpetual replenishments (at low doses). One more thing: I find that it's best to take vitamins and minerals with meals and not with medications and high-fiber foods or fiber supplements. For example, if you are taking thyroid medication and need iron supplementation, separate the two by 4 to 6 hours. If you are taking an antiseizure medication and therefore also need to take a folic acid supplement, again, separate these by hours. Don't pop all the pills at once.

DRUG MUGGERS:
How They Rob You

At least half of the drugs approved in the United States commonly deplete specific nutrients, creating the need for nutritional supplementation. More drugs probably deplete nutrients; we just don't have the data to prove it yet. The mechanisms by which drugs mug you can vary. Most people assume it's because the drug grabs hold of a nutrient in the gut and takes it out of the system through the gastrointestinal tract (called chelation). Certainly, a drug can mug you this way, but there are other ways, too.

- Altering the acidity in your gastrointestinal or urinary tract
- Stimulating or inhibiting enzymes involved in the transport of nutrients around your body
- Binding directly to the nutrient, thereby inactivating it
- Stimulating or inhibiting enzymes involved in activating nutrients or in transforming them into more usable substances

Also, certain drugs require specific nutrients in order to work; they might need to bind to a protein, for example, or perhaps they require a specific nutrient in order to be detoxified in your liver. So just by virtue of taking a certain drug, you may need more of a particular nutrient.

Let me put all this in perspective. You need concrete, nails, and wood to create a building. For the human body, you need the right building materials, too, such as carbohydrates, protein, and healthy fats. But this foundation will do you no good if you don't have the proper vitamins and minerals in it, because then your body can't synthesize new tissue or provide the cellular energy you need to move, breathe, and talk. Drugs can alter your body's ability to absorb, digest, transport, break down, or eliminate toxic compounds that you encounter every day, just by their ability to steal vital nutrients from you. The cascading effect affects your quality of life and may remain undiscovered for years as you get on a medication merry-go-round. Thankfully, the coming pages will shed some light on what may be happening to you.

COMMON DRUG MUGGERS

TYPES	COMMON DRUGS	INSTALL YOUR SECURITY SYSTEM
Acid blockers	Proton pump inhibitors, H_2 blockers	All nutrients, because these drugs alter the pH of the gut
Antibiotics	All	B vitamins, calcium, magnesium, iron, beneficial bacteria
Antidepressants	MAO inhibitors: selegiline (Eldepryl), phenelzine (Nardil), isocarboxazid (Marplan)	Vitamin B_6
	SSRIs: Paxil, Prozac	Iodine
	Tricyclics: amitriptyline (Elavil), desipramine (Norpramin), doxepin (Sinequan), clomipramine (Anafranil), imipramine (Tofranil), nortriptyline	CoQ10, riboflavin
Anxiety medications	Alprazolam (Xanax), clonazepam (Klonopin), diazepam (Valium), lorazepam (Ativan)	Melatonin
Blood pressure medications	ACE inhibitors: captopril (Capoten), enalapril (Vasotec), lisinopril (Zestril, Prinivil), quinapril (Accupril), ramipril (Altace), trandopril (Mavik), fosinopril (Monopril)	Zinc, magnesium, potassium, calcium
	Beta-blockers: atenolol (Tenormin), metoprolol (Toprol, Lopressor), timolol (Timoptic drops), nadolol (Corgard), sotalol (Betapace)	CoQ10, melatonin
	Calcium channel blockers: nifedipine (Procardia), felodipine (Plendil), verapamil (Calan, Isoptin), diltiazem (Cardizem), amlodipine (Norvasc)	Potassium, vitamin D, calcium, possibly CoQ10
	Clonidine (Catapres), methyldopa (Aldomet)	CoQ10
Breathing medications	Fluticasone (Flonase and Flovent)	Folic acid, most minerals, iodine

OR THESE COMPLICATIONS MAY RESULT

Heart disease, high homocysteine, fatigue, candida, irritable bowel syndrome, increased risk of cancer, poor vision, high blood pressure, anemia, brittle nails, tiredness, hair loss, hearing loss, tooth decay, higher risk of developing gluten sensitivity

Heart disease, high homocysteine, fatigue, candida, increased risk of cancer, irritable bowel syndrome, leg cramps, high blood pressure, fatigue, low thyroid, bone loss, weight gain

Heart disease, nerve pain, depression, mouth sores, fatigue, PMS, insomnia, dermatitis, fatigue

Hypothyroidism, depression, hair loss, weight gain, lowered immunity

Fatigue, headaches, heart failure, heart palpitations, leg cramps, skin and nerve problems, weight gain

Weight gain, insomnia, heart palpitations, lowered immunity, increased risk of autoimmune disorders

Loss of sex drive, prostate problems, loss of smell or taste, hair loss, slow wound healing, frequent infections, higher risk of cancer, leg cramps, high blood pressure, weight gain, bone loss

Heart disease, irregular heartbeat, memory loss, muscle cramps, insomnia, disrupted sleep, increased risk of cancer, autoimmune disorders

Heart disease, irregular or rapid heartbeat, bone loss, confusion, muscle weakness, thirst, leg cramps, frequent infections, high blood pressure, fatigue

Fatigue, weakness, muscle and leg cramps, memory loss, higher risk of cancer, frequent infection, liver damage, higher risk of heart attack

Hypothyroidism, depression, hair loss, weight gain, lowered immunity

(continued)

COMMON DRUG MUGGERS (CONT.)

TYPES	COMMON DRUGS	INSTALL YOUR SECURITY SYSTEM	
Cholesterol medications	Fibrates: fenofibrate (Tricor), ezetimibe (Zetia), gemfibrozil (Lopid), clofibrate (Atromid-S), colestipol (Colestid), cholestyramine (Questran)	Most minerals and B vitamins	
	Statins: atorvastatin (Lipitor), lovastatin (Mevacor), pravastatin (Pravachol)	CoQ10, vitamin D	
Diabetes medications	Glyburide (Diabeta, Glynase, Micronase)	CoQ10, B_{12}, folic acid	
	Metformin (Glucophage, Glucophage XR, Glumetza, Fortamet, Riomet), metformin and sitagliptin (Janumet), tolazamide (Tolinase), glipizide (Glucotrol)	CoQ10, B_6, B_{12}, folic acid	
Diuretics	Virtually all of them	B vitamins, vitamin C, zinc, calcium, magnesium, potassium	
Gout medications	Colchicine	Vitamin A, B_{12}, potassium, calcium	
Laxatives	Bisacodyl (Dulcolax)	Potassium, other minerals	
	Mineral oil	Vitamin A, calcium, vitamins D and E, most other nutrients	
NSAIDs	Ibuprofen (Motrin, Advil), naproxen (Aleve, Naprosyn, Anaprox), ketoprofen (Orudis), meloxicam (Mobic)	Vitamin C, folic acid, iron	
Oral contraceptives, hormone replacement therapy	All estrogen-containing hormone drugs used for contraception and menopause	Beneficial flora, magnesium, zinc, most minerals, B vitamins, vitamin C	
Salicylates	Aspirin, Percodan, Fiorinal	Vitamin C, calcium, iron, folic acid, pantethine, protein	
Thyroid medications	Levothyroxine, Synthroid, Armour	Iron, calcium	

OR THESE COMPLICATIONS MAY RESULT
Heart disease, high homocysteine, fatigue, candida, higher risk of cancer, irritable bowel syndrome, frequent infection, hair loss, muscle pain, weakness, cramps, insomnia, vision problems
Fatigue, weakness, muscle cramps, memory loss, shortness of breath, higher risk of cancer, frequent infections, liver damage, heart disease
Fatigue, weakness, muscle cramps, memory loss, higher risk of cancer, frequent infection, liver damage, heart disease
Heart disease, high homocysteine, frequent infection, fatigue, anemia, irregular heartbeat, memory loss, increased risk of cancer, muscle cramps
Osteoporosis, heart disease, slow wound healing, frequent infection, leg cramps, depression, memory loss, lowered immunity, vision problems, enlarged prostate, edema, weight gain, hair loss, high blood pressure, fatigue, mood swings
Lowered immunity, fatigue, muscle cramps and weakness, edema, weight gain, low appetite, heart disease, dehydration, vision loss
Vision problems, high blood pressure, bone loss, rickets, hearing loss, heart disease, muscle weakness and cramps
Irregular heartbeat, heart palpitations, muscle weakness and cramps, tiredness, water retention, weight gain
Heart disease, high homocysteine, cervical dysplasia, higher risk of cancer, higher risk of birth defects, depression, diarrhea, gray hair, mouth sores, anemia, frequent infections, hypothyroidism
Heart disease, fatigue, candida, increased risks of stroke and cancer, irritable bowel syndrome, depression, insomnia, lowered immunity, memory loss, irritability, nerve pain, hypothyroidism, inability to cope, higher risk of breast cancer
Fatigue, depression, osteoporosis, brittle nails, hair loss, edema, high cholesterol, high homocysteine, heart disease, high blood pressure
Anemia, weakness, brittle nails, irritability, fatigue, osteoporosis, tooth decay, high blood pressure, heart disease, insomnia, acid reflux, digestive problems, higher risk of cancer

SUPPLEMENTS TO BATTLE THE DRUG MUGGERS

SUPPLEMENT	NUTRIENTS	DRUG MUGGERS IT WILL BATTLE	
B_6	Vitamin B_6 (pyridoxine)	Antibiotics, diuretics, antidepressants, acid-reducing medications, estrogen-containing drugs, theophylline	
B_{12}	Vitamin B_{12} (methylcobalamin)	Antibiotics, diabetes medications, cholesterol medications, estrogen-containing drugs, diuretics, acid-blockers, gout medications	
Calcium	Calcium	Thyroid medications, salicylates, diuretics	
Calcium/ magnesium combination	Calcium, magnesium	Acid-reducing medications, blood pressure medications, salicylates, diuretics, thyroid medications, antibiotics, estrogen-containing drugs, laxatives	
CoQ10	Coenzyme Q10, ubiquinone, or ubiquinol	Blood pressure medications, diabetes medications, cholesterol medications, acid-reducing medications	
D_3	Vitamin D_3	Cholesterol medications, laxatives	
High-quality multivitamin	Men's or women's formula: vitamins A, C, D_3, E, K, B_6, B_{12}, thiamine, riboflavin, niacin, folic acid, biotin, pantothenic acid, calcium, iodine, magnesium, zinc, selenium, copper, manganese, chromium, molybdenum	Antibiotics, blood pressure medications, diabetes medications, acid-reducing medications, cholesterol medications, estrogen-containing drugs, salicylates, NSAIDs, diuretics, antidepressants, laxatives, gout medications, colchicine	
Iodoral and selenium	Iodine iodide, selenium	Breathing medications, fluoride toothpaste, vegetable oil, citrus-flavored soda	
Trace minerals	Boron, magnesium, copper, manganese, phosphorus, selenium	Blood pressure medications, diuretics, acid-reducing medications, estrogen-containing drugs	

BENEFITS*
Works with folic acid to break down homocysteine, supporting a healthy cardiovascular system; strengthens the immune system; promotes kidney health; helps prevent various nervous and skin disorders; acts as a natural diuretic; has antiaging properties; reduces dry mouth and urination problems caused by tricyclic antidepressants.
Supports red blood cell production and breakdown of homocysteine, strengthening the cardiovascular system; promotes energy production; maintains a healthy nervous system; properly utilizes fats, protein, and carbohydrates; enhances concentration, mood, memory, and balance; protects against secondhand cigarette smoke.
Boosts bone and oral health, cardiovascular health, digestive health, and immune function.
Helps maintain strong bones and healthy teeth; supports digestive tract function and colon health; boosts cardiovascular and nervous system health, healthy metabolism, and mental health.
Boosts heart health; efficiently breaks down fats, protein, and carbohydrates; acts as an antioxidant; promotes energy production.
Strengthens the immune system; supports bone, joint, muscle, and skin health; has antiaging properties; supports colon, pancreas, and stomach health; helps maintain healthy blood pressure and cardiovascular health; protects the brain and reproductive organs; decreases risk of diabetes and metabolic syndrome; improves mood.
Strengthens the immune system; promotes healthy vision and bone, skin, and nail strength; has antioxidant and antiaging properties; boosts digestive health, wound healing, and nervous system function; promotes metabolic function and cardiovascular health; prevents neural tube birth defects; promotes energy, sleep, mental health, and the list goes on!
Supports female reproductive health; boosts thyroid health; promotes metabolic function and energy production.
Supports bone health; strengthens immune system; promotes healthy blood pressure; maintains nervous system function; helps digestive system; boosts heart health and red blood cell production; has antioxidant properties; supports metabolic functions.

These statements have not been evaluated by the Food and Drug Administration. This book is not intended to diagnose, treat, cure, or prevent any disease.

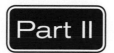

Vital Nutrients

5

Beta-Carotene and Vitamin A

A colorful, reddish-orange pigment, beta-carotene occurs naturally in the leaves of plants and in reddish-orange vegetables such as sweet potatoes, pumpkins, tomatoes, and carrots. Beta-carotene is actually one of many such pigments known as carotenoids. When the green chlorophyll in plants dies in the fall, it is the leftover beta-carotene that you see in the leaves imparting those beautiful autumn colors.

Once inside the body, beta-carotene is converted to vitamin A. Since vitamin A is a fat-soluble vitamin, it gets into fatty tissue—fat cells in your heart, brain, lungs, liver, and skin. That's a good thing. It may also help with asthma and lung function.

Vitamin A comes from two sources: a category of substances called retinoids, which are derived from animal sources and include retinol, and another group of molecules called carotenoids, which are derived from plants. As already mentioned, the carotenoids include beta-carotene and astaxanthin.

Among other benefits, vitamin A in the form of retinol is a powerful skin nutrient. When applied topically, it penetrates deep down and gets into the layers of collagen and elastin, the tissues that support the skin. This is where retinol begins to run damage control. It's a strong antioxidant, so it cleans up nasty, damaged cells and gunk that has accumulated in your skin. It's found in a gazillion skin care creams for women who want to diminish wrinkles and beautify their skin. If you buy a retinol-containing cream, make sure it says natural retinol on the label and is not made from a synthetic copycat.

Speaking of synthetics, did you know that the oral drug isotretinoin (Accutane, Sotret) is a morphed version of high-dose vitamin A? Introduced many years ago, this drug is often prescribed for teenagers with acne. My problem with Accutane (and also with high doses of vitamin A) is that it has been linked to birth defects. If you use this medication, make doubly sure that you are not pregnant or likely to become pregnant. Accutane was in the news more recently for its possible association with suicide. For real. As reported in the *British Medical Journal*, individuals treated with Accutane acne medication showed an almost twofold increase in suicide attempts. After drug treatment was stopped, the risk/incidence returned to normal.

We also have another vitamin A–derived skin cream in the pharmacy called Retin-A (tretinoin). It's a pricey medication that requires a prescription. As it's derived from vitamin A, it works on a similar principle and is helpful at smoothing skin and clearing acne. There are very few risks (if any) because this is applied to the skin, unlike Accutane, which is taken orally.

Excessive amounts of vitamin A in supplement form can be toxic, but beta-carotene is safer because your body will convert only as much vitamin A from beta-carotene as it needs. Vitamin A confers many health benefits, including supporting your eyesight, fertility, and immune function. It also supports healthy teeth, bones, and skin. One other fascinating benefit is that it acts as a kind of internal sunscreen and offers a little protection from the sun's rays.

Vitamin A is so important to skin that studies suggest it can protect against skin cancer as well as cancer of the mouth, bladder, breast, stomach, lungs, and cervix. It can be useful in treating myriad skin problems, including eczema, dermatitis, brown spots, and psoriasis.

The first signal of vitamin A deficiency shows up in the eyes. It may come in the form of poor night vision, dry eyes, vision loss, or cornea problems. It's also possible to experience an oddity such as gray patches in the whites of the eyes. These are called Bitot's spots. Blindness is also possible with long-term deficiency.

Because vitamin A protects the immune system from free radical damage, a deficiency increases your risk of infection and cancer. Some women develop cervical dysplasia, an abnormality in the cells of the cervix, in part because of vitamin A deficiency. Dry or rough skin can also signal a deficiency.

Drug Muggers of Vitamin A

Acid Blockers

Cimetidine (Tagamet)

Esomeprazole (Nexium)

Famotidine (Pepcid and Pepcid Complete)

Lansoprazole (Prevacid 24HR)

Nizatidine (Axid)

Omeprazole (Prilosec OTC)

Pantoprazole (Protonix)

Rabeprazole (Aciphex)

Ranitidine (Zantac)

Antacids

Aluminum and magnesium hydroxide (Maalox, Mylanta)

Aluminum carbonate gel (Basaljel)

Aluminum hydroxide (Amphojel, AlternaGEL)

Calcium carbonate (Tums, Titralac, Rolaids)

Magnesium hydroxide (Phillips' Milk of Magnesia)

Sodium bicarbonate (Alka-Seltzer, baking soda)

Antibiotics

Neomycin (eyedrops, eardrops, antibiotic ointments)

Antigout

Colchicine (Colcrys)

Cholesterol Agents

Cholestyramine resin (Questran)

Colesevalam (WelChol)

Colestipol (Colestid)

Corticosteroids (For some examples, see page 262.)

Lipase Inhibitors

Orlistat (Alli, Xenical)

Oral Contraceptives (Not a drug mugger; may lead to increases in plasma levels of vitamin A.)

Miscellaneous

Alcohol

Fat blockers sold as OTC diet aids (kidney bean extract or starch neutralizer, for example)

Malabsorption disorders like Celiac, Crohn's, IBS, pancreatic insufficiency

Mineral oil

Olestra (a fat substitute commonly found in light potato chips)

Beta-Carotene: Put This on Your Plate

Sweet potatoes, carrots, butternut squash, red peppers, tomatoes, pumpkin, spinach, collard greens, cantaloupe, apricots, peaches, and raw broccoli. Lightly sautéing or steaming vegetables seems to make it easier to absorb beta-carotene, unlike many other nutrients that are destroyed by light cooking. If you want vitamin A itself, good food sources include animal meats such as steak, liver, kidney, butter, dairy products, and eggs. If you think you need more vitamin A, drink my Apple Carrot Cocktail (page 371) every day.

An Absurdly Inexpensive Way to Feel Better

It's important to remember that beta-carotene is a precursor to vitamin A, but it is not actually vitamin A. The doses listed below are for beta-carotene.

For general health: About 5–15 mg (8–25,000 IU) per day

Drug mugger dose: 15–20 mg (25,000–33,340 IU) per day

Pregnant women: Follow your doctor's orders, but generally speaking, limit vitamin A to no more than 10,000 IU per day

Just So You Know

I prefer that you take beta-carotene rather than vitamin A unless your health-care provider specifically prescribes vitamin A. Beta-carotene is water soluble, so your body can convert it safely to vitamin A and excrete the rest, whereas vitamin A is fat soluble, so it's possible to accumulate too much.

Only buy natural forms. Synthetic forms don't offer antioxidant protection because they are not the real deal. Some experts (and I'm one of them) think that synthetic versions of beta-carotene are downright dangerous for you. Some forms appear to increase the risk of cancer in smokers, who often take the supplement. This was found in at least three research trials. That said, no study has checked to see whether natural beta-carotene could increase the death rate, but I'm going to bet it doesn't. A synthetic product will usually just say beta-carotene on the label and offer a dosage. The natural form will usually have these phrases on the label: "from *D. salina*" (for *Dunaliella salina,* an alga), "from an algae source," "natural beta-carotene," or "from a palm source."

You are getting too much beta-carotene if you start to develop diarrhea, a yellow-orange tinge to your skin that goes away on its own, easy bruising, or joint pain. Any of these things may occur with dosages of 50 mg (100,000 IU) per day or less if you are sensitive.

Install Your Nutrient Security System

Many delicious foods offer you a hefty dose of beta-carotene or vitamin A. Absorption of these nutrients is enhanced if you eat them along with some type of fat, such as a healthy oil. In my home, after I bake a sweet potato, I sprinkle it with a little cinnamon and cold-pressed flaxseed oil while it's still hot. I also sauté kale in grape seed oil and fresh garlic. The idea is to heat (or cook) these foods gently for a few minutes until the cell walls split open and the carotenes spill out into the fat (the oil), which easily totes the beta-carotene into your own cells. These nutrients have to penetrate your fatty cells for you to get the best effect. See Chapter 29 for delicious recipes to up your beta-carotene.

What's in My Cupboard?

Carrot Essence by Green Foods: This carrot powder combines beta-carotene from organically grown carrots along with vitamin C, another powerful antioxidant. The vitamin C is naturally derived from the acerola berry, so it's totally natural. The makers have not added sugar, salt, wheat, gluten, soy, or artificial colors. I've used this 100 percent pure brand in my home for years. It's easy to add a scoop to smoothies. If you want a quick pick-me-up, just add water to it. It contains 11,000 IU beta-carotene and 34 mg vitamin C per dose. I use this on days when I don't feel like breaking out my juicer and starting from scratch. See their entire product line of powdered natural foods and drinks at www.greenfoods.com.

BioAstin by Nutrex Hawaii: This carotenoid, astaxanthin, is 11 times more powerful than beta-carotene in terms of squashing free radical damage. It is also thought to be 550 times stronger than vitamin E. If you want a strong antioxidant, this newly discovered carotenoid is similar to beta-carotene but stronger. Sold at health food stores nationwide.

Natural Food Carotene Complex by Nutraceutical Sciences Institute (NSI): This product contains natural carotenes from the alga *D. salina* and spirulina extract, which I love because it's loaded with other nutrients and minerals. It is also gluten free and sugar free.

Oceanic Beta-Carotene 25,000 IU by Solgar: These softgels contain natural beta-carotene derived from *D. salina* along with other important carotenoids such as alpha-carotene, cryptoxanthin, zeaxanthin, and lutein for a synergistic blend of provitamin A substances (a blend of compounds that goes on to form vitamin A). It is free of all allergens and is sold at most health food stores.

Carotenoid Complex by Country Life: These softgels contain natural beta-carotene derived from *D. salina* as well as lutein, zeaxanthin, lycopene, broccoli and pumpkin concentrate, carrot seed oil, and astaxanthin (derived from krill). Each softgel delivers 25,000 IU beta-carotene.

Beta Carotene by Pure Encapsulations: This product can be purchased online or through your doctor. It contains a broad spectrum of natural carotenoids from *D. salina*, including zeaxanthin and lutein, among others. It's also gluten free and vegetarian. Contact information: www.purecaps.com.

Arctic Cod Liver Oil by Nordic Naturals: If you want a natural form of vitamin A itself instead of its precursor beta-carotene, then use cod liver oil. It's a fantastic source derived from an animal. This is the one I have tasted and liked. My mom swears by this one and has taken it for years. You can buy it in convenient softgels, which are tasteless, or in strawberry-, peach-, or orange-flavored liquids. It doesn't taste like fish! I always recommend this for people with neurodegenerative disorders, such as multiple sclerosis, amyotrophic lateral sclerosis (ALS), and arthritis; depression; memory problems; and especially heart disease and atherosclerosis. Contact information: www.nordicnaturals.com.

Allergy A and D$_3$ by Twinlab: This product was designed with people who don't eat fish in mind, or for those who are allergic to fish or fish oil products. The capsules contain 10,000 IU of a natural, preformed kind of vitamin A called retinyl acetate, along with 400 mg vitamin D$_3$. It is sold nationwide.

Lutein Lycopene Carotene Complex by Solgar: This multitasking product contains various carotenoids along with 10,000 IU beta-carotene in each softgel. The beta-carotene (and alpha-carotene) comes from pure carrot oil and *D. salina*. The lutein and zeaxanthin are derived from marigold flowers, and the lycopene comes from tomatoes.

Biotin

It's safe to say that biotin may make you more beautiful. If you have brittle nails or slow-growing, dull hair, there's a good chance you're deficient.

In one study published half a century ago in the *Journal of Nutrition*, researchers gave monkeys a combination of biotin and a few other B vitamins and found that natural hair color could be partially restored in old animals. The color transformation occurred by supplementing with natural forms of the nutrients (as found in animal feed), not by supplemental multivitamins. As exciting as this may be for silver-haired seniors, I must tell you that I've not been able to find a solid human or animal clinical trial that proves biotin restores hair color.

While it might not erase gray, there are plenty of studies that show biotin nourishes the skin and hair, as well as the liver, pancreas, and heart. So obviously its role goes way beyond beautification. Its most important one, in fact, is to help you break down food, namely carbohydrates, fats, and protein. It also helps regulate cholesterol and blood sugar.

Biotin, also known as vitamin B_7, belongs to the B complex family of vitamins, and like all vitamin Bs, it dissolves in water, not fatty tissue. But did you know that it is sometimes referred to as vitamin H? The "H" is for *haut*, which means "skin" in German.

The human intestinal tract can make some biotin. It is not made in the cells. The manufacture of small amounts of biotin in the gut happens thanks to the hard work of beneficial bacteria. A flourishing, natural, healthy camp of friendly bacteria is absolutely essential to making biotin. If you have poor gastrointestinal function, low amounts of healthy normal intestinal flora, or chronic diarrhea, you will become deficient in biotin. This explains why antibiotics are drug muggers of both probiotics and biotin. You can't make biotin without the presence of the good microorganisms that make up your intestinal flora, so please refer to Chapter 17, Probiotics. If you're out of those, you're out of biotin, too. In fact, biotin is produced naturally by all sorts of microorganisms such as bacteria, fungi, algae, and a few plants.

Symptoms of deficiency may include hair loss (alopecia), high cholesterol, blood sugar imbalances, liver enlargement, cardiac arrhythmias, depression, abnormal skin sensations (parasthesias), seborrheic dermatitis, low appetite, poor immunity, and muscle aches or pain. Children with low biotin may act withdrawn and show developmental delays. Because biotin works directly in the Krebs cycle (the chemical reactions in your body that release energy from food), it makes sense that a biotin deficiency could cause tiredness. Biotin also helps reduce symptoms of zinc deficiency because it extends the life span of zinc. People with diabetes often show deficiencies in both biotin and zinc. This is one of the safest and best B vitamins to take as a supplement.

Drug Muggers of Biotin (Vitamin B$_7$)

Acid Blockers

Cimetidine (Tagamet)

Esomeprazole (Nexium)

Famotidine (Pepcid and Pepcid Complete)

Lansoprazole (Prevacid 24HR)

Nizatidine (Axid)

Omeprazole (Prilosec OTC)

Pantoprazole (Protonix)

Rabeprazole (Aciphex)

Ranitidine (Zantac)

Analgesics

Butalbital-containing drugs (Fioricet, Fiorinal, Zebutal)

Antacids

Aluminum and magnesium hydroxide (Maalox, Mylanta)

Aluminum carbonate gel (Basaljel)

Aluminum hydroxide (AlternaGEL, Amphojel)

Calcium carbonate (Rolaids, Titralac, Tums)

Magnesium hydroxide (Phillips' Milk of Magnesia)

Sodium bicarbonate (Alka-Seltzer, baking soda)

Antibiotics (a few examples)

Amoxicillin (Amoxil)

Azithromycin (Z-Pak)

Cefaclor (Ceclor)

Cefdinir (Omnicef)

Cephalexin (Keflex)

Ciprofloxacin (Cipro)

Clarithromycin (Biaxin)

Doxycycline (Doryx)

Erythromycin (E.E.S.)

Levofloxacin (Levaquin)

Minocycline (Minocin)

Sulfamethoxazole and
   trimethoprim (Bactrim, Septra)

Tetracycline (Sumycin)

Anticonvulsants: When
supplementing for this
particular depletion, space your
vitamin at least 4 hours away
from the anticonvulsant
medication.

Carbamazepine (Carbatrol,
   Tegretol)

Oxcarbazepine (Trileptal)

Phenobarbital (Solfoton)

Phenytoin (Dilantin)

Primidone (Mysoline)

Zonisamide (Zonegran)

Antivirals

Delavirdine (Rescriptor)

Foscarnet (Foscavir)

Lamivudine (Epivir)

Nevirapine (Viramune)

Zidovudine, AZT (Retrovir)

Zidovudine and lamivudine
   (Combivir)

**Aromatase Inhibitors for breast
cancer**

Anastrozole (Arimidex)

**Hormone Replacement Therapy/
Oral Contraceptives**

Estradiol (Climara, CombiPatch,
   Estraderm, EstroGel, Menostar,
   and many others)

Estrogen-containing drugs (Estrace,
   Estring, Femring, Premarin)

Estrogen and progestrin (Activella)

Estrogens, conjugated (Prempro,
   Premphase)

Ethinyl estradiol (found in many
   birth control pills)

SERMs (Selective Estrogen Receptor
   Modulators—used for breast
   cancer)

Raloxifene (Evista)

Tamoxifen (Nolvadex)

Toremifene (Fareston)

Sulfonamides (Sulfa antibiotics,
   some diabetes medications)

Miscellaneous

Alcohol

Any drug that depletes beneficial
   bacteria in the gut is a drug
   mugger of biotin.

Estrogen dominance

Nicotine

Pregnancy

Raw egg whites

Biotin: Put This on Your Plate

Peanuts, hazelnuts, almonds, soy protein, cheese, beef liver, cauliflower, brewer's yeast, egg yolks, wheat germ, cashews, yogurt, sweet potatoes, spinach, Swiss chard, legumes, haddock, salmon, tomatoes, avocados, bananas, and canned tuna.

An Absurdly Inexpensive Way to Feel Better

For general health: 100–1,000 micrograms (mcg) per day

Drug mugger dose: 1,000–5,000 mcg per day

Just So You Know

Biotin is usually found in supplements as D-biotin, and this is just fine. There are high concentrations of this nutrient in royal jelly (a bee product) and brewer's yeast. Hair, skin, and nail formulas often contain 2,000 to 5,000 mcg. Excess biotin is eliminated in the urine, and this nutrient appears to be nontoxic, even when taken in high doses (up to 5,000 mcg per day). Biotin works best in conjunction with the rest of its family members, all found in a B complex. One more thing: Save your money on the shampoos that claim to include biotin for hair growth. It's fine if it's in there, but only nutritional supplements will allow you to get the active form of biotin into your gut and into your cells. In a shampoo, all of it swirls down the drain along with your money. Point: Take it by mouth; don't splash it on your head.

Install a Nutrient Security System

Biotin is found naturally in the protein in eggs. This protein contains a smaller peptide called avidin, which binds to the biotin like glue, keeping this B vitamin intact and preventing you from absorbing it. You want this love affair to break up so that the biotin becomes available to you for absorption. Cooking the eggs solves the avidin-biotin problem because the avidin hates heat. When you cook the egg, you break the "lovers" apart, which is why many experts suggest scrambled eggs as a source for biotin.

Not getting enough biotin when you think you have your bases covered is a big deal because biotin deficiency could suppress your level of IGF-1 (insulin-like growth factor 1), according to a 2009 study published in the *European Journal of Nutrition*. IGF-1 is a hormone (chemically speaking) but serves to promote youth and growth, help build muscles, and have an antiaging effect on the body. Besides keeping us youthful, these growth hormones protect against cardiovascular disease, arrhythmias, osteoporosis, wrinkling, gray hair, weight gain, depression, and muscle wasting. No wonder biotin keeps us beautiful, and now we have the science to prove it! In summary, the installation of a nutrient security system that includes biotin can make us beautiful inside and out. It works best in tandem with its sister B vitamins—B_1, B_6, folic acid, and the rest, so take your biotin along with a full-range B complex. And don't rely on eggs!

What's in My Cupboard?

Biotin by Nature Made: This product is easy to find and contains 2,500 mcg biotin in each softgel, which is free of artificial flavors, preservatives, and allergens such as yeast and gluten. The makers are very strict about quality control standards. Almost all Nature Made products are USP certified for potency and purity.

Dr. Ohhira's Probiotics by Essential Formulas: This is a fantastic combination of probiotics, along with many B vitamins, minerals, and amino acids. It contains a synergistic blend of beneficial bacteria along with biotin and other B vitamins, minerals, and amino acids. Since biotin is manufactured by intestinal microflora, it makes sense that a probiotic formula would enhance your body's own ability to produce normal levels of biotin. This brand is a capsule and is produced using non-GMO (that's short for genetically modified organism) ingredients. You can learn more about avoiding GMO foods in Chapter 29. *Note:* You need healthy bacteria in your gut in order to produce biotin.

For Longer Life Biotin 1% by Life Extension: This is a powder. You just mix up whatever dosage you like in water, juice, or a smoothie. This will go a long way because $1/8$ of a heaping teaspoon gives you 5,950 mcg daily.

Super Potency Biotin by Nature's Bounty: Each capsule gives you 5,000 mcg (or 5 mg) per dose.

Biotin by Swanson Health Products: This product contains 5,000 mcg per capsule.

Super Biotin by Puritan's Pride: Each capsule contains 5,000 mcg biotin.

Bluebonnet Ultimate Hair and Nail Formula: These vegetarian caps contain a comprehensive list of vitamins (including biotin), minerals, and amino acids all designed to support beauty and hair growth. The daily dose of 3 capsules contains 1,000 mcg of biotin.

Biotin by Natural Factors: Each tablet contains 300 mcg of biotin.

Biotin 1000 mcg by Nature's Way: These dissolvable lozenges contain 1,000 mcg of biotin. Biotin is helpful in creating normal skin and scalp secretions, so this is a tasty way to look pretty! It helps with dry scalp and seborrheic dermatitis.

Calcium

People think calcium is just for bones. Sure, it's needed for both bones and teeth, but it's also necessary for healthy blood pressure. Did you know that calcium also helps make your muscles work properly and more comfortably? If you have muscle cramps or spasms, you may be low in calcium. A deficiency could put you at greater risk for osteoporosis, tooth decay, high blood pressure, heart disease, insomnia, acid reflux, digestive problems, obesity, diabetes, and cancer.

Calcium is needed to keep weight off as well. If you have a calcium deficiency, your body will try to repair itself by sending messages to your parathyroid glands and your kidneys. In turn, these organs release parathyroid hormone and calcitriol. These hormones then increase the amount of calcium available in the body, but in doing so, they stimulate the production of fat and also help the body hold on to it very stubbornly. Simply put, low calcium means you store more fat on your butt or around your belly!

The calcitriol hormone I just mentioned is the active form of vitamin D, and it behaves as a hormone in this form. Calcitriol's effects on the body are usually beneficial. Like every good thing, however, it has a negative side. Too much calcitriol might squeeze your arteries, causing high blood pressure. Yep, that's right! Without being too technical, very low calcium triggers higher calcitriol, which in turn causes high blood pressure (to go with that spare tire on your belly). See, I told you, calcium is important. It's so much more than a bone builder!

If you're one of those women who feels like biting everybody's head off during your menstrual cycle, calcium can purge you of those devilish thoughts. It seems to control mood swings, calm feelings of irritability, lessen breast tenderness, and reduce cravings for sweets. Finally, it has a protective effect on the colon, preventing the formation of polyps, which may lead to colon cancer. Many people who don't get enough green veggies run out of calcium. Green vegetables have a lot of calcium—much more than milk. Does that surprise you? Where do you think the cows get their calcium from? It's in the grass they eat! Cows graze on greens all day, and I don't see any of them developing hip fractures and osteoporosis.

People who have suffered an unexplained bone fracture can bet that they're low in calcium and probably a lot of other minerals, especially magnesium. There's an interesting relationship between calcium and magnesium because magnesium is necessary for calcium absorption. Without enough magnesium, calcium can collect in soft tissues and cause joint pain. Not only does it collect in the soft tissues of people with arthritis, but the calcium levels in their blood and bones are reduced. You would think you'd need more calcium to counteract this problem, but taking calcium supplements only worsens the situation. Magnesium taken in proper dosages can actually solve the problem of calcium deficiency for these people and make calcium supplementation much safer. The magnesium pushes the calcium out of the soft tissue and into the bones where it's needed.

Taking calcium without enough magnesium throws the body out of kilter and may be harmful to some people, especially if they are also very acidic—meaning that their urine measures in the acid range according to urine test kits, such as litmus paper or Chemstrips. So the bottom line is that many supplements combine calcium and magnesium to enhance absorption and provide the benefits of both minerals. These combos are intelligent. Vitamin D is also crucial to help the body absorb calcium, so be sure to get enough sunlight each day or take a D_3 (cholecalciferol) supplement as well. Be warned, though, too much vitamin D and you will see a backlash of too much calcium in the blood.

While people with asthma, COPD, and chronic allergies often rely on inhaled steroids such as Flovent, these drugs may impair calcium absorption so significantly that over time your risk goes up for fracture. That's a shame, because the drugs are very helpful at opening airway passages and helping you breathe. Right now, I want you to realize that inhaled medications have a drug mugging effect and could be impacting the frailty of

your bones, causing more breakage. The articles I read on this topic sometimes say the link is controversial. Is it really? You decide.

A 2010 study on inhaled glucocorticoids (which is what Flovent is—
and, by the way, these drugs are also called inhaled corticosteroids) evaluated whether or not inhaled glucocorticoids or beta2-agonists (drugs like
albuterol, also used to treat respiratory issues) could influence bone
strength. The study assessed patients over the age of 50 and evaluated
vertebral fractures by X-ray and quantitative ultrasound. The scientists
found that people who took the highest dosages of medication (greater
than 1,500 mcg) of inhaled glucocorticoids experienced the highest risk of
spinal fracture and the most stiffness. The most severe cases of COPD
seemed to also have the highest risk of fracture. I'm guessing the ones with
the most severe cases were also taking the most medications. In this particular study, the beta2-agonist drugs came out smelling like a rose and
were not associated with increased fracture rates. The take-home point
from where I sit is that you should try to find out what is causing your
overreactive immune response, allergies, and asthma. Many of my readers
have gone dairy free or gluten free and enjoyed better breathing. Some
have quit smoking. If you can find out the trigger, remove it. That's so
much better than having to take drugs that can mug you and make your
bones break. And remember one more thing: When physicians find out
that your bones are more brittle, they usually won't suspect that it's your
breathing medication. They may only ask themselves which bisphosphonate they should prescribe to preserve their patient's bone mass. Then
you're on the medication merry-go-round, and it's a tough ride to get off.

Drug Muggers of Calcium

Acid Blockers

Cimetidine (Tagamet)

Esomeprazole (Nexium)

Famotidine (Pepcid and Pepcid
Complete)

Lansoprazole (Prevacid 24HR)

Nizatidine (Axid)

Omeprazole (Prilosec OTC)

Pantoprazole (Protonix)

Rabeprazole (Aciphex)

Ranitidine (Zantac)

Analgesics

Butalbital-containing drugs
(Fioricet, Fiorinal, Zebutal)

Antacids

Aluminum and magnesium
hydroxide (Maalox, Mylanta)

Aluminum carbonate gel (Basaljel)

Aluminum hydroxide (Amphojel,
AlternaGEL)

Calcium carbonate (Tums,
Titralac, Rolaids)

Magnesium hydroxide (Phillips'
Milk of Magnesia)

Sodium bicarbonate (Alka-Seltzer,
baking soda)

Antibiotics (a few examples)

Amoxicillin (Amoxil)

Azithromycin (Z-Pak)

Cefaclor (Ceclor)

Cefdinir (Omnicef)

Cephalexin (Keflex)

Ciprofloxacin (Cipro)

Clarithromycin (Biaxin)

Doxycycline (Doryx)

Erythromycin (E.E.S.)

Levofloxacin (Levaquin)

Minocycline (Minocin)

Sulfamethoxazole and
trimethoprim (Septra, Bactrim)

Tetracycline (Sumycin)

Anticonvulsants

Carbamazepine (Carbatrol,
Tegretol)

Ethosuximide (Zarontin)

Gabapentin (Gabarone)

Methsuximide (Celontin)

Oxcarbazepine (Trileptal)

Phenobarbital (Solfoton)

Phenytoin (Dilantin)

Primidone (Mysoline)

Valproic acid (Depakene)

Antigout

Colchicine (Colcrys)

Antiviral Agents

Delavirdine (Rescriptor)

Foscarnet (Foscavir)

Lamivudine (Epivir)

Nevirapine (Viramune)

Zidovudine, AZT (Retrovir)

Zidovudine and lamivudine
(Combivir)

**Aromatase Inhibitors for breast
cancer**

Anastrozole (Arimidex)

Bisphosphonates (bone-building
drugs)*

Alendronate (Fosamax)

Ibandronate (Boniva)

Risedronate (Actonel)

*But supplement the calcium at least 4
to 6 hours away from the medicine.

Blood Pressure Drugs

ACE inhibitor class:

Captopril (Capoten)

Enalapril (Vasotec)

Lisinopril (Prinivil, Zestril)

Quinapril (Accupril)

Angiotensin II receptor blockers:

Candesartan (Atacand)

Irbesartan (Avapro)

Losartan (Cozaar)

Olmesartan (Benicar)

Telmisartan (Micardis)

Valsartan (Diovan)

Calcium channel blockers: These may interfere with calcium supplements. The data is controversial, but it's best to take your calcium supplement at least 2 hours away from your medication. Examples of medications in this class include verapamil and any drug that ends in "dipine," like nifedipine, felodipine, amlodipine, and others.

Diuretics, loop:

Bumetanide (Bumex)

Ethacrynic acid (Edecrin)

Furosemide (Lasix)

Diuretics, thiazide:

Chlorothiazide (Diuril)

Chlorthalidone (Hygroton)

Hydrochlorothiazide or HCTZ (Hydrodiuril)

Methyclothiazide (Enduron)

Metolazone (Zaroxolyn)

Any combination drug that contains HCTZ or hydrochlorothiazide (dozens of drugs contain this)

Diuretics, sulfonamide:

Indapamide (Lozol)

Diuretics, potassium-sparing:

Amiloride (Midamor)

Spironolactone (Aldactone)

Triamterene (Dyrenium)

Cardiac Glycosides

Digoxin (Digitek, Lanoxicaps, Lanoxin) (High levels of calcium may increase the risk of digoxin toxicity, and low levels of calcium reduce digoxin's effectiveness. If you take digoxin, your doctor should monitor your calcium levels closely.)

Corticosteroids

Betamethasone (Diprolene, Luxiq)

Dexamethasone (Decadron)

Fluocinolone (Synalar topical)

Methylprednisolone (Medrol)

Prednisolone (Prednisol)

Prednisone (Deltasone)

Triamcinolone (Aricin)

Inhaled corticosteroids:

Budesonide (Rhinocort, Symbicort)

Flunisolide (Nasarel, Nasacort)

Fluticasone (Flonase)

Cholesterol Agents

Cholestyramine resin (Questran)

Hormone Replacement Therapy/ Oral Contraceptives

Estradiol (Activella, Climara, CombiPatch, Estrace, Estraderm, Estring, EstroGel, Menostar)

Estrogen-containing drugs (Femring) There are dozens!

Estrogens, conjugated (Prempro, Premphase)

Ethinyl estradiol (found in many birth control pills)

Laxatives that contain magnesium (like magnesium citrate or Milk of Magnesia)

Salicylates (Many substances, both drug and nondrug, contain this chemical. I've listed just a few here.)

Caffeine and aspirin (Fiorinal)

Magnesium salicylate (Mobidin)

Oxycodone and aspirin (Percodan)

Salicylic acid or aspirin (Bayer, Ecotrin, St. Joseph)

Salsalate (Disalcid)

SERMs (Selective Estrogen Receptor Modulators—used for breast cancer)

Raloxifene (Evista)

Tamoxifen (Nolvadex)

Toremifene (Fareston)

Sulfonamides (Sulfa antibiotics, some diabetes medications)

Thyroid Medications (Important: Separate calcium administration from thyroid medication by 4 hours or more.)

Levothyroxine (Synthroid, Levoxyl, Thyrolar)

Miscellaneous

Benzoates

Beta hydroxy acid

Estrogen dominance

Many artificial food colorings and flavorings

Mineral oil

Menthol

Mint, peppermint, and spearmint

Phenylethyl salicylate (a fragrance)

Calcium: Put This on Your Plate

Turnip greens, spinach, mustard greens, collard greens, basil, thyme, cinnamon, blackstrap molasses, Swiss chard, yogurt, kale, mozzarella cheese, cow's milk, sardines, celery, fennel, green beans, garlic, tofu, figs, and quinoa.

An Absurdly Inexpensive Way to Feel Better

For general health: 200–800 mg per day taken with food

Drug mugger dose: 600–1,200 mg per day taken with food

Just So You Know

Calcium citrate and calcium gluconate are ideal forms of supplemental calcium. Calcium carbonate is harder to digest and seems to create more acid in the stomach after it leaves, so I don't recommend calcium carbonate supplements for people with heartburn, reflux, gastroesophageal reflux

(GERD), or ulcers. Calcium supplements made from bone meal and dolomite may be high in elemental calcium, but on occasion, if they are of poor
quality, they may contain contaminants such as lead and other toxic metals. Most forms of commercial calcium on the market today are derived
from limestone, and do you think I recommend that you include rocks in
your diet? Of course not, so please invest a little bit more in your calcium
supplementation program and get the most bioavailable forms, the kind
that are easy on the stomach and actually get into your bones. Pretty labels
that promise to protect your bones and prevent osteoporosis don't always
contain the right form of calcium, and they can be a bit deceptive to the
naive consumer. Also remember that calcium is better absorbed when
you have a little magnesium, vitamin D_3, or vitamin K_2 on board. That's
why you'll find many commercial formulas in combination with one or
more of these nutrients.

I love calcium, and I want you to feel safe replenishing what the drug
mugger stole. However, like any good nutrient, too much is bad for you.
Studies have shown that prolonged supplementation with calcium salts or
consuming high dosages may cause calcium deposits to form in abnormal
locations—where there is no bone—and these calcifications are easily visible on X-rays. This may be an explanation for why so many postmenopausal women get breast calcifications. Remember, they are routinely told
to take calcium supplements after menopause to protect their bones.

If enough is deposited in your blood vessels, however, it apparently can
cause a condition called coronary artery calcification. This is exactly what
New Zealand researchers found during a study initially intended to evaluate the effects of calcium on bone health. The researchers combined and
analyzed data from 11 randomized trials in which patients took 500 mg or
more of calcium (without vitamin D). Turns out the risk for heart attack
was about $1^1/_2$ times greater in the group receiving the supplement than in
the placebo group. In fact, when everything was considered together,
stroke, sudden death, and heart attack were collectively more common in
those on supplements than on placebos, even after accounting for high
cholesterol, smoking, and high blood pressure.

Excessive calcium supplementation may elevate blood calcium levels and speed the calcification process in our fragile blood vessels, so if you do need calcium (because you take a drug mugger, for example), supplement safely by using high-quality bioavailable products and follow label directions for dosage or even take a little less.

Please know that the jury is still out about this; what you are reading is my opinion based on studies. There are certainly other studies that don't point to this problem. In a study published in the July 2010 issue of *Menopause*, for example, researchers concluded that moderate doses of calcium (with vitamin D_3) did not appear to alter the coronary artery calcified plaque burden in the 754 postmenopausal women who participated in the study. Whether higher or lower doses would alter the results remains to be seen.

A Mayo Clinic trial published in December 2009 similarly found no difference in aortic valve and coronary artery calcification in 262 older women who took calcium supplements over a 4-year period.

Prolonged consumption of high dosages of calcium carbonate or other forms of calcium can occasionally cause an individual to develop a triad of health problems—hypercalcemia (excess calcium in the blood), metabolic alkalosis, and kidney damage. This triad is called milk-alkali syndrome or Burnett's syndrome. This isn't new information, but it bears repeating because we are all hammered with the concept that the more calcium the merrier. As far back as 1995, I found a report in a Baltimore medical journal that opened as follows: "Milk-alkali syndrome can be caused by ingesting large amounts of calcium carbonate. Coincident with the promotion of calcium carbonate as treatment for both dyspepsia and osteoporosis, milk-alkali syndrome is now a common cause of hypercalcemia severe enough to require admission to the hospital."

The good news is that calcium carbonate is so poorly absorbed through the GI tract that it is unlikely to cause any systemic problem for the vast majority of people taking it, especially if you stick to label dosages and don't overdo it. On the other hand, calcium carbonate does bind with other minerals in the gut, inhibits digestive enzymes, and can cause constipation. This doesn't mean that you are free and clear of developing milk-alkali syndrome; I just want you to feel confident that for the most part, it is rare and more frequently associated with high dosages and chronic ingestion of calcium.

Certain people seem to have a higher risk of developing hypercalemia. They include individuals who have kidney insufficiency, excessive vitamin D intake, or hyperparathyroidism. You know you're taking excessive amounts of calcium if you have some of these early signs: constipation, anorexia, abdominal cramps, fatigue, nausea, headache, a metallic taste in your mouth, muscle weakness, muscle or bone pain, itching, dry mouth, kidney stones, iron deficiency anemia, or irregular heartbeat.

As calcium builds up, other late-stage symptoms sneak up on you, and they are so insidious that you may not even connect them to your dietary supplement. So be watchful for mental confusion, itchy skin, irregular heartbeat, frequent urination at night, severe thirst, coronary calcifications, and/or sudden onset of a seizure disorder.

Install a Nutrient Security System

There are several things you should do if you have concerns about building and maintaining your precious calcium stores. For one, include vitamin D in your regular daily supplement program. About 1,000 IU is all you need to boost vitamin D; however, you can take more if you also happen to take a drug mugger of vitamin D (see Chapter 23). Magnesium assists calcium in its job, too, so taking a multitasking formula that contains calcium, vitamin D, and magnesium might be perfect for you. There are many such products available at health food stores.

The other thing you should do is have your doctor do blood tests to evaluate your parathyroid and thyroid statuses. The parathyroid glands produce a hormone that tells the kidneys to conserve calcium and other minerals. When your thyroid gland is working well, it secretes another hormone called calcitonin that preserves calcium and other minerals and helps slow down the rate at which your bones break down. So healthy thyroids and parathyroids go a long way in preserving both your calcium stores and your bones!

What's in My Cupboard?

Bone Strength Take Care by New Chapter: This is a powerful blend of bone-building nutrients that include calcium derived from an alga (plant) source (*Lithothamnium calcareum*), which comes from pristine Icelandic shores. (I've been to Iceland, and everything there *is* pristine!) Best of all, our bodies understand how to incorporate this natural form of calcium. This is first on my calcium supplementation list. It offers genuine bone protection because it also contains other nutrients needed for bone health, such as strontium, magnesium, vitamin K_2, silica, and vitamin D_3.

Spirulina Pacifica by Nutrex Hawaii: Spirulina is a blue-green alga that occurs naturally in the ocean. This company is dedicated to the production of spirulina, which many experts call a superfood. Many people mistakenly think that the best source of calcium is milk, but as we've seen, that's not really true. Spirulina contains 300 percent more calcium than whole milk. To make this mineral-rich spirulina, Nutrex Hawaii uses ocean water drawn from a pipeline 2,000 feet deep in one of the world's cleanest oceans. It's available as a tablet or a powder, though people have a harder time getting used to the taste of the powder. You can mix it with apple juice, or just buy tablets. I take 3 to 6 tablets of this brand every day, and it makes my hair and nails grow like crazy.

Floradix Calcium Liquid by Flora: A lot of calcium supplements are the size of horse pills and are very hard to swallow. For this reason, I've included a liquid option that provides calcium in two excellent bio-available forms, calcium gluconate and calcium lactate. This liquid can be diluted in water or juice, if you prefer. It provides 200 mg per capful, so dosing is easy. I love the inactive ingredients that this company includes: carrots, roselle flowers, spinach leaves, rose hips, locust seed flour, and juices from pear, mango, and orange.

Calcium Citrate and Malate by Nutraceutical Sciences Institute (NSI): This product contains an intelligent form of calcium along with a healthy amount of malic acid, an extract from apples that helps prevent leg cramps and muscle soreness. Do you know why an apple a day keeps the doctor away? It's the malic acid. This combination goes a long way for people with muscle aches, fibromyalgia, and restless legs.

Calcium Magnesium Citramate by Thorne Research: This product contains calcium and magnesium in a 1:1 ratio, 80 mg of each. It also has 240 mg of malic acid and is completely free of allergens, fillers, and magnesium stearate.

Calcium Citrate by Solaray: These chewable calcium citrate tablets are great for people who cannot swallow easily. The product is naturally sweetened with orange juice powder and stevia, a natural sweetener.

Magic Minerals by Dr. Dave's Stages of Life: I like this brand and took it myself for about 2 years because it provides minerals in a highly absorbable form. It made my nails grow like crazy. The reason I like it is because minerals work best if ingested as chelates. A chelate is an organic salt. When minerals are in the chelated form, the GI tract is able to absorb them more easily. If they aren't chelated properly and in a balanced manner, the minerals in your supplement will compete for absorption in your body and you may not get the full effect. Absorption is enhanced when the minerals are properly balanced relative to each other. This particular brand is a full-spectrum mineral supplement and provides 300 mg of calcium along with vanadium, chromium, magnesium, potassium, zinc, and other cofactors needed to strengthen bones, lower blood pressure, and help with leg cramps.

Bone Strength Formula with KoAct by Life Extension: These capsules contain 300 mg of calcium (chelated as calcium collagen chelate, so it's bioavailable) along with vitamin D_3. This product is available from many GNC retailers, online retailers, and Life Extension.

Calcium Hydroxyapatite Microcrystalline by Solaray: This formula contains a unique multimineral supplement derived from freeze-dried calf bone. The freeze-drying process generally maintains intact the natural bone matrix, natually occuring proteins, and glycosaminoglycans, meaning that there is more calcium that is bioavailable and it is easier on your stomach. Four gluten-free capsules contain 1,000 mg of calcium, along with other bone builders such as phosphorus, magnesium, manganese, zinc, and chromium.

Coenzyme Q10

The powerful antioxidant coenzyme Q10 makes energy for you by sparking the production of the energy molecule ATP (adenosine triphosphate), which every single cell in your body needs in order to function. Among other things, ATP provides the energy that helps facilitate blood sugar regulation, muscle contraction, disease prevention, brain health, and proper heart function. In fact, coenzyme Q10 is most famous for its role in the heart.

Enzymes are substances that help make chemical reactions take place. A coenzyme is a substance that helps an enzyme do its job. Coenzyme Q10 is one of many coenzymes in the body, and it's a really important one. Without adequate amounts of coenzyme Q10, we would literally die within minutes.

Coenzyme Q10 is often shortened to CoQ10 or Q. It is ubiquitous, meaning it's found everywhere, in all plant and animal cells. This explains why it's sometimes referred to as ubiquinone. The active form is called ubiquinol; and if you buy that, it is absorbed more easily.

Unfortunately, as we age, the amount of CoQ10 the human body produces starts to dwindle. That's why taking a CoQ10 supplement can be so helpful. Indeed, no matter what your age, if your body is low in CoQ10, taking a supplement is helpful for many conditions. Multiple studies show that CoQ10 improves angina pectoris, arrhythmias, high blood pressure, shortness of breath, heart palpitations, and energy levels. It also protects cholesterol from harmful oxidation. This is a great supplement to take if you are fatigued or have heart disease or fibromyalgia. If you have suffered a stroke, it can help speed recovery and reduce damage from the stroke. It can also reduce your risk of Parkinson's disease.

CoQ10 can reduce your risk of—and reverse—congestive heart failure to some degree. It has been studied around the world, and there have been dozens of placebo-controlled studies on the treatment of heart disease with CoQ10. Many of them confirm its effectiveness. Ironically, this vital nutrient is depleted by the very medications used to treat heart disease. Are you with me on this, or am I the only one who thinks this is loony?

The depletion of CoQ10 is becoming epidemic primarily because of the popular cholesterol-lowering drugs called statins, which interfere with the body's natural metabolic pathway. When statins block an enzyme called HMG-CoA reductase, cholesterol production slows down dramatically. Unfortunately, this is the exact same pathway where CoQ10 is produced too, hence the drug mugging effect. What people may not know is that this effect is dose dependent, meaning that the higher the drug dosage the more depletion of CoQ10. The damaging effect of this drug–nutrient depletion is most often seen in people with heart failure or in the elderly. We know that low levels of CoQ10 cause muscle damage and may lead to leg cramps and muscles aches and pains, which is why you may have been told that you have leg cramps, restless legs syndrome, or chronic fatigue. Low CoQ10 isn't pretty; it hurts the muscles from head to toe. Need I remind you that your heart is a muscle, too, and you need that baby pumping 24/7, right?

I'll get to that shortly, but first let's talk more about the number one side effect of statins: muscle problems. The prevalence of muscle aches, spasms, and leg cramps is common among statin users. These phenomena can happen within weeks to months of beginning statin therapy. According to a double-blind study of 32 patients, it was shown that CoQ10 could ease this painful problem. This study included people who took either atorvastatin (Lipitor), lovastatin (Mevacor), pravastatin (Pravachol), or simvastatin (Zocor), allowing the researchers to evaluate a group of people who took different statins, not just one brand in particular. The participants were divided into two groups, one that received vitamin E and one that received CoQ10 for 30 days. No change in the pain intensity was noted in the vitamin E group between start and finish; however, in the group who took 100 mg of CoQ10, it was noted that "pain intensity had decreased significantly from baseline." Further, the researchers concluded that "the interference of pain with daily activities significantly improved with coenzyme Q10, whereas the vitamin E did not have a significant impact on this."

So there you have it, straight from the *American Journal of Cardiology,* proof that an inexpensive nutrient can help ease tremendous muscle discomfort.

And I don't need to read the literature to see how much CoQ10 (and ubiquinol) can improve muscle pain and cramps. I can read my own e-mails. When I reached out to readers of my syndicated health column, "Dear Pharmacist," and my Facebook fans, they inundated me with letters about how quickly their pain resolved with my tip about taking CoQ10. From Kathy Z.: "I read an article you wrote about statin drugs being drug muggers and causing leg cramps. I used to suffer from leg cramps like you can't imagine and my toes would feel like they wanted to climb over the top of one another. I took your advice and started taking CoQ10 (100 mg twice daily) and the leg cramps have stopped!"

CoQ10, also called ubiquinone, is absolutely, 100 percent, no-doubt-about-it, essential to healthy muscle function; a deficiency of it causes muscle damage, known technically as *myopathy.* Statin-induced CoQ10 depletion and myopathy are completely preventable. You just have to know that the drug is mugging you of this nutrient, then you can supplement with CoQ10 while still remaining compliant with your medication. You might say that a CoQ10 supplement is the side-effect solution to statin drugs.

Hundreds of research papers have been written on the benefits of using CoQ10 for treating heart failure without significant adverse effects. Much of this research has been done by Peter Langsjoen, MD, a cardiologist in Tyler, Texas, who has 30 years of experience treating heart disease with CoQ10.

When I interviewed Dr. Langsjoen for this book, he said that "patients with heart failure from any cause have low CoQ10 blood levels, and the CoQ10 level in both plasma and heart muscle is the lowest in those patients with the most severe heart failure. Supplementation of CoQ10 in these patients repletes this deficiency and brings about dramatic improvement in heart function and quality of life."

So there you have it. People with heart failure are often, if not always, deficient in CoQ10. That comes straight from the mouth of a leading world authority, and he should know! Do we make congestive heart failure (CHF) worse with statin cholesterol drugs? The literature suggests we do. Dr. Langsjoen had this to say about CHF. "We are currently in the midst of a congestive heart failure epidemic in the United States, the cause or causes of which are unclear. As physicians, it is our duty to be absolutely certain that we are not inadvertently doing harm to our patients by creating a widespread deficiency of a nutrient critically important for normal heart function."

We also know statins are associated with liver damage—this isn't a secret. It's the reason your doctor wants you to have your liver enzymes and liver function tested several times a year. You should do as your doctor asks if these tests are requested. But can CoQ10 supplementation prevent liver damage if you are on a statin? I believe so with all my heart. CoQ10 penetrates the liver because it has a fatty component to it, so it's one of those antioxidants that goes into the liver (and brain, too, just FYI). According to a 2007 study, researchers found that simvastatin caused a "moderately higher degree of cell death" and a reduction in CoQ10 in the mitochondria of liver cells, specifically HepG2 cells. I don't want to get too technical on you, but suffice it to say that the simvastatin damaged the DNA of the liver cells and affected the cells' ability to make ATP (to breathe). Basically, what I'm saying is that the statin drug squashed the CoQ10 right in the liver (and statin drugs are known to cause liver damage). The researchers were determined to see if CoQ10 supplementation could help, and indeed it could. It reduced the amount of cell death, which increased ATP synthesis (or the cells' ability to make energy). The researchers concluded that a deficiency of CoQ10 plays a role in liver damage and that CoQ10 supplements can protect the liver cells from this complication. Fab!

Coenzyme Q10 protects cells from DNA damage, so it makes sense that it may also have anticancer effects. It is such a powerful antioxidant and is very "slippery," so it goes into all of your cell membranes and even into the tiny energy-producing powerhouses (mitochondria) contained in each cell. That's right, CoQ10 actually penetrates into every cell in your body, including your brain cells. It makes sense that drugs that deplete CoQ10 may leave you with a higher risk of cancer and memory loss in addition to heart failure.

Anyone with cancer is, of course, at greater risk of dying than the general population. And, in fact, this is precisely what a recent study points to. It's not conclusive, but the cholesterol drug Vytorin (ezetimibe and simvastatin) is under scrutiny because a study suggests that users are more likely to die from cancer while taking the drug than those who don't take it are. It's worrisome, but it's not a surprise to me, given that Vytorin and similar drugs are muggers of CoQ10.

The trouble started for Vytorin when the ENHANCE trial, completed in March 2007, showed that the expensive combination drug did not do any better at unclogging arteries or preventing plaque buildup than the cheaper generic statin simvastatin, which is also known to be a drug mugger of CoQ10. Then, in 2009, the SEAS (Simvastatin and Ezetimibe in Aortic Stenosis) study published in *Heart, Lung and Circulation* reported a disturbing link between the cholesterol drug and cancer. It concluded that "cancer incidence and cancer deaths were more frequent in the simvastatin/ezetimibe group." The study found 1,873 patients with mild to moderate stenosis and was carried out in 173 clinical centers.

Ladies, pay attention: Several studies have looked at CoQ10 as a treatment for women with breast cancer, and there does appear to be some benefit.

One more important note: CoQ10 makes the body run more efficiently because it assists in hundreds of enzymatic reactions. So as your body's general health improves, you may be able to take a lower dosage of some medications or even discontinue them—with physician approval, of course. Your doctor may eventually reduce the dosage of your blood pressure meds, for example, because the CoQ10 kicks in and lowers it, too.

The take-home point is that CoQ10 can dramatically reduce the side effects you may get from statin cholesterol drugs and can protect your brain, liver, and heart as well.

You'll find CoQ10 in organ meats like kidney, heart, and liver. Food sources are not so appetizing to me, so I take supplements. Today, it's easy to find the nutrient in supplement form. There are many high-quality brands sold in health food stores and pharmacies nationwide.

Readers of my syndicated column often ask me whether CoQ10 will work just as well as ubiquinol, which is a more active version of CoQ10 and more effective in my opinion. I tell them that if they can afford ubiquinol, go ahead and get it since it is more readily taken up by the bloodstream, especially in the elderly and those with heart disease.

Just to be sure about the best form of the supplement to take, I asked Dr. Langsjoen, who has been busy researching these molecules for decades. He said, "Patients with end-stage heart failure do not absorb standard ubiquinone CoQ10 [the orange, oxidized formulation that has been in use since 1967]. These critically ill heart failure patients absorb the new ubiquinol formulation quite well, with lifesaving effect."

Did you hear that? "Lifesaving effect!" There isn't one medication that I can take off my pharmacy shelf and feel this confident about when it comes to treating your precious heart!

Drug Muggers of Coenzyme Q10

Acid Blockers

Cimetidine (Tagamet)

Esomeprazole (Nexium)

Famotidine (Pepcid and Pepcid Complete)

Lansoprazole (Prevacid 24HR)

Nizatidine (Axid)

Omeprazole (Prilosec OTC)

Pantoprazole (Protonix)

Rabeprazole (Aciphex)

Ranitidine (Zantac)

Antacids

Aluminum and magnesium hydroxide (Maalox, Mylanta)

Aluminum carbonate gel (Basaljel)

Aluminum hydroxide (Amphojel, AlternaGEL)

Calcium carbonate (Rolaids, Titralac, Tums)

Magnesium hydroxide (Phillips' Milk of Magnesia)

Sodium bicarbonate (Alka-Seltzer, baking soda)

Antiarrhythmics

Propafenone (Rythmol)

Sotalol (Betapace)

Antibiotics (a few examples)

Amoxicillin (Amoxil)

Azithromycin (Z-Pak)

Cefaclor (Ceclor)

Cefdinir (Omnicef)

Cephalexin (Keflex)

Ciprofloxacin (Cipro)

Clarithromycin (Biaxin)

Doxycycline (Doryx)

Erythromycin (E.E.S.)

Levofloxacin (Levaquin)

Minocycline (Minocin)

Sulfamethoxazole and trimethoprim (Septra, Bactrim)

Tetracycline (Sumycin)

Antidepressants, Tricyclic

Amitriptyline (Elavil)

Amoxapine (Asendin)

Clomipramine (Anafranil)

Desipramine (Norpramin)

Doxepin (Sinequan)

Imipramine (Tofranil)

Nortriptyline (Pamelor)

Protriptyline (Vivactil)

Antinausea Drugs

Promethazine (Phenergan)

Blood Thinner

Warfarin (Coumadin) (Talk to your doctor first, but CoQ10 may slightly reduce the effectiveness of this drug, so a higher dose may be needed. Taking CoQ10 still outweighs not taking it.)

Blood Pressure Drugs

Hydralazine (Apresoline)

Labetalol (Normodyne, Trandate)

Methyldopa (Aldomet)

ACE inhibitors:

Enalapril (Vasotec) (CoQ10 enhances this drug's effect.)

Angiotensin II receptor antagonists:

Candesartan (Atacand)

Candesartan and HCTZ (Atacand HCT)

Irbesartan (Avapro)

Losartan (Cozaar)

Telmisartan (Micardis)

Telmisartan and HCTZ (Micardis HCT)

Olmesartan (Benicar)

Valsartan (Diovan)

Beta-blockers:

Acebutolol (Sectral)

Atenolol (Tenormin)

Betaxolol (Kerlone)

Bisoprolol (Zebeta, Ziac, Cardicor)

Carvedilol (Coreg)

Metoprolol (Lopressor and Toprol XL) (CoQ10 enhances the benefits of this particular beta-blocker.)

Nadolol (Corgard)

Propranolol (Inderal)

Timolol (Timoptic eye drops)

Centrally acting alpha-agonist hypotensive agents:

Clonidine (Catapres)

Diuretic, sulfonamide:

HCTZ or hydrochlorothiazide (any of the dozens of drugs containing this, including Dyazide, Maxzide, Avapro HCT, Hyzaar, Micardis HCT)

Indapamide (Lozol)

Moexipril and HCTZ (Univasc)

Diuretics, thiazide:

Chlorothiazide (Diuril), chlorthalidone (Hygroton), hydrochlorothiazide or HCTZ (Hydrodiuril)

Methyclothiazide (Enduron)

Metolazone (Zaroxolyn)

Any combination drug that contains HCTZ or hydrochlorothiazide (dozens of drugs contain this)

Cancer Drugs

Doxorubicin (Adriamycin) (Pretreating yourself with CoQ10 can help reduce damage to the heart from this chemotherapy drug.)

Cholesterol Reducers

Fibrates:

Fenofibrate (Tricor)*

Gemfibrozil (Lopid)*

*These drugs are also drug muggers of vitamin E.

Statins:

Atorvastatin (Lipitor, Advicor)

Fluvastatin (Lescol)

Lovastatin (Mevacor, Altocor, Altoprev)

Pitavastatin (Livalo, Pitava)

Pravastatin (Pravachol, Lipostat, Selektine)

Rosuvastatin (Crestor)

Simvastatin (Zocor, Lipex)

Simvastatin and ezetimibe (Vytorin)

Simvastatin and niacin (Simcor)

Diabetes Medications

Acetohexamide (Dymelor)

Chlorpropamide (Diabinese)

Glimepiride (Amaryl)

Glipizide (Glucotrol)

Glyburide (Diabeta, Glynase, Micronase)

Glyburide and metformin (Glucovance)

Metformin (Fortamet, Glucophage, Glucophage XR, Glumetza, Riomet)

Metformin and sitagliptin (Janumet)

Pioglitazone (Actos)

Repaglinide (Prandin)

Rosiglitazone (Avandia)

Tolazamide (Tolinase)

Tolbutamide (Orinase)

HIV Drugs

Psychiatric Drugs

Chlorpromazine (Thorazine)

Droperidol (Inapsine)

Fluphenazine (Prolixin)

Haloperidol (Haldol)

Thioridazine (Mellaril)

Coenzyme Q10: Put This on Your Plate

Beef, chicken, soybean oil, rainbow trout, peanuts, sesame seeds, pistachios, broccoli, cauliflower, organ meats, fish (especially tuna, herring, mackerel, sardines, and salmon), whole grains, sesame oil, and spinach.

An Absurdly Inexpensive Way to Feel Better

For general health: 30–50 mg once daily (ubiquinol, 30–50 mg once daily)

Drug mugger dose: 100–200 mg once or twice daily (ubiquinol, 100 mg once daily)

For cancer or heart disease: 200 mg two to four times daily (ubiquinol, 100 mg two to four times daily) (Discuss with your doctor.)

Just So You Know

Look for a CoQ10 supplement suspended in rice bran oil or olive oil rather than a dry, powdered capsule form. The oil-suspended version seems to slip into the body's cells more easily, and some studies show that the powdered form is not as bioavailable. If you do choose to take capsules, make sure you take them with food to enhance absorption. The fat in your meal makes the powdered CoQ10 work better.

Generally speaking, CoQ10 made in Japan is superior to CoQ10 produced in China. If you can't find this information on the label, you can always call the company and ask where their CoQ10 comes from.

The better absorbed form of CoQ10 (ubiquinol) is sold under the brand name Kaneka QH; it is off-white in color. If you take something other than this top choice, I prefer that you get softgel forms that are orange in color, the natural color of CoQ10 (ubiquinone). It's hard to overdo CoQ10 as it is extraordinarily safe. Sensitive people may experience stomach upset, headache, insomnia, dizziness, or light-headedness at higher dosages.

Install Your Nutrient Security System

The synergistic combination of carnitine and coenzyme Q10 can't be beat when it comes to weight loss. The amino acid carnitine pushes fat out of your cells, and the CoQ10 acts like a taxi and delivers the fat to your muscles so you can burn it off as energy. Try 1,000 mg L-carnitine and 100 mg CoQ10 (or 50 mg ubiquinol) each morning with breakfast or at lunch.

What's in My Cupboard?

Ultimate Omega + CoQ10 by Nordic Naturals: The makers of this product have combined omega-3 fatty acids (which lower cholesterol and unclog arteries, according to some studies) with CoQ10 to give you more bang for your buck. This combination goes well together, like peanut butter and jelly. It contains 60 mg of CoQ10, some vitamin E to keep it fresh, and more than 1,200 mg total of omega-3s. It's so good that it surpasses all pharmaceutical standards for freshness and purity. It's gluten free, dairy free, and does not contain heavy metals, PCBs, or dioxins. This is first on my list because you can replenish what a drug mugger stole and simultaneously work to lower cholesterol and triglycerides, improve energy levels, and even normalize heart rhythm.

Kaneka QH by Kaneka Nutrients: This product is fermented from yeast rather than bacteria. It's bioidentical to human CoQ10 and free of the impurities often found in synthetic versions. This is the CoQ10 that is usually used in clinical trials, even those funded by the FDA and National Institutes of Health. It's non-GMO, and it's kosher and allergy free.

CoQ10 Gels by Healthy Origins: This brand is free of soy, dairy, gluten, yeast, and artificial colors and flavors. It is suspended in pure olive oil and contains no GMO ingredients. I like the fact that the CoQ10 is all natural and comes from Kaneka, the world's leading manufacturer of pure CoQ10. They also make another superior formula called **Ubiquinol,** which is better absorbed than the traditional oxidized ubiquinone form. After absorption, both forms are identical.

CoQmax CF by Xymogen: This product is sold online or through physicians' offices. When examined under a microscope, it is free of crystals. It has a special liquid carrier (patent pending) to help make the CoQ10 more bioavailable and usable than most other softgel and capsule formulas. This 50 mg formula is suitable for someone with digestive troubles. Your doctor can order it for you.

CoQ10 Liquid Softgel by Nature Made: Widely available, this is an affordable, pure version of CoQ10 with 200 mg per premium softgel.

CoQ10 + Food Complex by New Chapter: This is easy to digest, and it delivers CoQ10 and essential nutrients from cultured whole foods. Each dose offers an array of phytonutrients and antioxidants including beta glucan, glutathione, superoxide dismutase (SOD), lipoic acid, enzymes, and soy isoflavones.

Best Ubiquinol by Doctor's Best: Ubiquinol yields higher concentrations in the blood, so this product offers better antioxidant power. This brand is widely available and contains the reduced (active) form of CoQ10 that easily penetrates every cell in your body. Better absorption means more energy, too. It contains a little rosemary leaf extract to improve stability.

Ubiquinol CoQH by Source Naturals: This superior form of CoQ10 heightens absorption to yield higher concentrations of CoQ10 in the blood. Ubiquinol has been shown to provide a powerful antioxidant defense and also supports the body's cardiovascular and energy systems by aiding in the synthesis of ATP. The comprehensive benefits of ubiquinol also aid the liver, brain, and immune systems.

Cellular Active CoQ10 Ubiquinol by Bluebonnet: The name may be confusing, but it's pure ubiquinol, the body-ready form of this powerful antioxidant, at 200 mg per softgel.

MityQondria by Jarrow: This is a combination formula that contains 60 mg ubiquinol along with other nutrients that support mitochondrial health. These include alpha-lipoic acid, acetyl-L-carnitine, and creatine. This powerful blend can do a lot toward resuscitating your powerhouses (mitochondria) and playing a role in all the pathways needed to improve energy, muscle health, and heartbeat rhythm.

Folate (Vitamin B$_9$)

Folate gets its name from the Latin word *folium*, meaning "leaf." The naturally occurring nutrient is called folate, but when laboratories produce a synthetic form of this vitamin, it's referred to as folic acid. When you take a folic acid supplement, your body converts the folic acid back to an active form of folate. You can buy folic acid over the counter, or get higher dosages of it in prescription form.

Your body needs folate to make healthy red blood cells, which are necessary to shuttle oxygen all over your body. You also need folate to make healthy DNA—your genetic code—and I can't overstate the importance of this role. Folic acid is best known for helping to protect unborn babies from developing neural tube defects, serious birth defects that deform the spine or brain. That's why this nutrient is found in all prenatal vitamins.

Vitamin B$_9$ is so important that some anticancer regimens include folic acid in an effort to make tumors retreat. Even before a tumor develops, folic acid is useful. Let's take a look at just one instance: A deficiency of folic acid may contribute to problems in the cervix. If a woman goes to her gynecologist and gets an abnormal Pap test result, the doctor may tell her that she has cervical dysplasia. This is a precancerous condition of the cervix that can progress to cancer if it's not taken care of. Various treatments include medication and surgery, but many doctors overlook the fact that the problem may have occurred either because of a folate deficiency or because of the woman's genetic inability to activate the nutrient when it is consumed—what I call folate misbehavior.

The problem is that when you have this inability to activate folate and use it properly, your level of homocysteine goes up. High homocysteine has been studied and found to increase a person's risk for cancer, including cervical and uterine cancer. Folate also plays an important role in a basic detoxification reaction known as methylation. When we methylate a compound, we help deactivate it and clear it from the body. So for a couple of reasons low folate means more toxins in the body. It's that simple, but it's huge in terms of health. DNA methylation helps to slow down the vigorous and dangerous activity of about 1,700 cancer-promoting genes. You need to methylate, but some people can't do it properly because of their genes. People with a defect in the gene responsible for using folate efficiently require extra amounts of vitamin B$_9$, whether or not they take a drug mugger.

A simple blood test for homocysteine will help determine whether your folate levels are optimal. You want it to be less than 7 micromoles per liter of blood. Homocysteine levels above 13 are a risk factor for heart attack, stroke, inflammation, Alzheimer's and Parkinson's diseases, autoimmune disorders, pain, and several other diseases. Elevated homocysteine levels also mean that you have trouble with methylation reactions and therefore have more damage to DNA and thus a higher risk of cancer.

I'm betting that many women have undergone cone biopsies or hysterectomies because they did not know that they were simply deficient in folate. How many women could have avoided surgery if only they realized the important role folate plays in reproductive health? Please put my book in the hands of every woman you love. Even if you ingest enough folic acid, you can develop cervical dysplasia if you are genetically incapable of fully utilizing folate. Just in case you're wondering, the heavily promoted Gardisil vaccine against human papillomavirus (HPV) does nothing to replenish folate. A young woman who gets this vaccine may feel that she's better protected from HPV and therefore from cervical cancer, but cervical problems could occur anyway because of a folate deficiency, among other things. A 2009 study published in *Cancer Epidemiology, Biomarkers and Prevention* confirmed this. The researchers concluded, "These findings are compatible with a role for folate in modulating the risk of cervical cancer, possibly through an influence over high-risk HPV infection."

Folate deficiency can also cause atherosclerosis, depression, irritability, pale skin, and megaloblastic anemia, a condition in which red blood cells become larger or uneven in size. When you run out of folate, you run out of energy as well. Confusion, forgetfulness, and diarrhea may set in. Sounds like many elderly folks, doesn't it? I think many of our seniors are clean out of this B vitamin. A deficiency could certainly account for those embarrassing "senior moments"—forgetting why you went to a particular room or what you were trying to say when you began a sentence. Sound like you? Keep reading.

Folate deficiency can occur fairly easily since the vitamin is water soluble. Because water-soluble vitamins are not stored in the body, they're only good for a relatively short period of time. Your body takes what it needs into the cells and tissues, and then you urinate the rest out. Because your body fails to store this nutrient, you have to be vigilant about replenishing anything that a drug mugger steals.

When people think of folate deficiency, they often think of birth defects. That's why pregnant women supplement with folate, and it's included in all the prenatal vitamins. But folate deficiency can also cause depression. It's that simple. And just look at the list on page 142 to see how many drugs deplete it from your body. If you are feeling blue, it could be your medicine. In a study conducted in 1997, 213 patients with major depressive disorder took 20 mg fluoxetine (Prozac) for 8 weeks. The researchers found that people with the lowest folate levels were *more* likely to have depression and *less* likely to respond to their antidepressant medication because folic acid, in and of itself, is an antidepressant. It works by increasing levels of a natural amino acid in your body called SAMe (S-adenosyl-L-methionine). This SAMe improves your emotional well-being and feelings of joy.

Guess why else folic acid is important to our mood? Because folic acid helps to lower an inflammatory chemical called homocysteine, which most of you know is tied to heart disease. But homocysteine also makes a person unhappy! In 2007, researchers hypothesized that high homocysteine levels cause cerebral vascular disease as well as a deficiency of key neurotransmitters that are considered "happy" brain chemicals. It makes sense to me because homocysteine is known to dampen levels of dopamine. Low dopamine makes a person very depressed. It can also cause Parkinson's disease. Low folic acid leads to low serotonin, another brain chemical needed to feel joy. See how many awful conditions can happen by the loss of just one lovely nutrient? You have to keep the vitamin robbers from stealing the life out of you. If you take any of the drug muggers on pages 142–45, please supplement with folic acid and try some of the folate recipes from Chapter 29, which help arrest the vitamin robbers and give your body what it's hungry for.

NSAIDs (such as sulindac, naproxen, indomethacin, ibuprofen, salicylic acid, piroxicam, and mefenamic acid) have the ability to suppress the body's absorption and utilization of folic acid, an important B vitamin that participates in hundreds of biochemical reactions that support optimal health. The NSAID drugs are very popular and effective at relieving pain. Does the folic acid depletion mean you should stop taking your medication? No; if you need it for pain relief, I completely support your taking it. Just take folic acid also to replenish your stores.

A 1992 study in the *Biochemical Journal* showed just how the depletion takes place. The study found that NSAIDs inhibit the effects of enzymes that allow your body to make folate. Simply put, the drug pushes its way into a chemical reaction, pretending to be what it's not, and your body just allows it in. It's sort of like a suave and debonair thief who cuts in and asks for a dance and you comply. Then he picks your pockets! Get the picture? For physicians who really want to understand this, what I'm saying is that NSAID drugs are competitive inhibitors of phosphoribosylaminoimidazole carboxamide formyltransferase and dihydrofolate reductase; and when they interfere, your ability to form and activate folic acid is reduced. The effect is cumulative over time.

One more thing: NSAIDs also interfere with another enzyme system that uses folate and makes serine in the body. Serine is needed to protect the brain and nervous system. It may be a stretch, but I suspect that peripheral neuropathy in some people may be driven by the folate-depletion impact of drug muggers, which, over time, reduces healthy levels of serine in the body. By the way, you can buy phosphatidylserine supplements at any health food store, and I recommend that you do so if you have nerve pain or neuropathy. If you need to take an NSAID, and I don't mind if you do (I actually tote Advil around in my purse), then consider taking a little folic acid as a supplement. The two together (the NSAID and the folic acid) are better because you get the safety *and* the benefits of both compounds. NSAIDs are famous for their ability to upset the gastrointestinal system and increase risk of GI bleeding. There's a way around that, too, if you need to take the medication. Try licorice root, an extract known as glycyrrhizin (not licorice root candy, though). A 1998 study showed that licorice might protect the stomach against NSAID damage.

Folate also plays an important role in cardiovascular disease. The National Institutes of Health has identified many risk factors for cardiovascular disease, including an elevated LDL cholesterol level, high blood pressure, a low HDL cholesterol level, obesity, diabetes, and, most recently, an elevated level of homocysteine. This is where folate comes into play, because, as we've seen, folate reduces the level of homocysteine, especially when combined with vitamin B_6 and B_{12} (methylcobalamin). Listen carefully, because folate, coenzyme Q10, and many B vitamins can protect your heart. If you run out of any of those nutrients, your heart suffers.

Some drug muggers rob your body of multiple nutrients, leaving you very susceptible to a heart attack and high blood pressure. Is this far-fetched? I think not. If you look at the drug mugger list for folate, you'll see a very popular diabetes drug called Avandia (rosiglitazone). I'm going to spend some time on this subject because it made so many headlines over the past 3 years, when people died while taking it. Even if you don't take this medication, the following information is crucial. And even if you don't have diabetes, it's likely that someone you love does. Avandia controls blood sugar, and there are other medications that are just like it, including the most popular one, Actos. Avandia and Actos are drug muggers for folate, B_{12}, and CoQ10.

These nutrients are essential to your good health. If you run out of all three of them, you will more than likely develop heart trouble and possibly liver trouble. Would it surprise you to know that a study published in the *Journal of the American Medical Association* in July 2008 found that people who took Avandia had a 60 percent higher risk of heart failure and a 40 percent higher risk of heart attack? They also displayed a 30 percent higher chance of dying during the study period than patients given other oral diabetes medications. The scientists analyzed data from 227,571 patients who began taking Avandia (or Actos) between July 2006 and June 2009. Their conclusion? Avandia is riskier than Actos, a similar drug in the same category for diabetes. This isn't the first negative study on Avandia, nor is it the first problem with diabetes medication. In the late 1990s, the drug Rezulin was taken off the market as a result of fatalities. The problem with Rezulin was liver failure. But the makers made millions of dollars before they decided to recall it. Oops, did I just say that out loud? My bad.

In May 2008, a study published in the *New England Journal of Medicine* reported more dangers. The heart problems were so blatantly obvious that it compelled the FDA to force the makers of the drug to post a black box warning on Avandia so that doctors could weed out which patients should get the medicine and which ones shouldn't. Remember, a black box warning is the strongest warning a drug can carry before it is yanked off the market.

Now here's the part where I just fell out of my chair. Scientists ultimately concluded that the evidence for heart trouble in correlation with this drug was inconclusive. Go to the funeral of someone who died while taking the drug and tell that to the family. Inconclusive? I'm not a brain surgeon, but you don't have to hit me over the head with the evidence. Here is my bigger concern, though. It's not only about Avandia. It's about all the medications out there just like it that people take. Is nobody but me (and now you!) making the connection between side effects and drug muggers?

If you take Avandia and run out of folate, B_{12}, and CoQ10 because of its drug mugging effect, you are asking for heart (and liver) trouble. The black box warning is just an alert that trouble could occur in certain patients. But warnings don't offer a solution for avoiding heart trouble in the first place. These warnings are for doctors to read. It isn't always on your drug information sheet. Unless your doctor tells you, you may not even know, unless, of course, you are reading this book.

I'm often asked whether Actos (pioglitazone) is as risky as Avandia. According to a study published in August 2009 in the *British Medical Journal*, Actos still appeared to be safer, but there are serious health complications possible. The study detailed hospitalization and death rates of almost 40,000 patients, 66 years or older. For the patients taking Avandia, 6.9 percent died or were hospitalized; for patients on Actos, 5.3 percent died or were hospitalized. Specifically, researchers concluded, "Among older patients with diabetes, pioglitazone is associated with a significantly lower risk of heart failure and death than is rosiglitazone. Given that rosiglitazone lacks a distinct clinical advantage over pioglitazone, continued use of rosiglitazone may not be justified." So there you have it. Avandia appears to be more dangerous than Actos. And another 2009 study in the *Archives of Internal Medicine* reported that Actos increased fractures in women by 77 percent and in men by 61 percent; the study included 84,000 people with type 2 diabetes. Before we leave the subject of these two medications, I'd like to tell you that you can find natural ways to help yourself and possibly get off your diabetes medications if you read my other book, *Diabetes without Drugs*.

And, of course, if your doctor tells you that you must take either Avandia or Actos, you can protect your heart yourself by taking drug mugger doses of vitamin B_{12}, coenzyme Q10, and folic acid. Some drug companies get it. Beyaz and Safyral (estrogen/progestin and folate) are two different birth control pills from the same drug maker. The two pill packs use different ingredients for oral contraception, but they share one cool thing. Both Beyaz and Safyral are fortified with a form of folic acid. As you saw in Chapter 1, estrogen-containing drugs are notorious for reducing folate levels, which may raise your risk for heart disease. It's outstanding to see a drug company replenish what the drug mugger stole, patenting a product that minimizes side effects for you. If you choose to take oral contraceptives, these are better choices.

The following list of drug muggers contains some very popular medications including birth control pills, steroids, anticonvulsants, and diabetes medicine.

Drug Muggers of Folate (Vitamin B_9)

Acid Blockers

Cimetidine (Tagamet)

Esomeprazole (Nexium)

Famotidine (Pepcid and Pepcid Complete)

Lansoprazole (Prevacid 24HR)

Nizatidine (Axid)

Omeprazole (Prilosec OTC)

Pantoprazole (Protonix)

Rabeprazole (Aciphex)

Ranitidine (Zantac)

Analgesics

Hydrocodone and acetaminophen (Lortab, Lorcet, Vicodin)

Hydrocodone and aspirin (Lortab ASA, Alor)

Oxycodone and aspirin (Percodan)

Antacids

Aluminum and magnesium
  hydroxide (Maalox, Mylanta)

Aluminum carbonate gel (Basaljel)

Aluminum hydroxide (Amphojel,
  AlternaGEL)

Calcium carbonate (Tums,
  Titralac, Rolaids)

Magnesium hydroxide (Phillips'
  Milk of Magnesia)

Sodium bicarbonate (Alka-Seltzer,
  baking soda)

Antibiotics (a few examples)

Amoxicillin (Amoxil)

Azithromycin (Z-Pak)

Cefaclor (Ceclor)

Cefdinir (Omnicef)

Cephalexin (Keflex)

Ciprofloxacin (Cipro)

Clarithromycin (Biaxin)

Doxycycline (Doryx)

Erythromycin (E.E.S.)

Levofloxacin (Levaquin)

Minocycline (Minocin)

Sulfamethoxazole and
  trimethoprim (Bactrim, Septra)

Tetracycline (Sumycin)

Anticonvulsants

Carbamazepine (Carbatrol)

Ethosuximide (Zarontin)

Gabapentin (Neurontin)

Phenobarbital (Solfoton)

Phenytoin (Phenytek, Dilantin)

Primidone (Mysoline)

Valproic acid (Depakene, Depakote)

Anti-Inflammatory Drugs

Celecoxib (Celebrex)

Diclofenac (Voltaren)

Etodolac (Lodine)

Ibuprofen (Motrin, Advil)

Indomethacin (Indocin)

Ketoprofen (Orudis)

Lodine (Etodolac)

Nabumetone (Relafen)

Naproxen (Aleve, Anaprox,
  Naprosyn)

Piroxicam (Feldene)

Sulfasalazine (Azulfidine)

Sulindac (Clinoril)

Antimetabolites (for psoriasis)

Methotrexate (Rheumatrex,
  Trexall)

Antivirals

Delavirdine (Rescriptor)

Foscarnet (Foscavir)

Lamivudine (Epivir)

Nevirapine (Viramune)

Zidovudine, AZT (Retrovir)

Zidovudine and lamivudine
  (Combivir)

Aromatase Inhibitors for breast cancer

Anastrozole (Arimidex)

Barbiturates

Amobarbital (Amytal)

Butalbital (Fiorinal, Fioricet,
  Zebutal)

Pentobarbital (Nembutal)

Secobarbital (Seconal)

Secobarbital and amobarbital
(Tuinal)

Thiopental (Pentothal)

Blood Pressure Drugs

Diuretics, loop:

Bumetanide (Bumex)

Ethacrynic acid (Edecrin)

Furosemide (Lasix)

Diuretics, potassium-sparing:

Spironolactone (Aldactone)

Triamterene (Dyazide, Dyrenium,
Maxzide)

Diuretics, sulfonamide:

Indapamide (Lozol)

Diuretics, thiazide:

Any combination drug that
contains HCTZ or
hydrochlorothiazide (dozens of
drugs contain this)

Chlorothiazide (Diuril)

Chlorthalidone (Hygroton)

Hydrochlorothiazide or HCTZ
(Hydrodiuril)

Methyclothiazide (Enduron)

Metolazone (Zaroxolyn)

Cholesterol Agents

Cholestyramine (Questran)

Colestipol (Colestid)

Corticosteroids

Betamethasone (Diprolene,
Luxiq)

Dexamethasone (Decadron)

Hydrocortisone (Cortef)

Methylprednisone (Medrol)

Prednisone (Prednisol)

Inhaled corticosteroid:

Fluticasone (Flonase)

Diabetes Medications

Glimepiride (Amaryl)

Glipizide (Glucotrol)

Glyburide (Diabeta, Glynase,
Micronase)

Glyburide and metformin
(Glucovance)

Metformin (Fortamet, Glucophage,
Glucophage XR, Glumetza,
Riomet)

Metformin and sitagliptin (Janumet)

Pioglitazone (Actos)

Rosiglitazone (Avandia)

Tolazamide (Tolinase)

**Hormone Replacement Therapy/
Oral Contraceptives**

Estrogen-containing drugs
(hormone replacement therapy
and birth control)

Estrogens, conjugated (Prempro,
Premphase)

Levonorgestrel (found in many
birth control pills)

Muscle Relaxant

Carisoprodol (Soma)

Salicylates

Aspirin (Bufferin, Bayer)

SERMs (Selective Estrogen Receptor
Modulators—used for breast cancer)

Raloxifene (Evista)

Tamoxifen (Nolvadex)

Toremifene (Fareston)

SSRI Antidepressants

   Fluoxetine (Prozac)

   Paroxetine (Paxil)

   Sertraline (Zoloft)

Sulfonamides (Sulfa antibiotics, some diabetes medications)

Miscellaneous

   Alcohol

   Estrogen dominance

Folate: Put This on Your Plate

Romaine lettuce, kale, spinach, asparagus, turnip greens, mustard greens, collard greens, broccoli, cauliflower, celery, parsley, beets (boiled), lentils, pinto beans, black beans, chickpeas, summer squash, cucumbers, papaya, lima beans, strawberries, and flaxseed. Drink my Detox on the Rocks, page 362, on Day 2 for a quick dose of folate. It's green, but you'll feel better within minutes.

An Absurdly Inexpensive Way to Feel Better

The B vitamins are interdependent. In other words, it's very easy to tip your Bs out of balance. If you take too much folic acid, you may become deficient in your other B vitamins. So whenever you take a single B vitamin, it may be wise to also take a B complex so that the other Bs are on board.

   For general health: 400–800 mcg once daily

   Drug mugger dose: 400–800 mcg two or three times daily

Just So You Know

Folic acid is a synthetic form of folate that is made in the lab. Many experts say that it's just fine and that your body (and some stomach acid) will convert it to an active, usable form. But you can actually buy the active form found in nature and save your body the work. These active forms are actually the way we find folate in food. Names to look for include 5-methyltetrahydrofolate (5-MTHF), calcium folinate, and folinic acid.

   Folate is eliminated from the urine like most B vitamins. That's why many people can take up to 5 mg (5,000 mcg) per day for a few months without any long-term ill effect. However, I do not recommend this type of dosing for more than 3 to 6 months. I think that this is a huge dose, and it will tilt your other B vitamins off-kilter. I realize that some doctors are folate happy and order 5 mg dosages like this (and even higher, sometimes up to 20 mg for people with tumors). But for the general public, 5 mg dosages given daily are just too high.

Cutting-edge research shows that the anticancer effects of folate backfire when you take too much and may even propel the growth of cancer. This paradox is what prompts me to tell you to keep your dosage appropriate to your specific needs. As I said, high doses of folic acid will tilt all of your B vitamins out of healthy ratios and contribute to a B_{12} deficiency. This could cause all sorts of problems. Typically, you know you are getting too much folic acid if you develop nausea, flatulence, abdominal distension, or kidney stones.

Install a Nutrient Security System

Taking supplements of folic acid provides your body with the precursor for making 5-MTHF, which is important because 5-MTHF is the most biologically active form of this B vitamin. If you are one of those people who has difficulty converting folic acid to this active form, you can go ahead and take a supplement of 5-MTHF instead of folic acid. This active form of the nutrient has been proposed as a treatment for cardiovascular disease and advanced cancers, including breast, colon, and rectal cancers. To find out if you have trouble converting it, there's a pricey blood test you can take that assesses your genes. A cheaper way to determine your ability to make 5-MTHF is to just evaluate your homocysteine level. If it's high, you may be one of those people who can't activate it properly.

To install the tightest security system possible, take vitamin B_{12} along with your 5-MTHF. Vitamin B_{12} is a methyl donor just like 5-MTHF. The tag team of B_{12} and folic acid helps support nervous system function, cardiovascular health, normal cell division, and gum health. It also offers protection against cancer.

What's in My Cupboard?

Folic Acid 800 mcg by Solaray: Each capsule provides 800 mcg of folic acid.

Folic Acid with DHA by Nature Made: This is a unique combination product that contains 600 mcg folic acid along with 50 mg DHA (an extract from fish oils that is thought to protect the nervous system). Think of this supplement as brain food because both folic acid and DHA are known to protect the brain, improve mood, and nourish nerve cells. I'd take 1 softgel daily with a meal.

B Complex Phosphorylated by Metabolic Maintenance: This formula contains a full range of B vitamins, including folic acid, with 800 mcg per capsule. I like the combination of B vitamins in this formula because some of them are active and body ready. For example, the form of B$_{12}$ used in this formula is readily available to the body as methylcobalamin (versus cyanocobalamin, which is fine, but has to undergo conversion); the riboflavin 5'-phosphate (R5P) is also bioavailable immediately, versus its inactive form riboflavin (found in most dietary supplements). It's not that the precursor vitamins are bad; they are found in millions of high-quality products. Just so you understand, though, they (cyanocobalamin, riboflavin, folic acid, pyridoxine, and others) have to undergo conversion in your body in order to become available to your cells. This brand provides the B vitamins to you in their body-ready forms—basically on a silver platter. While it's not necessary, it certainly is helpful to people who have malabsorption issues, digestive trouble (like celiac or Crohn's disease or irritable bowel syndrome), or low acid (a condition called hypochlorhydria).

5-MTHF by Thorne Research: 5-MTHF is the body-ready type of folic acid, which means you can take it up easily and use it along with B$_{12}$ to improve your cardiovascular and nervous systems. This company also produces an excellent form of B complex called **Basic B Complex** that provides a full range of all the vitamin Bs in their active, body-ready forms, including 200 mcg folinic acid and 200 mg 5-MTHF per capsule.

10

Glutathione and N-Acetylcysteine

Glutathione, a powerful antioxidant with a funny name, ranks high on my list as a powerful detoxifier. Like other antioxidants, glutathione (sometimes referred to as GSH) sweeps up dangerous free radicals, the naturally occurring molecules that damage the body. GSH helps boost the immune system and reduce your risk of cancer.

Think "liver" when you think of glutathione, because your liver cells need a lot of it on board to break down your breakfast of scrambled eggs, sausage, biscuits, and coffee, as well as all the other meals of the day. Realize that you pretty much use up your body's stores of glutathione just for eating, never mind dealing with drug muggers and lifestyle choices, such as drinking alcohol, that further deplete it. Remember, the liver is your body's filter for toxins. Without a finely tuned and well-functioning liver, you would die very quickly. Glutathione helps your liver do its job.

Glutathione is also needed for healthy joints and cartilage, so I find it paradoxical that acetaminophen (the generic name for Tylenol) depletes this nutrient, as it is often used for joint pain. Acetaminophen is sold over the counter in the United States and overseas (where it is called paracetamol).

I asked Walter Crinnion, ND, one of the world's leading experts in environmental medicine and author of *Clean, Green and Lean,* about glutathione's role in helping to keep our bodies running efficiently. He explained how important this nutrient is and why it might help you: "Glutathione can help remove harmful toxins other than heavy metals, such as pesticides and dry-cleaning solvents, transforming them in such a way that the body can excrete them more easily. This becomes very important for people who suffer with neurological disorders, such as multiple sclerosis or

Parkinson's, sometimes thought to be connected to heavy metal toxicity or solvent poisoning from childhood."

With the rise of these diseases, I think that keeping glutathione levels high is crucial to your health.

The nutrient glutathione has a hard time getting into your cells because it's so big and bulky. It doesn't fit through the doorway, the cell membrane. Because glutathione is so large and hard to assimilate, taking it as a stand-alone supplement isn't normally my recommendation, although it's safe to do so if you wish to. I'd prefer that your cells be given the right elements to make their own glutathione. Think of it as a recipe. You don't start out with a cake; you have to mix up all the ingredients, and the magic happens in the oven. It's the same concept with glutathione. You need to cook it in your cells, so to speak. It's far more effective for you to take the precursor nutrients that go easily through your cells' doorways. Once inside, they happily join together and create glutathione right where you want it.

The recipe for creating glutathione calls for a good B complex formula, because B complex supplies important B vitamins such as B_6, B_{12}, niacin, and riboflavin, which you need to drive the reaction. You also need three amino acids. I've listed them here along with their primary benefits to your body.

L-glycine: Protects the prostate gland and helps build muscles
L-glutamine: Helps digestion and the immune system
L-cysteine: Detoxifies the body while protecting the liver

These three important amino acids (and many others) are found in protein powders that are available at health food stores nationwide. There are so many types of protein mixes that it's almost dizzying to shop for one of them. I prefer protein powders in this order: hemp, rice, whey, and egg. I like hemp the best because it's a protein that is derived from a vegetable, and it contains a great deal of omega-3 fatty acids per serving. Hemp seeds are considered a superfood, so protein derived from hemp (which, by the way, does not cause a buzz like marijuana) is incredibly healthful. It's quite possibly the single most important health supplement you can take on a daily basis. Hemp protein gives you large amounts of zinc, iron, and magnesium, three minerals you need for healthy mood, energy production, and blood sugar control.

Rice, whey, and egg protein supplements are also available, and all these products come in different flavors, like vanilla and chocolate. Don't worry that much about the taste, though. Concern yourself with the fact that these supplements are a quick and easy way to get all the glutathione precursors you need. That is the gift that they offer. You can always throw a scoop into the blender and mix it up with some fruit and water for a delicious pick-me-up that also helps build muscle. I drink protein shakes right before I go to Zumba dance class, so I have all the items on board to build muscle and feel energetic. See Chapter 28, The Total Body Tune-Up, for recipes that include whey.

While shopping for a protein supplement, you will quickly see that the most popular is whey. This animal-derived protein is a good source of glutathione precursors. Some people feel well and do well on the dosages recommended on the label, but others who have higher requirements for glutathione (because of heavy metal toxicity or intensive workout sessions) need more than recommended. They might need four scoops instead of one or two per day. Don't make this decision on your own, please; consult with your health-care provider about the right dose for you.

Why the concern? Not only does doubling the amount exceed label directions for commercial products, but whey protein also is animal-derived, and high amounts of animal proteins (even from steak) can raise your uric acid levels, a condition known as hyperuricemia that is associated with kidney stones, bladder cancer, and gout. Big meat eaters and bodybuilders who take too much whey may have to deal with these problems. The condition happens when a collection of uric acid crystals settles somewhere. With gout, they generally wind up in the joints of your toes or fingers and can cause a great deal of pain. When this happens in the kidney, it can cause kidney stones. In a 2006 study published in the *American Journal of Clinical Nutrition* that analyzed data from two large studies tracked over 22 years, men and women with high intake of bacon (more than 5 servings a week) had a higher risk for bladder cancer.

So should you take a vegetable-derived protein supplement such as hemp or rice instead? Go ahead if you want to. But variety is also fine with me. You can alternate your protein supplements from day to day or month to month. I've taken whey myself over the years, but I alternate my protein supplement. The best kinds of whey supplements are those that say "undenatured." This means that the protein has not been destroyed and all the ingredients are still active. Whey protein that has been exposed to high heat in the manufacturing process will not increase your glutathione levels, so stick with those products that are produced with high pressure instead of high heat.

The three amino acids I mentioned above—L-glycine, L-glutamine, and L-cysteine —are present in very small amounts in all the protein options I've mentioned. They each have an important role to play in the body. Protein supplements are a rich source of all the amino acids you need, so you don't have to take supplements of each one, although you certainly could. I believe that protein supplements are the fastest way to drive up your glutathione levels. Of the trio, L-cysteine is by far the most important, which is why it is often sold as a stand-alone supplement for increasing glutathione. In fact, it's very easy to buy supplements of cysteine or its derivatives at any health food store.

In particular, one stable commercial derivative of cysteine known as N-acetylcysteine (NAC) is sold as a stand-alone supplement at most health food stores. NAC undergoes a couple of chemical reactions to help you make reduced glutathione in your body—"reduced" means that the glutathione is active, and that's what you want. Many holistic doctors recommend that their patients take NAC for the express purpose of building up levels of glutathione because this nutrient is so important in detoxifying our bodies of dangerous toxins, used-up drugs and hormones, and some heavy metals. Doctors recommend NAC because glutathione itself is too bulky to get into the cells. NAC slips right in.

NAC (and obviously its offspring glutathione) can help you deal with respiratory problems, emphysema, congestive heart failure, HIV, epilepsy, heart disease, and heavy metal toxicity. It also seems to help smokers in their quest to quit.

People who have eye problems resulting from the autoimmune condition called Sjögren's syndrome may also benefit from glutathione. This was shown in one double-blind, placebo-controlled study using dosages of 200 mg three times per day.

Caution: If you have diabetes, you need to be aware that NAC can help to lower blood sugar. This is a good thing, but if you happen to take medication or insulin shots to keep your blood sugar tightly controlled, then NAC may alter the amount of medication you need. I recommend careful blood sugar monitoring if you opt to take this supplement. Your doctor can make appropriate changes to your medications should it become necessary.

You should also be aware that NAC, like the protein supplements discussed above, may spark the formation of kidney stones. You'll need to take about two or three times as much vitamin C as NAC. The added vitamin C helps minimize the formation of stones. NAC helps you to get rid of your body's load of toxic metals, such as mercury, lead, cadmium, and arsenic, but there is disagreement about whether NAC affects other minerals in the body. A few experts think that NAC can't distinguish between the dangerous metals and some of the essential ones such as copper and zinc, and they suggest taking a low-dose copper-and-zinc formula each day to counter the loss of these minerals. Most people, including me, take NAC without supplementing with copper and zinc and do just fine.

The combination of vitamin C and NAC is fantastic for many people. It has been shown to stop the spread of prostate cancer and lymphoma in animal studies. NAC and glutathione recycle other antioxidants in your body, giving them a second go-round. So if you take this supplement, instead of an antioxidant having just one chance to clean you up, it gets two or three chances. NAC and glutathione recycle vitamins C, A, and E, so they better protect you and therefore you have a lower risk of cancer. You might say that these nutrients do a great housekeeping job on your cells.

There is some debate about which is better: taking protein supplements, which provide the precursors to glutathione, or taking NAC. Dr. Crinnion weighed in on this for me: "NAC is much better for boosting glutathione levels than whey. It is both less expensive and faster at building up the levels. NAC boosts glutathione levels in the body quickly, and this helps the body to excrete more heavy metals. Most people are impressed when they learn that glutathione also helps the kidneys excrete methylmercury, which comes from fish. NAC is a great way to boost glutathione levels, and it doesn't redistribute the heavy metals, it just takes them out of the body."

Certainly glutathione can help you if you have any form of liver damage or infection. Besides loving your liver, the list of what glutathione can do goes on and on. If you have a serious condition that could benefit from glutathione (Parkinson's, multiple sclerosis, amyotrophic lateral sclerosis [ALS, or Lou Gehrig's disease], or heavy metal poisoning), you can ask your doctor for glutathione injections. They are given intravenously and take just a few minutes. Taking an oral supplement is cheaper and easier, but it's good to know that the IV form is available for those who need it, and injectable forms are probably better utilized than oral forms.

Glutathione improves your sensitivity to circulating dopamine, a happy brain chemical, which explains why severely depressed people can increase their intake of whey protein and suddenly find their outlook on life more hopeful. Kids with autism may also benefit from glutathione.

In my opinion, glutathione, in tandem with other minerals and vitamins, can boost brain function and improve mood in a safer way than expensive pharmaceuticals. Our current arsenal of antidepressant drugs can cause an array of side effects, including aggression, insomnia, heart palpitations, and even thoughts of self-harm, so glutathione comes as a welcome relief. It can be taken along with medications, too.

The following list outlines drug muggers of glutathione, and it's relatively short. I wish I could list the hundreds of medications that are processed by the liver. The liver uses glutathione to metabolize all the medications you take and remove them from the body once their purpose has been served. Without glutathione, you simply wouldn't be able to clear drugs and toxins from your blood, so it's critical.

Let's take a look at the popular OTC painkiller acetaminophen as an example. If you have enough glutathione on board, your body renders the acetaminophen metabolite nontoxic and then excretes it. If you take too much acetaminophen, or too many other medications that the liver must process, it can overtax your body's store of glutathione. Do you see? If you can no longer metabolize the acetaminophen well enough, it (or its metabolites) becomes toxic to your cells. That can actually kill liver cells and prove fatal in sensitive people. I'm not exaggerating. It is interesting that doctors use NAC in the hospital to save the lives of acetaminophen-poisoning victims, usually kids. I once worked in a poison control center and saw this treatment used myself. Yep, NAC is *the* antidote to Tylenol poisoning because it rescues the liver.

Any medication, whether it's listed here or not, that goes through your liver can increase your requirements for this nutrient. If a med goes through your liver, it's taxing it, so you need a liver-loving nutrient like NAC or glutathione. In fact, anything that taxes your liver (smoking, coffee, alcohol, diet pills, herbal remedies, and so on) may cause you to need more glutathione, so consider a protein or NAC supplement to provide the amino acids that allow your body to make glutathione from scratch.

The following list is only a fraction of the hundreds of drugs that are processed (metabolized) by the liver. I haven't listed other drugs because there aren't any nutrient-depletion studies on those drugs.

Drug Muggers of Glutathione

Acid Blockers

Cimetidine (Tagamet)

Esomeprazole (Nexium)

Famotidine (Pepcid and Pepcid
   Complete)

Lansoprazole (Prevacid 24HR)

Nizatidine (Axid)

Omeprazole (Prilosec OTC)

Pantoprazole (Protonix)

Rabeprazole (Aciphex)

Ranitidine (Zantac)

Analgesics

Acetaminophen and codeine (Tylenol 3)

Acetaminophen or paracetamol (Tylenol and others)

Butalbital-containing drugs (Fiorinal, Fioricet, Zebutal)

Hydrocodone and acetaminophen (Lortab, Norco, Vicodin, Lorcet)

Oxycodone and acetaminophen (Endocet, Percocet, Roxicet, Tylox)

Propoxyphene and acetaminophen (Darvocet)

Antacids

Aluminum and magnesium hydroxide (Maalox, Mylanta)

Aluminum carbonate gel (Basaljel)

Aluminum hydroxide (Amphojel, AlternaGEL)

Calcium carbonate (Tums, Titralac, Rolaids)

Magnesium hydroxide (Phillips' Milk of Magnesia)

Sodium bicarbonate (Alka-Seltzer, baking soda)

Antibiotics (a few examples)

Amoxicillin (Amoxil)

Azithromycin (Z-Pak)

Cefaclor (Ceclor)

Cefdinir (Omnicef)

Cephalexin (Keflex)

Ciprofloxacin (Cipro)

Clarithromycin (Biaxin)

Doxycycline (Doryx)

Erythromycin (E.E.S.)

Levofloxacin (Levaquin)

Minocycline (Minocin)

Sulfamethoxazole and trimethoprim (Bactrim Septra)

Tetracycline (Sumycin)

Antidepressants, Tricyclic

Clomipramine (Anafranil)

Desipramine (Norpramin) and others

Antivirals

Foscarnet (Foscavir)

Lamivudine (Epivir)

Zidovudine, AZT (Retrovir)

Zidovudine and lamivudine (Combivir)

Miscellaneous

Alcohol

Any drug mugger of thiamine

Any drug mugger of vitamin B_6, B_{12}, niacin, or riboflavin, because these are needed to make glutathione

Any drug mugger of vitamin C (because C is needed to make glutathione)

Any medication that goes through the liver (there are hundreds)

Hypochlorhydria

Nicotine

Glutathione: Put This on Your Plate

Glutathione is manufactured inside the cells. Therefore, you have to eat foods that contain its precursor amino acids so that your body can convert the amino acids into glutathione inside the cells. Protein supplements and foods containing amino acids are sources of these precursors. Foods rich in these amino acids include fruits, fish, meats, and whey. Good sources also include greens, chlorella algae, asparagus, broccoli, cabbage, brussels sprouts, cauliflower, kale, watermelon, avocados, walnuts, grapefruit, oranges, cantaloupes, acorn squash, peaches, zucchini, spinach, and eggs. It's also good to spice up with turmeric. Eating fresh, raw cilantro or parsley is a fantastic way of upping levels very quickly.

An Absurdly Inexpensive Way to Feel Better

For general health: NAC, 400–800 mg per day

Drug mugger dose: NAC, 600–1,200 mg per day

Chemotherapy: NAC, 1,800 mg per day to reduce nausea and vomiting. Check with your doctor.

Just So You Know

Protein powders (such as whey, rice, egg, and hemp protein mixes) are a quick way to boost glutathione levels. Take one scoop once or twice daily. Buy whey protein "concentrate" rather than "isolate" because isolates acidify the body and turn the natural L-isomer of the protein molecule into a dangerous D-isomer that may harm your brain and nervous system. The other way to get glutathione is to take NAC supplements. You know you are getting too much NAC if you start to get an upset stomach, heartburn, or increased appetite. If this happens, cut back on the dose. Be careful about getting too much NAC (or cysteine) because it is a gentle heavy metal chelator. This means that it has the capacity to pull out mercury, lead, cadmium, and cesium. If you do not have good digestive abilities and you are always constipated, these metals just get loosened up from various organs, combine with the cysteine, and get redeposited elsewhere. In other words, shaking up your metals without getting them out is not good for you, so first and foremost, fix your digestion. Like any good thing, you want to use NAC (and cysteine supplements) in moderation, and take the dosages suggested here or on your label.

Install a Nutrient Security System

The widely available herb milk thistle works hand in hand with glutathione. Detoxification occurs mostly in the liver, which has a big job on its hands. Milk thistle (or its active ingredient, silymarin) is known for its ability to protect the liver and enhance detoxification. It also can raise levels of glutathione in the liver by as much as 50 percent in rats, according to a study published in 1989 in *Planta Medica*. Milk thistle and glutathione working together in the body form an amazing team, especially in terms of helping you rid yourself of unwanted chemicals, poisons, used-up drugs, and heavy metals. Talk about a tight security system!

What's in My Cupboard?

Cysteplus by Thorne Research: These capsules contain 500 mg N-acetylcysteine and will help protect the liver, support the immune system, and promote detoxification. Thorne products are free of magnesium stearate and all other additives.

Warrior Food by Warrior Power Nutritional (HealthForce): I love this product because it's a complete food that combines both sprouted organic rice and organic hemp protein, and it's also enhanced with organic phycocyanin extract from Klamath algae for kidney support and with enzymes like bromelain, papain, other proteases, lipase, and amylase, which help digestion and improve assimilation. It's vegan, raw, and gluten free. I love the texture and flavor of this food.

Certified Organic Hemp Pro Fiber by Manitoba Harvest: This is a hemp protein powder that is USDA-certified organic and cold milled. It contains all 10 essential amino acids, including glutathione precursors, as well as 400 mg omega-3 fatty acids and 11 grams of fiber per serving. It is sweetened with organic, fair trade cane juice, nothing artificial. It is free of soy, gluten, and preservatives.

Organic Hemp Protein by Nutiva: This is USDA-certified organic and easy to find at health food stores. It has a nice flavor, a fine texture, and is great mixed in smoothies, water, juice, or hemp milk. It is free of all allergens.

Glutathione by ReadiSorb: In a patented process, the manufacturer places reduced glutathione into liposomes—liquid bubbles made from essential phospholipids, a beneficial form of fat. Wrapping the glutathione in fat helps ensure better bioavailability, making for a better chance that the bulky glutathione will actually slide into your body's cells, where it needs to go to do its job. The supplement smells like sulfur (all glutathione does), but tastes almost like water. I just drink it without inhaling. You only need a tiny amount, like a teaspoon.

Superberry by LivingFuel: This is an all-in-one concentrated, optimized whole meal superfood that delivers 300 mg of NAC in each serving along with excellent amounts of vitamins, minerals, proteins, essential fats, enzymes, coenzymes, herbs, botanical extracts, and soluble plant fiber. It's a convenient way to get the amino acids that form glutathione, and it also can improve your general health in many other ways. I like this product as a substitute for food when I'm in a hurry and don't have time to eat.

Immunocal by Immunotec: This form is made of bioactive whey protein from organic milk. It's lactose and fat free and delivers cysteine to your cells, where your body converts it to NAC and glutathione. You have to blend it with milk or juice—ideally orange juice so you get the added benefit of vitamin C. Use a whisk or Aerolatte hand blender, not a strong blender. It foams a little bit, and you can drink the foam. This product is useful for people with autoimmune disorders, depression, chronic fatigue, fibromyalgia, immune deficiency, and other problems. I buy mine online from numerous sources because it's not sold in stores.

NanoPro by BioPharma Scientific: This is natural whey protein that also contains colostrum extract, polypeptides, and reduced glutathione. The product is highly absorbable and tastes like a vanilla shake, even when mixed with water. I've taken this a lot because I like the taste so much. The company uses nanotechnology to get the particles to survive the harsh environment in your stomach. Its rich polypeptides help balance the immune system and provide growth factors to support repair and regeneration. Contact information: www.biopharmasci.com or 877-772-4362.

OxiCell Cream by Apex Energetics: This is a transdermal cream that contains glutathione along with other powerful anti-inflammatories such as CoQ10, vitamin E, superoxide dismutase (SOD), alphalipoic acid, zinc, niacin, ashwaganda root, arnica, and astragalus root. It raises energy while improving cellular metabolism, and improves immunity. It may be helpful in cancer and liver disease because it neutralizes free radicals and improves phase II detoxification. I never go a day without this product.

Apply ¼ to ½ teaspoon to the skin twice daily. The product is sold online at many Internet retailers. The manufacturer's Web site is www. apexenergetics.com.

Whey to Go by Solgar: Sold at health food stores nationwide, this whey protein powder is pure, easy to find, and very affordable.

Egg White Protein by Jay Robb: This protein supplement comes from egg whites, not whey, hemp, or rice. It tastes great and is free of casein, lactose, sugar, gluten, and artificial anything. It's sweetened with stevia. It is available unflavored or in chocolate, vanilla, and strawberry flavors. Contact information: www.jayrobb.com.

B Complex: I've already discussed the need for B vitamins if you are trying to make glutathione out of NAC. B vitamins work as a team, so it's a good idea to take them together in a single supplement. B complex is sold nationwide, it's easy to find, and there are many brands from which to choose. Look for capsules (because they're easier to absorb than tablets), and stick to dosages of around 50 mg (as in B complex 50). Take a B complex daily with your NAC, and it will help you "cook" glutathione in your cells.

Iron

Iron is sold over the counter in supplement form, but it's a naturally occurring mineral found in many foods. Even though the World Health Organization considers iron deficiency the number one nutritional deficiency in the world, I don't frequently recommend iron supplements for people complaining of fatigue because most US citizens have an adequate supply. Iron can be hard on the gut, causing nausea, cramping, and diarrhea or constipation. That said, if you have a blood test that shows that you are deficient in iron or if your doctor recommends an iron supplement, then by all means please take it.

Your body must have iron in order to make a protein called hemoglobin, which acts like a tow truck and lugs oxygen all over your body. It's amazing that humans can stash away some iron until it's needed again, so you might say it's recyclable. And speaking of going green, your stool can turn this color when you take iron supplements of any type. They can also simply darken, or even turn almost black. It's easy to overdo iron since it accumulates, making it particularly dangerous to tots. So if you do take an iron supplement, make sure to lock it up in your medicine cabinet.

In addition to fatigue, a number of other symptoms could signal an iron deficiency. For example, you may feel cranky or depressed and have trouble concentrating. Or you may be cold all the time. Pale skin and a pale or sore tongue are dead giveaways. You might have brittle nails or be prone to infections as a result of a weakened immune system. And your heart may beat like crazy upon very little exertion. Other conditions and nutritional deficiencies paint the same picture, so teasing out iron deficiency from other health issues is not always easy, but it's incredibly important if you ever want to build up your energy reserves.

Iron is so important to your energy level that without enough of this metal, you will develop hypothyroidism (low thyroid hormone). So if you've been told that you have low thyroid, it may stem from an iron deficiency. You need adequate amounts of iron for your inactive precursor thyroid hormone (T_4) to be converted into your active, energizing thyroid hormone (T_3). Iron also helps carry T_3 across cell membranes so it can do its energy-producing job inside the cells. In fact, iron deficiency anemia is one commonly overlooked cause of hypothyroidism. It makes me sad that many people receive a prescription for Synthroid or Armour Thyroid that they need to take for the rest of their lives (and have to increase the dose over time) when what they really need is iron! It's important to note that you should not make a decision to switch from your prescription medication to an iron supplement on your own. You need appropriate testing and your doctor's expertise to determine whether you fall into this category.

Doctors utilize many tests to determine iron levels. Two fairly reliable ones are the serum ferritin and transferrin saturation ratio tests. If appropriate blood testing finds that you are legitimately deficient in iron, then this nutrient will breathe life back into you very quickly—in about 3 to 6 months. Please note, though, that some people can take iron supplements orally for many months and not respond, meaning their blood levels stay low or they still feel very tired or have hypothyroidism. This may be the result of undiagnosed leaky gut, which I'll explain momentarily.

By the way, if you must take both a prescription thyroid hormone and an iron supplement, do not take them together. Separate the iron from the thyroid by 4 to 6 hours, or they could cancel each other out. Drug interactions aren't the only situation that will cause you to not absorb the iron. It can occur for other reasons related to medical conditions, like low stomach acid or a leaky gut. Leaky gut is the term used when the intestinal lining becomes damaged and large openings develop in the gut wall as a result. Normally, the walls of the colon remain tightly sealed to protect you from reabsorbing waste that is about to get eliminated. Some of the toxic debris (such as undigested food particles and toxins) breaks through the walls of the gut, hence the syndrome is called leaky gut. It's not well recognized by conventional physicians; however, the condition definitely exists, and having leaky gut may be the cause of hundreds of diseases because the toxins that leak through your gut can lodge in any organ of your body and cause symptoms. Most people understand that a gluten allergy results from wheat proteins that leak out of the gut; this is, perhaps, the most common example of damage done by a leaky gut. Also, the yeast known as *Candida albicans* is a common result of leaky gut, which may occur after months of chronic medication intake, especially antibiotics and female hormones. This fungus is the cause of hundreds of diseases.

Finally, people who are allergic to milk may be allergic because the casein protein has found its way into their bloodstreams from their leaky guts! Are you getting the picture? Holes in your colon will cause you to leak out toxins that make mayhem in your body. Leaky gut syndrome prevents proper absorption of vitamins and minerals, iron included.

In my book, leaky gut is a known drug mugger for all sorts of nutrients because it causes malabsorption. Hypochlorhydria, or low stomach acid, will also cause iron deficiency. It's easy enough to test for low stomach acid; your doctor can order a blood test known as a gastrin test. If the test shows that you need acid, you can buy healthy digestive acids variously labeled trimethylglycine, betaine HCl, or betaine hydrochloride at any health food store. Follow the label directions closely to enjoy the benefits without getting heartburn. Testing for leaky gut can be done through either Genova Diagnostics or Metametrix Clinical Laboratory. (See information about these companies in the Resources section on page 448.)

Certain groups of people seem to run out of iron most easily. They include:

- Vegetarians
- People who have recently had surgery
- People who take drug muggers of iron
- Women who experience heavy periods
- People who have a minor perforation in the GI tract such as an ulcer that can cause a slow and steady leak of blood
- Pregnant women
- People with leaky gut, Crohn's disease, celiac disease, or irritable bowel syndrome

- People undergoing chelation therapy
- People with a riboflavin deficiency (see Chapter 19)
- People with kidney disease

You can see that there are a lot of people who can become iron deficient. When I interviewed oncologist John Lohrey, MD, a physician who has experience with patients suffering from anemia and who practices in Tulsa, Oklahoma, he had a lot to share with my readers. He makes this great point in regard to iron: "Anyone besides a menstruating female who is iron deficient should have a colonoscopy in order to rule out colon cancer. It doesn't matter if the stools don't show blood in them, as bleeding can be very slight or noncontinuous."

Having this test done could save your life because it could detect colon cancer early on. If a premenopausal woman finds blood in her stool, she should have a colonoscopy, too, according to Dr. Lohrey. "A less common place to lose blood is the genitourinary tract," he says. "Iron-deficient patients should also have a urinalysis to rule out blood in the urine as well."

People with kidney disease (especially if they are undergoing dialysis) tend to run out of iron because their kidneys are no longer able to create a hormone (erythropoietin) that forms red blood cells. People who drink a lot of dark grape juice or red wine also need additional iron.

Unless your doctor advises taking a supplement, you may be able to replenish your iron stores simply by eating iron-rich foods such as clams, oysters, mussels, liver, beans, lentils, and pumpkin seeds. And do drink some orange juice along with these foods, as the vitamin C bolsters iron absorption.

One more note of caution: There is a new theory on multiple sclerosis that suggests that iron accumulation in the brain causes lesions and symptoms. If you have MS, please watch my video "Suzy Cohen Discusses the Liberation Treatment for MS & CCSVI," which is posted at www.youtube.com, and read my article "New Discovery: Liberation Treatment for Multiple Sclerosis," which is posted at my Web site, www.dearpharmacist.com. Iron supplementation in this group of people should perhaps be avoided.

Drug Muggers of Iron

Acid Blockers

Cimetidine (Tagamet)

Esomeprazole (Nexium)

Famotidine (Pepcid and Pepcid Complete)

Nizatidine (Axid)

Omeprazole (Prilosec OTC)

Pantoprazole (Protonix)

Rabeprazole (Aciphex)

Ranitidine (Zantac)

Analgesics

Butalbital-containing drugs (Fiorinal, Fioricet, Zebutal)

Carisoprodal and aspirin (Soma Compound)

Hydrocodone and acetaminophen (Lortab, Lorcet, Norco, Vicodin)

Hydrocodone and aspirin (Lortab ASA, Alor 5/500)

Oxycodone and aspirin (Percodan)

Antacids

Aluminum and magnesium hydroxide (Maalox, Mylanta)

Aluminum carbonate gel (Basaljel)

Aluminum hydroxide (Amphojel, AlternaGEL)

Calcium carbonate (Tums, Titralac, Rolaids)

Magnesium hydroxide (Phillips' Milk of Magnesia)

Sodium bicarbonate (Alka-Seltzer, baking soda)

Antibiotics (a few examples)

Amoxicillin (Amoxil)

Azithromycin (Z-Pak)

Cefaclor (Ceclor)

Cefdinir (Omnicef)

Cephalexin (Keflex)

Ciprofloxacin (Cipro)

Clarithromycin (Biaxin)

Doxycycline (Doryx)

Erythromycin (E.E.S.)

Levofloxacin (Levaquin)

Minocycline (Minocin)

Neomycin (found in some eyedrops, eardrops, and antibiotic ointments)

Sulfamethoxazole and trimethoprim (Bactrim Septra)

Tetracycline (Sumycin)

Anti-Inflammatory Drugs (NSAIDs)

Celecoxib (Celebrex)

Diclofenac (Voltaren)

Ibuprofen (Motrin, Advil)

Indomethacin (Indocin)

Ketoprofen (Orudis)

Methocarbamol and aspirin (Robaxisal)

Naproxen (Aleve, Anaprox, Naprosyn)

Sulindac (Clinoril)

Antivirals

Delavirdine (Rescriptor)

Foscarnet (Foscavir)

Lamivudine (Epivir)

Nevirapine (Viramune)

Zidovudine, AZT (Retrovir)

Zidovudine and lamivudine
(Combivir)

**Bisphosphonate Bone-Building
Drugs** (Iron can prevent their
absorption, so an iron supplement
should be taken 2 to 4 hours later.)

Alendronate (Fosamax)

Etidronate (Didronel)

Risedronate (Actonel)

Tiludronate (Skelid)

Blood Pressure Drugs

Methyldopa (Aldomet)

Diuretics, loop:

Bumetanide (Bumex)

Ethacrynic acid (Edecrin)

Furosemide (Lasix)

Diuretics, potassium-sparing:

Amiloride (Midamor)

Spironolactone (Aldactone)

Triamterene (Dyazide, Dyrenium.
Maxzide)

Diuretics, sulfonamide:

Indapamide (Lozol) (This is a
"sulfonamide" medication, and
those types of drugs deplete iron;
however, there is not a direct
study for this medication and the
depletion effect.)

Chelating Agent

Penicillamine (Cuprimine)

Cholesterol Agents

Cholestyramine resin (Questran)

Colestipol (Colestid)

Parkinson's Drugs

Levodopa (L-dopa or Larodopa)

Levodopa and carbidopa (Sinemet)

Levodopa, carbidopa, and
entacapone (Stalevo) (Stalevo has
not been shown to deplete iron;
however, it contains levodopa as
one of its ingredients.)

Salicylates

Aspirin (Bayer, Ecotrin, St. Joseph)

Aspirin and dipyridamole (Aggrenox)

Sulfonamides (Sulfa antibiotics,
some diabetes medications)

Thyroid Medicine (Separate iron
supplements from thyroid
medication by 4 to 6 hours.)

Armour Thyroid (thyroid hormone)

Levothyroxine (Levoxyl, Synthroid,
Unithroid)

Miscellaneous

Alcohol

Allopurinol (Not a drug mugger; it
boosts absorption of iron.)

Coffee and tea (even decaf!) (It's okay
to drink coffee or tea, but separate
the beverage from your iron
supplement by a couple of hours.)

Dairy products (These reduce
absorption of iron supplements.)

Excess zinc supplementation (Zinc
and iron have to stay in balance;
excess zinc inhibits iron uptake.)

Hypochlorhydria (low levels of
   stomach acid)
Grape juice
Low ferritin levels

Red wine
Riboflavin muggers (See
   Chapter 19.)

Iron: Put This on Your Plate

Meat, poultry, and fish all contain iron in a form that's easy to absorb. Other sources include Swiss chard, spinach, thyme, turmeric, dill weed, cinnamon, parsley, rosemary, blackstrap molasses, mustard greens, turnip greens, green beans, shiitake mushrooms, asparagus, chickpeas, leeks, tofu, olives, lentils, kelp, and sesame seeds. Tea may reduce the absorption of iron from fruits and vegetables, so drink it 1 to 2 hours away from eating produce.

An Absurdly Inexpensive Way to Feel Better

For general health: Just eat iron-rich foods because excessive iron supplementation can backfire and turn into free radicals, which then have a toxic oxidative effect on tissues, especially the lining of your blood vessels. This is one of those moments when too much of a good thing turns bad, so unless you are known to be deficient in iron as measured by a serum ferritin blood test, don't supplement for longer than 3 months. Men need approximately 10 to 20 mg per day, whereas menstruating, pregnant, or lactating women tend to need more, approximately 20 to 30 mg per day.

Drug mugger dose: About 20–30 mg elemental iron each day for up to 3 months. Don't take your iron supplement within 2 hours of other minerals (like calcium or dairy products). It may take several weeks to months before optimal benefits are seen. A harmless discoloration of the stool often occurs, turning it dark green or black. This is normal and caused by iron that fails to get absorbed. Remember, the mineral itself is very dark.

Just So You Know

Don't take your iron with dairy products. Typical side effects of most iron supplements include stomach upset, gas, constipation (or diarrhea), heartburn, cramps, and nausea. These problems can be minimized or eliminated altogether by taking your supplement in the form of iron bisglycinate, iron glycinate, or ferrous bisglycinate. These are chelated forms of iron, which means that amino acids are attached to the mineral. In these examples, two molecules of the amino acid glycine are bound to one molecule of iron. This unique form is absorbed through the intestinal tract like any other amino acid without the usual irritation and constipation that most forms of iron cause. This is why I often recommend taking minerals in chelated form. Generally, this type is taken up easily and causes fewer side effects.

The human body appears to have a built-in limit for chelated iron bisglycinate and won't take up more than you need. So you are also safer when you take iron bisglycinate. This is important since iron is toxic in large quantities and is one of the leading causes of poisoning and death in young children. In adults, excessive amounts can cause oxidative damage because it can form free radicals.

While various brands of iron bisglycinate may be found in many health food stores and doctors' offices, the average family physician or pharmacist may not have heard of it. There is plenty of research regarding its safety and efficacy available on the Internet, and I prefer this form myself, having taken iron on and off for more than a year. I noticed that my nails grew like crazy and became beautiful for the first time in my life. I have since switched to spirulina tablets, a superfood that is rich in iron, as well as other minerals, because I did not want to develop a relative deficiency of other minerals.

It's ideal to take iron supplements on an empty stomach, but minerals are irritating to the gut, so if it upsets your stomach, take it with food. The bisglycinate form should not affect you, however. With any type of iron supplement, don't take it within 2 hours before or after consuming antacids, eggs, whole grain breads, milk, cereal, tea, or coffee. With most OTC brands of iron sold in pharmacies (i.e., ferrous sulfate, ferrous gluconate, ferrous fumarate, and others), it's relatively easy to get too much, unlike with iron bisglycinate. As noted earlier, you are safer with iron bisglycinate because it is nonconstipating and also because your body has a mechanism to keep you from absorbing too much. Nevertheless, I hardly ever recommend taking an iron supplement unless blood tests confirm that you are deficient and your symptoms support the test results.

There are a few instances in which supplementation is safe and advised, when the right amount can make a tremendous difference in your life. For example, if you are being mugged by a drug, if you are truly iron deficient, or if you are a regular blood donor or have heavy periods, then I feel it's okay to supplement with low doses for a short period of time. Remember, if you have children, be especially vigilant about your medicine cabinet because iron overdose is extremely dangerous to kids.

Install a Nutrient Security System

Although orange juice does not contain iron, it is considered helpful to drink a glass of orange juice each day to help boost the amount of iron your body absorbs; the vitamin C in OJ increases the absorption rate. Drinking OJ may not be enough for some individuals who need a real boost. If your doctor really wants you to drive the iron into your body, he or she may suggest vitamin C supplements instead of juice. In this case (and it's not for everyone), take about 200 mg of vitamin C along with your 20 to 30 mg elemental iron dose. I'm not recommending supplemental vitamin C for everyone, though, because it increases the side effects of iron, but if you are trying to install a tight security system, this is one way.

The other way is to take the supplement betaine hydrochloride or trimethylglycine (sold at health food stores) with your meals and your iron supplement. Take them all together. This supplement provides a little stomach acid. Many people today have low stomach acid (hypochlorhydria), so they don't assimilate their iron well and they burp a lot after eating. This supplement improves digestion and iron absorption for most people.

There should be no side effects, but if you develop heartburn after doing this, you may not need the betaine after all. And if you take an acid blocker, naturally you'll want to avoid the acid these supplements provide. (That opens up another can of worms because many people who take acid blockers actually need acid. For more information about this, you'll have to read my article "Heartburn? My Gut Feeling Is That You Need More Acid," which is posted on my Web site.)

What's in My Cupboard?

Iron 18 mg Capsules: Non Constipating Iron Bisglycinate by Bluebonnet: These are easy-to-swallow, small, tasteless capsules that provide elemental iron in the nonconstipating chelated form. You can find this product at health food stores.

Iron Glycinate by Xymogen: This brand is sold in doctors' offices. It provides 29 mg of pharmaceutical-grade iron per capsule. You'll have to ask your physician to order it for you.

Comfort Iron (Iron Bisglycinate) by Vitamin Shoppe: This product can be found at Vitamin Shoppes nationwide. It is called Comfort Iron because it is the iron bisglycinate form. Each veggie cap provides 25 mg elemental iron.

Easy Iron by Country Life: This is another easy-to-find brand of iron bisglycinate. Like the others, it is a pure form of bioavailable iron, so it's easy on the tummy.

Ferrochel Iron with B Vitamins by Nutraceutical Sciences Institute (NSI): This brand of iron bisglycinate is sold at Vitacost.com. I like it because it also contains all the B vitamins—thiamine, riboflavin, niacin, folic acid, pyridoxine, and B_{12} (as methylcobalamin). This product could be extremely helpful if you are anemic and stressed out, because the iron helps the anemia and the B vitamins help you cope by supporting your adrenal glands. Remember, the Bs are called stress vitamins for a reason. It's a powerful combination. Contact information: www.vitacost.com.

Energizing Iron with Eleuthero by Enzymatic Therapy: This product contains a highly absorbable form of iron derived from beef liver, along with the right amounts of B_{12} and trace minerals to help you absorb it. The herb eleuthero is great for energy. Even though this iron is animal derived, it's absorbable and does not raise your cholesterol.

Polysaccharide Iron by Niferex, Nu-Iron, or a store brand: This form of iron is slightly better tolerated than ferrous sulfate, and it's easy to find at pharmacies. If it's not in the vitamin aisle, ask the technician because sometimes these brands are kept behind the pharmacy counter. One capsule offers 150 mg polysaccharide iron complex. I like this brand, but it's not quite as digestible as the bisglycinate forms.

Spirulina Pacifica by Nutrex Hawaii: Spirulina is a blue-green alga that occurs naturally in the ocean, and it's one of those supplements I take every day because it is so energizing and detoxifying. This company is dedicated to production of spirulina, which many experts call a superfood. They offer both tasteless tablets or a powder that can be mixed in water or juice (because it has a unique flavor). Spirulina contains a lot of iron along with other minerals and proteins that work in a synergistic manner. To produce this product, the company uses pristine water that is rich in minerals from the lava beds. They are the only spirulina farm in the world to use only 100 percent potable municipal water and deep seawater. Other farms use river or irrigation water.

This brand has approximately 40 percent more total carotenoids than their competitors, as well as double the amount of natural vitamin B_{12}. It has 8 mg iron compared with its competitor's spirulina, which has a meager 1 mg per equivalent serving size (3 g).

Spirulina is believed to have anticancer effects, plus it acts as an antihistamine, antiviral, and anti-inflammatory agent. It protects against stroke, too. See why I take it every day?

Ocean's Alive Marine Phytoplankton by Sunfood: This is concentrated raw food containing phytoplankton straight from the ocean, and it will give you amazing nutritional benefits. The intense chlorophyll content detoxifies the body, neutralizes (chelates) heavy metals, sends fuel to the muscles, and increases energy, heart health, and mental clarity. Although it does not contain a large amount of iron, the combination of all the minerals together in their live forms is synergistic. I take a dropperful in water each day when I'm not taking spirulina. It's completely tasteless. You can do one or the other each day (spirulina or phytoplankton) to provide the minerals you need in order to keep your electrolytes (your electrical system) running in tiptop shape.

Magnesium

Magnesium has to be one of my all-time favorite minerals because it has beneficial effects all over the body. Think of it as your chill pill because it makes you relax from your head down to your toes. Magnesium is important for a good mood, first and foremost, but most people don't realize it's also necessary for stabilizing blood pressure. Without enough magnesium, your blood pressure rises. You need the mineral to keep your heart beating in perfect rhythm and to keep your pancreas functioning optimally. Deficiencies of magnesium can lead to cardiac arrhythmias and high blood sugar.

Western societies are short on magnesium in part as a result of soil depletion and the processing of food. I believe this is one reason why we are seeing so much heart disease, depression, and diabetes. Magnesium is not as chic as calcium. You don't see people wearing magnesium mustaches, do you? If you did, they'd be green, since magnesium is found in a lot of green foods, including seaweed, spinach, kale, and spirulina. It would not be pretty.

I feel that magnesium is so important that without enough of it in your system, you will suffer more diseases in your lifetime and die sooner than if you had normal, healthy levels. Seriously, it's that important.

Magnesium deficiency can cause muscle weakness, tremor, and spasm. Your heart is a muscle. If you get a spasm or tremor in your heart, you're in trouble. In fact, magnesium deficiency can cause arrhythmias such as atrial fibrillation, irregular contraction, and rapid heart rate. Some studies show that magnesium also benefits people with asthma by preventing bronchospasm.

Magnesium is so protective of the brain that when you run low, you are more prone to migraines, insomnia, anxiety, phobias, brain fog, depression, and suicidal thoughts.

A deficiency of this mighty mineral could result in more frequent headaches, migraines, fasciculation (twitching), muscle pain, fibromyalgia, poor nail growth, and asthma. And if that's not bad enough, you could also develop leg cramps, tenderness all over your body, a weak heart, high blood pressure, and thicker, stickier blood.

Since magnesium is married to calcium and used to build bone, a magnesium deficiency could cause bone brittleness (osteoporosis), a condition more likely to occur in women. In fact, women have a particularly hard time of it when they run low on magnesium. In addition to osteoporosis, we see a lot more emotional instability and PMS symptoms such as tearfulness, cramps, mood swings, and irritability—even panic attacks.

Kids need magnesium for healthy brain function. Studies have shown that low magnesium can cause attention deficit problems. In fact, medical researchers have known about this effect for quite some time. One study done in 1997 found that 95 percent of kids with ADHD (attention-deficit/hyperactivity disorder) were deficient in magnesium. In 1997, another trial included 75 magnesium-deficient children with ADHD who were randomly assigned to receive either magnesium along with their standard treatment (200 mg of magnesium given once daily) or just their standard treatment alone for 6 months. Those who received magnesium showed a significant improvement in personality and behavior, while the control group exhibited worsening behavior over the study period.

This explains why many natural supplements for ADHD contain magnesium. The mineral helps relax the brain and allow more focus.

This book is for adults, not children, so the doses I suggest throughout the book are adult doses. But it seems necessary to include appropriate daily children's doses here: For children 1 to 3 years old, 80 mg; for children 4 to 8, 130 mg; and for children 9 to 13, 240 mg. Make sure you let your child's pediatrician know about the supplement. If your child takes medication, you'll want to get the doctor's approval before starting.

Furosemide is one of the most commonly prescribed diuretics, or water pills, in the world, often ordered for high blood pressure and edema. It is sold under various brand names including Lasix in the United States. This diuretic drug is known to deplete magnesium levels. It happens because the diuretics cause the kidneys to filter out (meaning, lose) more magnesium than they should. Magnesium is known to participate in more than 300 biochemical reactions in the body. Let's talk about magnesium for just a moment, because if you don't have enough, you probably have some kind of heart disease. And I want to spend a moment here because I suspect your levels of magnesium are not being measured accurately. Who am I to say and why on Earth would I say such a preposterous thing? Because most doctors are ordering blood tests to check your magnesium levels, but less than 1 percent of the body's magnesium is located in the blood (outside of your cells). So when you measure your blood magnesium levels, it doesn't correlate to what's inside your body because your body stashes the mineral *inside* the blood cells. So unless your doctor orders an RBC magnesium level, you will never know if you have enough of it or not. You might be able to tell from symptoms. For example, if you have low magnesium you may have depression, high blood pressure, muscle cramps, or any of numerous problems with your heart. Heart rhythm irregularities are common and are often covered with drugs when the problem is low mag. Muscle tremors, muscle weakness, twitches of any sort, and brain fog are quite common. So if you take a diuretic, make sure you are checking your red blood cell magnesium level (RBC mag). You'll have to specify exactly what you want with your physician because they may not be familiar with this information.

I often recommend magnesium to people with depression (for mood stability), fibromyalgia (because it reduces muscle pain), and anger management problems and for aggressive personalities (for its calming effects). Make no mistake, if you are married to a Tasmanian devil who blows his or her fuse at the sight of dirty dishes, magnesium won't do a thing for it. It's really for people who want to chill out a bit more, stop being worrywarts, feel more content, or reduce the frequency of panic attacks.

Some experts think magnesium has a place in treating suicidal depression, and I happen to agree. Anyone with serious depression should, of course, be under a doctor's care. But do ask the doctor about adding a magnesium supplement to the treatment regimen. It goes without saying that it's a good bet for milder forms of depression as well. Many of my readers have taken magnesium for this reason with good results after reading a syndicated column that I wrote on the subject, "Natural Ways to Ease Depression and Reduce Anxiety." It is now posted on my Web site, www. dearpharmacist.com.

I've saved the best surprise of all for last: One bar of exceptionally dark chocolate contains about 300 mg of magnesium. I've drawn the conclusion that chocolate is not only good for your soul, it's also good for your brain! Sweet.

Drug Muggers of Magnesium

Acid Blockers

Cimetidine (Tagamet)

Esomeprazole (Nexium)

Famotidine (Pepcid and Pepcid Complete)

Nizatidine (Axid)

Omeprazole (Prilosec OTC)

Pantoprazole (Protonix)

Ranitidine (Zantac)

Rabeprazole (Aciphex)

Ranitidine (Zantac)

Antacids

Aluminum and magnesium hydroxide (Maalox, Mylanta)

Aluminum carbonate gel (Basaljel)

Aluminum hydroxide (Amphojel, AlternaGEL)

Calcium carbonate (Tums, Titralac, Rolaids)

Magnesium hydroxide (Phillips' Milk of Magnesia)

Sodium bicarbonate (Alka-Seltzer, baking soda)

Antibiotics (a few examples)

Amoxicillin (Amoxil)

Azithromycin (Z-Pak)

Cefaclor (Ceclor)

Cefdinir (Omnicef)

Cephalexin (Keflex)

Ciprofloxacin (Cipro)

Clarithromycin (Biaxin)

Doxycycline (Doryx)

Erythromycin (E.E.S.)

Levofloxacin (Levaquin)

Minocycline (Minocin)

Sulfamethoxazole and trimethoprim (Bactrim, Septra)

Tetracycline (Sumycin)

Antiviral Agents

Delavirdine (Rescriptor)

Foscarnet (Foscavir)

Lamivudine (Epivir)

Nevirapine (Viramune)

Zidovudine, AZT (Retrovir)

Zidovudine and lamivudine (Combivir)

Aromatase Inhibitors for breast cancer

Anastrozole (Arimidex)

Bisphosphonates (bone-building drugs)*

Alendronate (Fosamax)

Ibandronate (Boniva)

Risedronate (Actonel)

*But supplement the calcium at least 4 to 6 hours away from the medicine.

Blood Pressure Drugs

Hydralazine (Apresoline)

ACE inhibitors:

Enalapril and HCTZ (Vaseretic)

Angiotensin II receptor blockers:

Candesartan (Atacand)

Valsartan (Diovan)

Valsartan and HCTZ (Diovan HCT)

Diuretics, loop:

Bumetanide (Bumex)

Ethacrynic acid (Edecrin)

Furosemide (Lasix)

Torsemide (Demadex)

Diuretics, thiazide (and any combination drug that contains HCTZ or hydrochlorothiazide— dozens of drugs contain this)

Candesartan and HCTZ (Atacand HCT)

Chlorothiazide (Diuril)

Chlorthalidone (Hygroton)

Hydrochlorothiazide or HCTZ (Hydrodiuril)

Methyclothiazide (Enduron)

Metolazone (Zaroxolyn)

Diuretics, potassium-sparing:

Possibly the potassium-sparing diuretics; however, this is not conclusive.

Diuretics, sulfonamide:

Indapamide (Lozol)

Cardiac Glycoside

Digoxin (Digitek, Lanoxicaps, Lanoxin)

Central Nervous System (CNS) Stimulants

Methylphenidate (Metadate, Ritalin)

Cholesterol Agents

Cholestyramine (Questran)

Colestipol (Colestid)

Corticosteroids

Betamethasone (Diprolene, Luxiq)

Dexamethasone (Decadron)

Hydrocortisone (Cortef)

Methylprednisolone (Medrol)

Mometasone (Elocon)

Prednisolone (Pediapred Liquid)

Prednisone (Deltasone, Liquid Pred, Sterapred)

Triamcinolone (Aristocort cream)

Inhaled corticosteroids:

Flunisolide (Nasarel, Nasalide)

Futicasone (Flonase)

Triamcinolone (Azmacort inhaler)

Hormone Replacement Therapy/ Oral Contraceptives

Diethylstilbestrol (DES)

Estradiol (Activella, Climara, Combipatch, Estrace, Estraderm,

Estring, EstroGel, Femring,
Menostar, and many others)

Estrogen-containing drugs
(hormone replacement therapy
and birth control)

Estrogens, conjugated (Premphase,
Prempro)

Estrogens, esterified (Estratab)

Estropipate (Ogen)

Ethinyl estradiol (found in many
birth control pills)

Levonorgstrel (found in many birth
control pills)

Immunosuppressants

Cyclosporine (Sandimmune,
Neoral)

Tacrolimus (Prograf)

SERMs (Selective Estrogen
Receptor Modulators—used
for breast cancer)

Raloxifene (Evista)

Tamoxifen (Nolvadex)

Toremifene (Fareston)

Sulfonamides (Sulfa antibiotics,
some diabetes medications)

Miscellaneous

Alcohol

Calcium supplementation
(prolonged or in excess)

Coffee

Estrogen dominance

High cortisol levels

High-sugar diet (glucose, fructose,
sucrose)

Malabsorption of any sort
(celiac or Crohn's disease,
pancreatitis, crash dieting,
anorexia)

Mineral oil

Magnesium: Put This on Your Plate

Swiss chard, spinach, kelp, tofu, legumes, chocolate, baked potato with skin, oatmeal, whole grains, summer squash, turnip greens, pumpkin seeds, broccoli, halibut, flaxseeds, ginger, sunflower seeds, sesame seeds, quinoa, buckwheat, tomatoes, beets, brussels sprouts, scallops, yellowfin tuna, asparagus, mushrooms, tempeh, brown rice, oats, lima beans.

An Absurdly Inexpensive Way to Feel Better

For general health: 100–200 mg once or twice daily

Drug mugger dose: 200–400 mg two or three times daily

Just So You Know

You should be aware that many physicians aren't yet using the best test for diagnosing an underlying magnesium deficiency. You could be having all kinds of problems related to low magnesium and still be told your levels are fine. Let me emphasize it here: *Magnesium level has to be measured in the red blood cells, not the blood serum.* Your doctor needs to know what your RBC magnesium level is, *not* your serum magnesium level. Otherwise you could have heart palpitations or scary arrhythmias, for example, that don't get diagnosed properly, and ultimately have a heart attack. So make sure your doctor measures your magnesium properly.

It may be a good idea to get about twice as much calcium as magnesium; however, the data are not clear on this. Some experts feel that it's best to consume a 1:1 ratio rather than a 2:1 ratio. Formulas are made with these ratios in mind, so you can always try a product and see how you feel. The best forms of magnesium are the amino acid chelate or glycinate forms, or any form bound to an amino acid such as aspartate, malate, and so on. When you read the label, you may see it designated as magnesium chelate, magnesium amino acid chelate, or magnesium glycinate. These forms are less likely to cause diarrhea. Many brands of magnesium sold at pharmacies are magnesium oxide, but I don't recommend this kind because it is hard on the stomach and seems to cause diarrhea.

Another readily available form is concentrated liquid magnesium citrate. I know you've seen this type at the pharmacy. It comes in a bottle that lines the bottom shelf of the laxative aisle. This type of magnesium is used to relieve constipation. I promise you, this is not what you want! A few swigs of magnesium citrate from one of these bottles could elicit an explosive bowel movement whether you want one or not. Do not drink this before getting on the bus, please. Or a taxi, airplane, subway, or anywhere public! Reserve these drinks for required bowel evacuations, like right before your colonoscopy or other gastric procedure.

And do get naked with magnesium. Why not? I mean, take a bath with it, silly! I'm talking about Epsom salts, a product that contains a hefty helping of magnesium. Pour 2 cups of Epsom salts in hot bathwater and relax. Magnesium goes right through your skin because it's absorbed through your pores, or transdermally. If you recall, I said magnesium is very relaxing. It makes your muscle cells take a deep sigh of relief and release their tension. Add some soft music and candlelight and you have the perfect antidote to a long, hard day. If there's no time for a bath, you can spray magnesium right onto your skin. (See page 180 for more on this mineral spray.)

You should be aware that magnesium can accumulate in the body, especially if you have reduced liver or kidney function. And if you take too much, you may develop heart palpitations and arrhythmias. As a general rule, what's important is not how much magnesium you take, but the ratio of magnesium to the other minerals in your body, such as calcium, iron, potassium, selenium, and so on. Monitoring your mineral levels isn't that hard with SpectraCell Laboratories, Metametrix Clinical Labs, or Genova Diagnostics. (See page 448, Resources, for more information about these labs.)

People who have suppressed thyroid function or take lithium tend to develop an overload of magnesium more easily. You'll know you're getting too much if you develop nausea, appetite loss, diarrhea, drowsiness, weakness, irregular heartbeat, or very low blood pressure. Magnesium interacts with many medications and can make certain antibiotics (like tetracycline, Cipro, and Levaquin) less effective, so avoid magnesium while on these medications and for 3 days thereafter.

Install a Nutrient Security System

One of the most common problems that people suffer with is intestinal yeast overgrowth with *Candida albicans*. This could cause difficulties in absorption of magnesium. It bothers me that most conventional physicians dismiss *C. albicans*, but in my book it is a common cause of mineral deficiency, especially magnesium. To install the best security system, eliminate sugary foods (which feed the *C. albicans*) and take healthy probiotics and yeasts (see Chapter 17 for how to do that). Then, when you take a good brand of magnesium, your body will be better able to take it up so it can help soothe your muscles, nervous system, and cardiovascular system.

What's in My Cupboard?

Energy Boost 70 by Morningstar Minerals: This is a liquid product that contains easily digested and bioavailable organic mineral complexes. These minerals are all plant-derived "fulvic acid mineral complexes," which may help your endocrine system, lower high blood pressure, and rebuild your immune system. It's tasteless and can be mixed with juice or water, plus it can be dosed according to your needs because it is a liquid. These minerals also improve metabolism, energy, and cellular repair. Contact information: www.msminerals.com or 866-898-4467.

Calcium Magnesium Citrate by Bluebonnet: This formula is great because each capsule comes complete with vitamin D and minerals in a highly bioavailable form. It integrates 1,000 IU of cholecalciferol (vitamin D) with 1,000 mg calcium citrate and 400 mg magnesium citrate aspartate.

Marine Minerals by Seagate: Each capsule contains 75 minerals, including magnesium, calcium, iodine, zinc, selenium, and copper. It is a pure seaweed- and fish-based form of minerals, mainly from sardines. It contains omega-3 essential fatty acids and all the marine minerals because it's derived from the ocean. You may not like sardines, but those critters are nature's own concentrator's of sea minerals. Contact information: www.seagateproducts.com or 888-505-4283.

Calcium and Magnesium Mineral Complex by Nature's Way: The combination of calcium and magnesium in this product is provided in various forms, allowing for enhanced absorption. Each capsule contains calcium and magnesium in a 2:1 ratio (500 mg calcium to 250 mg magnesium).

Aspartic-Mag by Nutri-West: This vegetarian tablet provides the body with a highly absorbable form of magnesium that is bound to aspartate. When it comes apart in the body, the aspartic portion works its way into the biochemical pathways to help you produce more energy, while the magnesium works on the cellular level. It's an intelligent combination. Each tablet supplies 70 mg of elemental magnesium (from 500 mg of magnesium aspartate) and 430 mg of L-aspartic acid. To buy a Nutri-West product, ask your physician to order it for you or look online. They are not sold in health food stores.

Spirulina by Nutrex-Hawaii: This spirulina provides more antioxidant power than five servings of fruits and vegetables. It contains magnesium, calcium, and all 94 trace elements to support your body with key nutrients. This can help with cholesterol, vision, energy, and infections.

Broad Spectrum Magnesium by Stephen Sinatra, MD/ Advanced BioSolutions: Each capsule provides 100 mg of magnesium (as citrate, glycinate, orotate, and taurinate salts) and is very absorbable. Contact information: www.drsinatra.com.

High Absorption 100 Chelated Magnesium Mineral Supplement with BioPerine by Doctor's Best: This product is a chelated magnesium bound to two amino acids, glycine and lysine. The BioPerine (a black-pepper extract) helps it get into your cells. I like that it contains glycine, an efficient carrier for minerals through the intestinal tract. The body uses glycine to form collagen, a key protein in cartilage and connective tissue. Lysine is an essential amino acid that assists gastric function. Each vegetarian tablet provides 100 mg elemental magnesium.

Magnesium Aspartate by Thorne Research: These vegetarian capsules provide magnesium intelligently, because it is bound to aspartate. When the compound comes apart in your body, the aspartic acid portion jumps into your Krebs cycle to help you make energy, while the magnesium goes to work on your muscles, nerves, and mood. Each capsule provides 90 mg.

Ultra Pure Magnesium Oil by Ancient Minerals: You spray this clear liquid onto your skin. It's a little tingly, but that is minor. The direct application allows the magnesium to enter directly into your bloodstream, bypassing your gut, which is good if you have malabsorption issues, a sensitive stomach, or have trouble swallowing pills. I've asked my massage therapist to spray a little of this on areas of pain, along with the massage oil, right after a particularly hard workout. Contact information: www.ancient-minerals.com.

Epsom salts: This product, which contains magnesium, goes right through the skin and into your body when you add it to your bathwater. It's not enough to give you a therapeutic level if you are deficient, but it's a nice aid. It is sold at pharmacies and health food stores.

Melatonin

Think of melatonin as nightfall in a pill. Melatonin is your sleep hormone, and it plays a pivotal role in both sleep and immune function. You make this hormone naturally; it is secreted by your pineal gland, which functions as your body's master clock. When night falls and it gets dark outside, melatonin leaks out of your pineal gland, your brain becomes flooded with the potent sleep hormone GABA (gamma-aminobutyric acid), and voila! You drift off to la-la land. Melatonin is thought to amplify the effects of GABA. When the sun rises, all the melatonin scurries away and you wake up. Even though it's not quite that simple, I think you get the gist.

Night-shift workers have to overcome the urge to sleep at nightfall and must reverse their sleep cycles. Many of them rely on melatonin supplements to help. When you take supplements of this hormone, you might say that you're taking nature's sleeping pill. Since melatonin helps you sleep, it gives your mind a mini vacation. This goes a long way in rejuvenating your body, healing your damaged cells, and refreshing your spirit for the next day.

Melatonin actually sets the biological rhythm of every cell in your body. It supports your immune system while you sleep by producing immune-boosting and anticancer substances that prevent infection and reduce signs of aging. Healthy adults usually secrete about 5 to 25 mcg of melatonin during the night, which is about 80 times less than is in the widely available 2 mg over-the-counter tablets. It doesn't take much. The problem is that when we get older, our melatonin level—like everything else—begins to decline.

This is why as you age you begin to awaken earlier and earlier. This is also why your 60-year-old mother-in-law phones you at 6:00 a.m. to remind you that she will be arriving for dinner at 5:00! (Sheesh, go back to sleep like the rest of the world, would ya?) Melatonin is secreted only while you sleep, so the minute you open the fridge for that 2:00 a.m. ice cream binge, your melatonin production screeches to a halt. Melatonin is suppressed during daylight hours. This is one of the ways it helps with our natural sleep/wake cycle and biological rhythm. I recommend using a flashlight (instead of bright lights) for that 4:00 a.m. potty break, too, so your melatonin level doesn't drop so drastically, making it more difficult to go back to sleep. People with insomnia have lower levels of melatonin than good sleepers. And obviously teenagers have high levels of melatonin; my teens never crawled out of bed before noon.

Melatonin's most important role is to enhance production of youthful growth hormones. The antiaging benefits of this hormone occur with natural secretion, as well as with dietary supplementation. On the surface, this makes sense, right? Without adequate melatonin, you suffer from sleep deprivation, and everyone knows how bad that is for the body. But it goes much deeper than that.

Melatonin's ability to increase natural growth hormones in the body has been examined in several studies, and in one particular study, published in *Clinical Endocrinology* in 1993, melatonin administration produced an approximate twofold increase in levels of growth hormone in men. This makes sense to me; we all know that as we age, levels of melatonin and growth hormone decline, almost in sync with one another. Perhaps the reason is in part because the melatonin is responsible for the growth hormone release. And both of these hormones are known to scavenge free radicals, thereby protecting our cells and organs from damage and dysfunction.

Why is this such a big deal? Because when your growth hormone declines, you start to lose muscle mass, strength, energy, passion, skin tone, hair, hearing, and so forth. Your risk of disease increases, too. As years go by, your age starts to show. So maintaining an adequate level of melatonin may help you maintain some youthfulness.

In other words, just because your kids think you are over the hill doesn't mean that you can't take melatonin supplements and cheat Father Time a little.

Now, if you're a young person who happens to take a drug mugger, melatonin depletion occurs—the same kind of depletion that aging people experience. Stress and all-nighters also make you run low on melatonin. Melatonin deficiency actually poses a bigger problem than missing a good night's sleep. This important hormone has anticancer properties because it is a very good antioxidant. Melatonin is especially important for protecting the DNA inside our cells against dangerous chemicals called peroxynitrites, which damage the cells' energy powerhouses (mitochondria) and kill cells. This will shock you, so I hope you're sitting down. Peroxynitrites are formed in the body from nitrites. Certain foods, namely cured meats, are high in these nitrites, which are added to protect their pink color. Cured meats have, in fact, been implicated in most neurological disorders, including Parkinson's disease, as well as chronic obstructive pulmonary disease, cancer, and diabetes. So if you like bacon, hot dogs, salami, and bologna, you are probably producing lots more peroxynitrites than you want to, and I'd recommend antioxidants for you (as well as a change in diet!). Can melatonin repair bologna damage? No, but melatonin does play a strong neuroprotective role in the body and suppresses the formation of dangerous peroxynitrites.

Studies show that women with low levels of this sleep hormone tend to have higher rates of breast cancer. According to some recent and well-designed trials, bringing in a melatonin supplement might halt the growth of breast cancer cells. One of these studies was published in the *International Journal of Cancer* in January 2006. Scientists found that melatonin acted like a weak aromatase inhibitor similar to a type of drug (Femara, Arimidex, Aromasin, or Evista) used to prevent or treat early breast cancer. Aromatase inhibitors act by controlling and slowing down the production of estrogen. Less estrogen equals slower tumor growth. The study concluded that "melatonin could exert its antitumoral effects on hormone-dependent mammary tumors by inhibiting the aromatase activity of the tumoral tissue." Simply put, melatonin acted as a weak but effective antiestrogen.

One study was conducted at Harvard, where scientists evaluated 147 women with invasive breast cancer and 291 without cancer. Melatonin was measured using morning urine samples. What they found is incredibly important to women. Basically, women who had the highest levels of melatonin had the lowest risk of cancer! Has your physician told you about this?

And this is also amazing: A meta-analysis that pooled data from 10 studies was conducted by scientists at McMaster University in Canada. The researchers examined data from studies on people who had solid tumors and looked at their survival rate after 1 year. They found that melatonin reduced the risk of death, regardless of the type of cancer, and there were no reported serious adverse effects.

All this doesn't surprise me, because melatonin regulates your hormones and seeks to balance them. I happen to think that what's good for Betty is also good for Bob in this case! Supplements that help with breast cancer can also help with prostate cancer because these cancers are often driven by the estrogen hormone. The prostate actually contains melatonin receptors, so melatonin is needed for a healthy prostate.

Back in 1998 a German study found that men with prostate cancer showed extremely low melatonin levels and therefore altered circadian rhythms, causing poor sleep. Circadian rhythm is the scientific name given to your internal body clock, which includes all the biological processes that regulate a 24-hour cycle. Both plants and animals have their own circadian rhythms. In people, this normal biorhythm can be disrupted by events like chronic illness, stress, grief, and traveling across time zones, just to name a few. There have, in fact, been many studies on laboratory animals showing that melatonin in varying doses could shrink the prostate and lower prostate weight. Melatonin has a place in the prevention and management of prostate tumors, not just mammary ones. I believe that melatonin may improve survival for some men, especially when the hormone is combined with other anticancer compounds or treatments.

Some of the best cancer-protective substances include medicinal mushrooms, antioxidants, B vitamins, minerals, and a diet rich in fresh organic herbs, vegetables, and fruits. I know you try hard to protect your precious cells from negative environmental and dietary influences. There is more on the subject of hormones as they relate to cancer in my new *Breast Cancer Protection* e-book available on my Web site. You should also read the section in this book beginning on page 11 regarding menopause to find out what nutrients you need if you are taking a prescribed hormone drug.

Melatonin levels may be suppressed after using common antianxiety drugs, such as alprazolam, lorazepam, diazepam, and others in the benzodiazepine class of medications; these are also popular medications for insomnia. With long-term use of these drugs, however, I worry that your ability to fall asleep naturally and feel refreshed in the morning will be affected.

According to a study published in *Chronobiology International*, alprazolam (Xanax) can suppress the levels of natural melatonin in the brain. And taking it one step further, low melatonin leads to poor sleep. So chemically speaking, you may be asleep because you've taken the drug, but physiologically, your body doesn't have enough sleep hormone going on. Over time, I suspect you may be laying there with your eyes closed, but you're not truly sleeping like you should. Six otherwise healthy folks were given 2 mg of alprazolam at 9:00 p.m. Every hour, blood samples were collected until the following 8:00 a.m. (I don't know about you, but getting up every hour to get stuck with a needle for a blood draw may very well cause insomnia to begin with, but let's find out what the study concluded.) This study showed that melatonin concentrations in the blood were dramatically suppressed by the drug, beginning at 11:00 p.m. and onward through the wee hours. Interestingly, cortisol concentrations were also suppressed. Cortisol is a natural hormone in your body that is produced by the adrenal glands in response to stress. The significance of this proves that long-term administration of benzodiazepine drugs could very well deplete a person's natural stash of melatonin, a healthy life-sustaining nutrient. I want you to know this because if you need the medication, you may also need some melatonin, too. And as you've already learned in this chapter, melatonin in and of itself can make you fall asleep, too. Could that be all you need? For more on how to fall asleep and stay asleep, please refer to my book *The 24-Hour Pharmacist.* I have a whole chapter on sleep with all sorts of natural remedies.

Finally, it's worth mentioning that melatonin can be helpful in dealing with the discomforts of jet lag. Jet lag doesn't rank up there with the serious conditions just discussed, but many people fly internationally, and crossing six time zones, for example, is no picnic. It's hard for your body to adjust to the new hours of daylight and nightfall, which makes it difficult to conduct business meetings, give a lecture, or simply enjoy a vacation. Your body doesn't know whether to sleep or stay awake, because all of a sudden you're in bright daylight in a hustling, bustling city when your body thinks it's 4:00 a.m. and you are sleepy. Fortunately, melatonin is universally accepted as a safe remedy.

Simply take 2 to 5 mg at nighttime in the time zone you have arrived in. If you are still on the plane when nighttime occurs in the location to which you are headed, take the first dose while still in the air. How many nights should you take it? Divide the number of time zones you've crossed by half. For example, if you've crossed six time zones, take the melatonin each night for 3 nights. If the opposite occurs, that is, you land in broad daylight but it's 4:00 a.m. where you came from, I would skip the melatonin. Just check in at your hotel, take a catnap, and then wake up with the rest of the country, find a nice café, and get yourself a large mocha latte! The whole idea is to minimize the confusion in your body and quickly adapt to the time zone you're in.

Drug Muggers of Melatonin

Acid Blockers

Cimetidine (Tagamet)

Esomeprazole (Nexium)

Famotidine (Pepcid and Pepcid Complete)

Lansoprazole (Prevacid 24HR)

Nizatidine (Axid)

Omeprazole (Prilosec OTC)

Pantoprazole (Protonix)

Rabeprazole (Aciphex)

Ranitidine (Zantac)

Analgesics

Aspirin (Bayer, Bufferin)

Ibuprofen (Advil, Motrin)

Naproxen (Aleve, Naprosyn)

Oxycodone (Oxycontin)

Hydrocodone-containing drugs
(Vicodin, Lortab)

Antacids

Aluminum and magnesium
hydroxide (Maalox, Mylanta)

Aluminum carbonate gel
(Basaljel)

Aluminum hydroxide (Amphojel,
AlternaGEL)

Calcium carbonate (Tums,
Titralac, Rolaids)

Magnesium hydroxide (Phillips'
Milk of Magnesia)

Sodium bicarbonate (Alka-Seltzer,
baking soda)

Antianxiety Medications

Alprazolam (Xanax)

Clonazepam (Klonopin)

Diazepam (Valium)

Lorazepam (Ativan)

Triazolam (Halcion)

Antidepressants, SSRIs

Fluoxetine (Prozac)

Paroxetine (Paxil)

Sertraline (Zoloft)

Antidepressants, Tricyclic

Desipramine (Norpramin, for
example, is not a drug mugger, but
it increases levels of melatonin.)

Antihistamines

Hydroxyzine (Atarax, Vistaril)

Anti-Inflammatory Drugs
(NSAIDs)

Celecoxib (Celebrex)

Diclofenac (Voltaren)

Etodolac (Lodine)

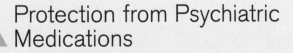

Protection from Psychiatric Medications

Psychiatric medications can cause a dreadful and usually irreversible side effect called tardive dyskinesia. It is usually seen with drugs that treat schizophrenia, but also sometimes with others. This side effect causes a person to perform involuntary, purposeless movements, such as tongue rolling, lip smacking, and grimacing, or wild movements of the arms and legs. One study suggests that melatonin supplements can reduce symptoms. This treatment is worth discussing with your doctor.

Ibuprofen (Advil, Motrin)

Indomethacin (Indocin)

Ketoprofen (Orudis)

Naproxen (Aleve, Anaprox, Naprosyn)

Sulindac (Clinoril)

Antipsychotics

Chlorpromazine (Thorazine)

Fluphenazine (Prolixin)

Haloperidol (Haldol)

Thioridazine (Mellaril)

Blood Thinners

Warfarin (Coumadin) (Not a drug mugger; melatonin may potentiate the effect of this blood thinner, and too much blood-thinning increases the risk of bruising or bleeding.)

Blood Pressure Drugs

Adrenergic receptor agonist:

Methoxamine (Vasoxyl)

Beta-blockers:

Atenolol (Tenormin)

Bisoprolol (Cardicor, Zebeta, Ziac)

Carvedilol (Coreg)

Metoprolol (Lopressor and Toprol XL)

Nadolol (Corgard)

Propranolol (Inderal)

Sotalol (Betapace)

Calcium channel blockers:

Amlodipine (Norvasc)

Diltiazem (Cardizem)

Felodipine (Plendil)

Nifedipine (Procardia) This combination is not recommended. (Melatonin may reduce effectiveness of the drug.)

Nisoldipine (Sular)

Verapamil (Calan, Isoptin)

Centrally acting alpha-agonist hypotensive agents:

Clonidine (Catapres)

Cancer Drugs

Tamoxifen (Nolvadex) (Not a drug mugger, but the combination of melatonin with this breast cancer drug may enhance the effect.)

Corticosteroids (all of them)

Betamethasone (Diprolene, Luxiq)

Cortisone (Cortone Acetate)

Dexamethasone (Decadron)

Fluocinolone (Synalar topical)

Halobetasol (Ultravate topical)

Mometasone (Elocon)

Methylprednisolone (Medrol)

Prednisolone (Pediapred and Orapred liquid)

Triamcinolone (Aristocort)

Inhaled corticosteroids:

Budesonide (Rhinocort)

Flunisolide (Nasacort, Nasalide, Nasarel)

Fluticasone (Flonase)

Fluticasone and salmeterol (Advair)

Inhibitory Hormones/ Somatostatins

Octreotide (Sandostatin)

MAO Inhibitors

Phenelzine (Nardil)

Tranylcypromine (Parnate) and others increase melatonin levels.

Sleep Medications

Eszopiclone (Lunesta)

Temazepam (Restoril)

Zaleplon (Sonata) and others

Zolpidem (Ambien)

Miscellaneous

Alcohol

Any drug mugger of niacin, B_1, B_6, calcium, or magnesium because you need those nutrients to make melatonin.

Caffeine

Hypochlorhydria (because you need stomach acid to convert proteins in your food into key amino acids, which ultimately form melatonin)

Marijuana (Cannabis) (can increase levels of melatonin)

Niacin muggers

Nicotine (tobacco)

St. John's wort (can increase melatonin levels)

Smoking cessation patches, lozenges, or gum

Sunlight, lamps, fluorescent light

Vitamin B_6 muggers

Melatonin: Put This on Your Plate

Oats, corn, rice, ginger, tomatoes, banana, barley, tart cherries, spirulina, seaweed, soybeans, chicken liver, pumpkin seeds, turkey, chicken, almonds, peanuts, walnuts, brewer's yeast, and dairy products.

An Absurdly Inexpensive Way to Feel Better

For general health: For insomnia, 0.5–1 mg at bedtime (may increase to 2 or 3 mg if no effect after 1 month)

Drug mugger dose: 1–3 mg at bedtime (ask your physician if 4 or 5 mg is okay if no effect after 1 month)

For cluster headaches: 6 mg at bedtime

For cancer or autoimmune disorders: Doctors suggest 5–20 mg per night (I am not recommending that you take it unless your doctor approves it. You can have your melatonin level assessed through urine or saliva testing.)

Dose for jet lag: 2–5 mg at nighttime in your new location

Just So You Know

This is one of those rare instances when I prefer a synthetic brand to a natural one. Synthetic melatonin is better than natural melatonin because the natural type is extracted from cows' brains and some people are sensitive to proteins and potential viruses from the animals. Synthetic is cleaner in this case. That's what I take when I need it for jet lag.

Melatonin is not for everyone, though. Women who are trying to conceive a baby may want to give it a pass, as this hormone may hinder the ovulation process.

You may be getting too much melatonin if you have trouble rolling out of bed and fully waking up—sort of like a morning hangover. Excessive melatonin will also cause wild and crazy dreams that frighten you, increased daytime agitation, sweating, and heart palpitations. It might also suppress the level of estrogen or progesterone.

Some people have adrenal exhaustion (low levels of the hormone cortisol). As a result, they are constantly fatigued, feel faint when standing up, or have trouble coping with little annoyances. Taking melatonin in these cases may be inappropriate because it can further reduce cortisol levels. You can measure your hormone levels and get a good baseline level with a simple saliva test from ZRT Laboratory (www.zrtlab.com) or urine tests offered by Genova Diagnostics. I also suggest that your doctor measure prolactin (an important hormone) levels, which may increase if you take excessive amounts of melatonin.

Install a Nutrient Security System

As a result of an age-related decline of melatonin, most older people respond to melatonin in a positive way because it increases their youthful growth hormones. One big benefit of melatonin is that it helps you fall asleep faster and stay asleep a little longer. If you could see the complex metabolic pathway on which melatonin is made, you would know that protein is important to that process. Most people get enough protein in their diets, unless they are vegetarian. If you are vegetarian or if you suspect that you don't get enough protein, consider protein supplements like hemp or rice protein and make yourself a shake every morning. See Chapter 10 on glutathione for more about these supplements. This is even more important: The B vitamins play an important role in the production of melatonin in the human body, particularly B_3 (niacin) and B_6 (pyridoxine). If you take a B complex supplement during the day and take your melatonin supplement at night, you can rest easy because you've installed the tightest security system possible. This is a good time to tell you that melatonin increases non-REM sleep, which can lead to vivid, bizarre, or frightening dreams. So one potential problem is that you just might create too tight a system by producing a little too much melatonin. If this happens to you, reduce your dosage of melatonin or stop taking it altogether for a few weeks. It's okay with me if you want to continue with your protein shakes and B complex, though.

What's in My Cupboard?

Melatonin (Sublingual) by Source Naturals: These 1 mg melatonin tablets are formulated to allow for a gradual release of the active ingredient over an approximate 6-hour period. This provides the body with more even absorption of melatonin through the night. Contact information: www.sourcenaturals.com.

Melatonin 500 mcg by Life Extension: This is a pure product containing a very small but physiologically appropriate dose of melatonin. It is free of all allergens and preservatives. You take it 30 to 60 minutes before bedtime. This company also makes a 3 mg lozenge, which you dissolve in your mouth at bedtime.

Melatonin Forte with L-Theanine by Vitaline: This is a natural sleep aid that combines melatonin with the amino acid theanine, the relaxing chemical found in green tea. Each tablet delivers 3 mg melatonin and 40 mg theanine.

Melatonin 3 mg by Nature's Bounty: Affordable and easy to find, each tablet delivers 3 mg melatonin.

Melatonin 3 by GNC: Each tablet delivers 3 mg melatonin plus vitamin B_6 to help it work faster. It is free of all allergens, gluten, and artificial chemicals.

Melatonin 3 mg by KAL: This 100 percent pure vegetarian form of melatonin offers a 2- to 4-hour sustained-release action. This brand is easy to find at health food stores nationwide.

Melatonin Caps by Twinlab: This easy-to-find supplement contains 3 mg melatonin delivered to the body over the course of a few hours. It's an easy-to-swallow capsule, and just as with all Twinlab formulas, quality control is assured.

Melatonin by Source Naturals: This company produces three strengths, 1 mg, 2 mg, and 3 mg, and they are timed-release formulas, so they should have a longer action in the body. This product is sold at health food stores.

Melatonin 1 mg Liquid by Natrol: This comes with a dropper so you can gauge your dosage and adjust it up or down as needed. You take it 20 minutes before bedtime and combine it with water or juice. The product is naturally sweetened with raspberry and vanilla flavors.

Melatonin 3 mg by Nature Made: This is easy to find in pharmacies and health food stores nationwide. The company has USP certification on all of their supplements. Their melatonin is free of artificial colors, flavors, preservatives, yeast, and gluten.

Methylcobalamin (Vitamin B_{12})

Vitamin B_{12} is a term that includes a group of compounds called *cobalamins*, and it's important for energy, sleep, and your nervous system. In fact, vitamin B_{12} has so many virtues that I can't wait to get to all the good stuff—the stuff that will really help people suffering from autoimmune conditions and serious health problems.

But first, a brief history lesson: The complete molecular structure for B_{12} wasn't discovered until the 1960s. Way back in the 1930s, scientists knew that a substance could help people with pernicious anemia. Pernicious anemia causes damage to red blood cells and occurs when the body cannot properly absorb vitamin B_{12} from the gastrointestinal tract. This can result from poor gut health, from taking drug muggers, from having certain infections, or from a lack of intestinal flora (probiotics). People who have pernicious anemia feel tired, short of breath, confused, and off balance. To this day, vitamin B_{12} is still recommended for this purpose, and what's so lovely is that many forms of B_{12} are available over the counter.

Vitamin B_{12} is water soluble and naturally present in some foods. It's added to other foods. It's available as a dietary supplement as well as a prescription medication given by intramuscular injection. No matter what the form, vitamin B_{12} contains the mineral cobalt, so any naturally occurring compounds with vitamin B_{12} activity are collectively called cobalamins. Methylcobalamin and adenosylcobalamin are the two primary active forms of natural vitamin B_{12}. There is a synthetic version called cyanocobalamin that is used widely in foods and dietary supplements sold in health food stores. Cyanocobalamin has to be converted by the body to methylcobalamin before it can be utilized.

One of the most intriguing facts about B_{12} is that plants and animals can't manufacture it on their own. Most vitamins are made by plants or animals, but only microorganisms—yeasts, molds, algae, and bacteria—can make B_{12}. That's important for humans because our digestive tracts contain friendly yeast and bacteria that manufacture this vital nutrient. For that reason, true deficiency is rare, but a deficiency based on having a poor camp of healthy microorganisms in the gut is quite common. In any case, you seriously need to be getting sufficient vitamin B_{12} for a number of reasons. For one thing, it helps you make red blood cells, and you need those for your very survival. A good store of red blood cells helps you create energy. Plus, red blood cells make up your blood!

One really cool thing about B_{12} (specifically, methylcobalamin) is that it provokes faster release of the sleep hormone melatonin, so you can get to sleep easier. It also happens to sensitize you to waking up earlier by causing the melatonin to retreat as soon as light shines into your room. So this is a good vitamin if you have sleep problems, although it may not work for everyone. Melatonin regulates sleep, and many older people who run out of B_{12} have trouble sleeping. You could be sleeping poorly because you are short on B_{12}. If you take a drug mugger for B_{12}, you could end up suffering with insomnia because, again, B_{12} provokes the release of your melatonin sleep hormone.

To treat insomnia, doctors generally prescribe conventional (and usually addictive) sleeping pills. Before you say yes to them, it's worth giving a vitamin B_{12} supplement a try and adding in a little melatonin as well. (See Chapter 13 on melatonin for more information about supplementing with this hormone.) I'm so happy to share that secret with you! You'll likely get your doctor's blessing on this approach. Studies have even shown that B_{12} supplementation not only helps people with sleep disorders get to sleep, but also improves the quality of their sleep and allows them to wake up feeling more refreshed.

Now the good stuff that I promised you at the beginning of the chapter. I'm going to focus on autoimmune conditions because millions of you are suffering, and conventional drugs are expensive and often ineffective. If you have any sort of pins-and-needles sensations, numbness, nerve pain, or neuralgia (including trigeminal neuralgia), I want you to pay especially close attention right now.

If you have a history of autoimmune disease, rheumatoid arthritis, diabetic neuropathy, multiple sclerosis (MS), amyotrophic lateral sclerosis (ALS, or Lou Gehrig's disease), or chronic neuralgia, then getting enough vitamin B$_{12}$ is crucial for you, particularly methylcobalamin or hydroxocobalimin. These are two natural, body-ready forms of B$_{12}$. These conditions are so hard to treat and so disabling that I'm delighted to tell you about this secret little B vitamin that I believe can help you.

Let's focus on multiple sclerosis first. Some physicians realize that stress, nutritional deficiency, and exposure to solvents, pesticides, mercury, and other heavy metals play a role in MS and neurological disabilities. In people who have MS, the thin coating around the nerve fibers, known as the myelin sheath, starts to unravel and deteriorate. This process, called demyelination, strips away the protection the nerve fibers need and worsens over time. Understandably, the nerves become extremely sensitive. Imagine an electrical wire that has lost its insulation and outer coating. This is why people with demyelination disorders have chronic pain, numbness, tingling, burning, muscle cramps, and other weird sensations.

There are many theories about why the myelin breaks down. One possible reason that I believe is worth paying attention to is wheat protein (gluten) allergy, the autoimmune version of the disease called celiac disease. I think people with MS should stay away from gluten just as a safety measure. That means no more pizza, bagels, and a bunch of other goodies unless they are baked with gluten-free flours. It's worth paying that price, in my opinion. It's not that hard to go gluten free, and I've posted some information on my Web site, www.dearpharmacist.com, to help you. Studies show that when people with MS go on gluten-free diets, they often improve. I found an article published in *Neurologia* in 2009 that discussed remission in an MS patient who went on a gluten-free diet. While studies conflict, there are many experts who connect autoimmune disorders to gluten allergy.

Anyway, if your myelin sheath deteriorates, you start to feel pain, tingling, numbness, burning sensations, and so on. You may even be diagnosed with MS or another serious neurodegenerative condition. B$_{12}$ can help you repair it.

That's a hefty statement if you are one of those people who happen to suffer the painful consequences of myelin degeneration, so I am going to elaborate. I will refer to both methylcobalamin and methyl B_{12}, which are the same thing, because you see it referred to both ways if you search studies in the literature. You can skip the science if you want to. I'm including it so that you know just how important B_{12} is if you have MS. Bear with me here.

The subject of myelin sheath degeneration could fill a book, and by no means do I mean to oversimplify this painful condition. Methyl B_{12} works hard in the body to reduce the amount of a pain-causing (and myelin-destroying) compound called methylmalonic acid.

Experts widely accept that the condition is an autoimmune process in which the white blood cells attack the myelin sheath. Methylcobalamin donates methyl groups to the myelin sheath that insulate nerve fibers and regenerate damaged neurons. But it goes much deeper than that, because methyl groups are not the only things that methyl B_{12} offers your myelin.

If you consume too much of an excitatory chemical called glutamate (yes, you get that from the MSG in thousands of food products), your nerve cells die. Methylcobalamin has been shown (you could even say proven!) to protect against glutamate-induced excitotoxic neuronal damage.

The cells most often affected by a B_{12} deficiency are called astrocytes and microglial cells. These are very interesting cells because they are highly reactive and can amplify immune mechanisms throughout the central nervous system, meaning that if it's a good reaction, these cells break out their megaphones and tell the rest of the body, and if it's a bad reaction, likewise. Trillions of cells in your body hear whatever these cells are saying. These astrocytes and microglial cells also help to clear glutamate, and without proper clearance the excess glutamate damages myelin. We always want to make nice with these cells and try our best to avoid irritating them. When we run out of B_{12}, we irritate them.

There is a strong correlation between B_{12} deficiency and damage in the central nervous system because the deficiency sparks an inflammatory response and allows excessive glutamate to stay where it is. According to researchers at the University of Milan, animal studies suggest that the process goes something like this (and I've just cut to the chase here for reading ease):

A person becomes severely deficient in vitamin B$_{12}$. Chemicals called cytokines are produced in greater amounts in the cerebrospinal fluid. These cytokines then attack and destroy the fragile myelin sheath. These myelinotoxic cytokines include TNF-alpha (tumor necrosis factor-alpha) and sCD40, another chemical related to TNF-alpha. Boom! Lesions form on the myelin, or it may start to unravel or decay. With continued production of inflammatory chemicals, this process progresses and sclerosis (scarring) occurs and the degeneration may spread along the spinal cord.

As if that's not bad enough, this animal study also showed that the good stuff that helps myelin form was not being produced in high enough quantities. The researchers found a reduced synthesis of two neurotrophic agents, interleukin-6 and EGF (epidermal growth factor). This imbalance was also a result of cobalamin deficiency. Remember, B$_{12}$ is a cobalamin. It's methylcobalamin, to be exact.

The bottom line here is that you should never underestimate simple remedies. Our nerves don't start to hurt because we suddenly run low on Vicodin or Lyrica (although these meds may be incredibly helpful and necessary at times). My point is that our nerves hurt because of neurochemical imbalances that trigger inflammatory chemicals. Vitamin B$_{12}$ plays an important role in improving the metabolic pathways that form your myelin.

Some of the research I've been elaborating on was published in *Progress in Neurobiology* in 2009. The researchers made it clear that a deficiency of B$_{12}$ leads to an increase in toxic chemicals that damage myelin. High levels of pain-causing chemicals and low levels of healthy growth factors were confirmed in people with severe B$_{12}$ deficiency.

I've actually saved the best for last. In a 2005 paper published in the *Journal of the Neurological Sciences*, Israeli researchers stated it best when they said this: "Multiple sclerosis and vitamin B$_{12}$ deficiency share common inflammatory and neurodegenerative pathophysiological characteristics. Due to similarities in the clinical presentations and MRI findings, the differential diagnosis between vitamin B_{12} deficiency and MS may be difficult. Additionally, low or decreased levels of vitamin B_{12} have been demonstrated in MS patients. Moreover, recent studies suggest that vitamin B_{12}, in addition to its known role as a co-factor in myelin formation, has important immunomodulatory and neurotrophic effects. These observations raise the questions of possible causal relationship between the two disorders, and suggest further studies of the need [for] close monitoring of vitamin B_{12} levels as well as the potential requirement for supplementation of vitamin B_{12} alone or in combination with the immunotherapies for MS patients."

Aren't you glad you learned that? Now you have the knowledge to protect your precious nerve fibers. And B_{12} won't interact with any of your medications either. It's as natural to you as green is to plants! Physicians often prescribe antiseizure medications, narcotic pain relievers, and interferon to treat neurological disorders, neuralgia, and nerve pain. But in my book, nothing is wrong with adding vitamin B_{12} (specifically, methylcobalamin) to help you rebuild the coating around your nerves.

Many doctors still say that it's impossible to regenerate human nerve cells and improve painful neuropathies associated with myelin degeneration. Yet a Japanese study in the *Journal of the Neurological Sciences* published way back in 1994 found that methylcobalamin could trigger nerve regeneration in lab rats. The rats were divided into three groups (ultrahigh dose of 500 mcg B_{12}, low dose of 50 mcg per kg body weight, and a control group receiving saline injections). The rats that received ultrahigh doses showed significantly faster nerve and muscle recovery.

And back in 1983 a study published in the Russian journal *Farmakolologia i Toksikologiia* showed that the daily administration of methylcobalamin to rats markedly activated the regeneration of mechanically damaged neurons. Finally, two studies published in 1976 in the Japanese journal *Nippon Yakurigaku Zasshi* showed that B_{12} administration resulted in greater protein synthesis and neural regeneration.

Okay, I'm done with the studies for now. That was a lot of science to absorb, but it was important to include it here because so many doctors maintain that vitamins will not help something like MS. Given that these studies showing otherwise are out there, and that vitamin B$_{12}$ is safe, it makes sense to make this nutrient a part of the treatment plan for MS.

I also think it can help people with trigeminal neuralgia, shingles, neuropathies, problems with visual accommodation, neurological disorders, painful mouth sores, memory loss, and other autoimmune diseases (besides MS) in which demyelination is the underlying problem. Cyanocobalamin won't help these conditions to the extent that methylcobalamin will, so if you are going to supplement, use the superior form.

Vitamin B$_{12}$ is also useful in preventing heart disease. In Chapter 9 on vitamin B$_9$, or folate, I discussed how B$_9$ helps reduce homocysteine, an inflammatory substance that contributes to heart attack risk. B$_{12}$ also reduces the homocysteine level, but only in the methyl form. These two Bs work better together to lower homocysteine.

I've also seen vitamin B$_{12}$ supplements cure depression and memory loss. B$_{12}$ deficiency can cause symptoms that look exactly like Alzheimer's disease, primarily because the deficiency affects those astrocytes and microglial cells I told you about earlier. These cells get upset and create all those inflammatory chemicals that damage the cells in the brain that are responsible for memory. I'm not saying that myelin breakdown is the cause of Alzheimer's, but it may contribute to it. Memory loss, fatigue, and mental confusion are usually the first signs of a vitamin B$_{12}$ deficiency.

This reminds me of a story my friend Bill Shafer told me. Bill was one of the primary anchors for WESH TV news in Orlando for many years. He's best known for his sense of humor and compassion. Now he and Marc Middleton head up a unique site for boomers, http://growingbolder. com. Since he's very articulate, I've decided to let him tell you the story himself. Take it away, Bill.

> My 87-year-old mother-in-law suddenly started having delusions. Before we knew what hit us, we were told that she had Alzheimer's disease, and she was slammed into the mental ward of a psychiatric hospital for evaluation. Can you imagine how horrified and frightened she was?

My wife, Mary, was told to find a nursing home for her mother. Fortunately, she's a voracious Internet researcher and a Suzy Cohen disciple. Something didn't seem right. Mary saw that her mother's B_{12} level was 202. Normal range is considered to be 200 to 900, but as we age, many believe, that number should be as close to the high end as possible. All of her doctors dismissed this lab value, then Mary found one who absolutely confirmed her suspicions. Her mother was prescribed daily, then weekly injections of methylcobalamin, and within a few short weeks her psychiatric symptoms and delusions completely disappeared. I'm happy to report that Mary's mom is back at home, healthy, happy, and loving life. All because of B_{12}.

When you run low on B_{12}, you feel tired and could even experience profound fatigue and weakness, especially in the arms and legs. You may become depressed, and you could develop tongue, mouth, or gum sores, as well as pale skin and lips. Other deficiency symptoms include low appetite, confusion, and forgetfulness. A B_{12} shortage may also lead to easy bruising and peripheral neuropathy, a feeling of vibration or buzzing in the legs, and a pins-and-needles sensation in your hands and feet, like little bee stings everywhere but not quite that intense.

Vegetarians and vegans may become deficient in B_{12} because they do not eat meat, which is a source of B_{12}. Anyone who drinks alcohol, deals with prolonged stress, or has had gastrointestinal surgery, nerve pain, chronic fatigue, or digestive disorders could also benefit from additional B_{12}.

Many people run out of B_{12} because they are taking drug muggers of this nutrient. Junk food and refined white sugar also strip your gut of essential components that you need to make or absorb B_{12}.

Acid blockers in the proton pump inhibitor class may affect the proper absorption of vitamin B_{12}, beta-carotene, and iron, according to a 1996 study published in the *Journal of Internal Medicine*. These medications are used to reduce acid secretion in the stomach. They work directly on the parietal cells of the gastric mucosa, which are the cells that produce acid. The drugs bind (like glue) to the parietal cells in the stomach lining and then block the action of hydrogen-potassium ATPase, which is an enzyme that normally pumps protons into the gastric lumen in exchange for potassium ions, creating more gastric acid. When these drugs are given, the effects of this enzyme are suppressed and so is the gastric acid secretion in the parietal cells. This, in turn, interferes with protein absorption, which requires a little digestive acid. How does that affect B$_{12}$ and lower it? Because B$_{12}$ is a B vitamin that is protein-bound, so a deficiency in protein causes the deficiency in B$_{12}$.

Drug Muggers of B$_{12}$ (Methylcobalamin)

Acid Blockers

Cimetidine (Tagamet)

Esomeprazole (Nexium)

Famotidine (Pepcid and Pepcid Complete)

Lansoprazole (Prevacid 24HR)

Nizatidine (Axid)

Omeprazole (Prilosec OTC)

Pantoprazole (Protonix)

Rabeprazole (Aciphex)

Ranitidine (Zantac)

Antacids

Aluminum and magnesium hydroxide (Maalox, Mylanta)

Aluminum carbonate gel (Basaljel)

Aluminum hydroxide (Amphojel, AlternaGEL)

Calcium carbonate (Tums, Titralac, Rolaids)

Magnesium hydroxide (Phillips' Milk of Magnesia)

Sodium bicarbonate (Alka-Seltzer, baking soda)

Antibiotics (just a few examples here, although there are many others)

Amoxicillin (Amoxil)

Azithromycin (Z-Pak)

Cefaclor (Ceclor)

Cefdinir (Omnicef)

Cephalexin (Keflex)

Ciprofloxacin (Cipro)

Clarithromycin (Biaxin)

Dicloxacillin (Dynapen)

Doxycycline (Doryx)

Erythromycin (E.E.S.)

Levofloxacin (Levaquin)

Minocycline (Minocin)

Sulfamethoxazole and trimethoprim (Bactrim Septra)

Tetracycline (Sumycin)

Anticonvulsants

Phenobarbital (Solfoton)

Phenytoin (Dilantin) (Space supplement at least 2 hours away from anticonvulsant medication.)

Primidone (Mysoline)

Antigout

Colchicine (Colcrys)

Antimetabolites

Methotrexate (Rheumatrex, Trexall)

Antivirals

Foscarnet (Foscavir)

Lamivudine (Epivir)

Stavudine (Zerit)

Zidovudine, AZT (Retrovir)

Zidovudine and lamivudine (Combivir)

Aromatase Inhibitors for breast cancer

Anastrozole (Arimidex)

Blood Pressure Drugs

Methyldopa (Aldomet)

Cholesterol Medicine

Fibrate cholesterol medicine:

Clofibrate (Atromid-S)

Ezetimibe (Zetia)

Fenofibrate (Tricor)

Gemfibrozil (Lopid)

Bile acid sequestrant medicine:

Cholestyramine resin (Questran)

Colestipol (Colestid)

Colesevelam (Welchol)

Corticosteroids (all of them)

Betamethasone (Diprolene, Luxiq)

Cortisone (Cortone Acetate)

Dexamethasone (Decadron)

Fluocinolone (Synalar topical)

Halobetasol (Ultravate topical)

Mometasone (Elocon)

Methylprednisolone (Medrol)

Prednisolone (Pediapred and Orapred liquid)

Triamcinolone (Aristocort)

Inhaled corticosteroids:

Budesonide (Rhinocort)

Flunisolide (Nasacort, Nasalide, Nasarel)

Fluticasone (Flonase)

Fluticasone and salmeterol (Advair)

Diabetes Medications

Glimepiride (Amaryl)

Glipizide (Glucotrol)

Glyburide (Diabeta, Glynase, Micronase)

Glyburide and metformin (Glucovance)

Metformin (Fortamet, Glucophage, Glucophage XR, Glumetza, Riomet)

Metformin and sitagliptin (Janumet)

Pioglitazone (Actos)

Rosiglitazone (Avandia)

Hormone Replacement Therapy/ Oral Contraceptives

Estradiol (Activella, Climara, CombiPatch, Estraderm, Estring, EstroGel, Menostar, and many others)

Estrogen-containing drugs (Estrace, Femring)

Estrogens, conjugated (Prempro, Premphase)

Ethinyl estradiol (found in many birth control pills)

Norethindrone (Aygestin)

Parkinson's Drugs

Levodopa/carbidopa (Sinemet)

Psychiatric Drugs

Chlorpromazine (Thorazine)

Fluphenazine (Prolixin)

Haloperidol (Haldol)

Thioridazine (Mellaril)

SERMs (Selective Estrogen Receptor Modulators—used for breast cancer)

Raloxifene (Evista)

Tamoxifen (Nolvadex)

Toremifene (Fareston)

Miscellaneous

Alcohol

Any drug mugger of beneficial bacteria

Estrogen dominance

Hypochlorhydria (low stomach acid)

Infection with *H. pylori* bacteria

Potassium supplements and drugs (Micro-K, Slow-K)

Vegetarian or vegan diet

Vitamin B$_{12}$: Put This on Your Plate

Primarily animal foods: beef liver, liverwurst, snapper, venison, shrimp (cooked), scallops, salmon, beef, lamb, cod, oysters, sardines, clams, flounder, halibut, yogurt, cow's milk, blue cheese, and eggs. Other sources: spirulina, brewer's yeast, tempeh, miso, and tofu.

An Absurdly Inexpensive Way to Feel Better

For general health: 250–500 mcg per day

Drug mugger dose and vegetarians: 1,000–5,000 mcg methylcobalamin per day (reduce dose after 1 or 2 months), along with a B complex to give you the full range of benefits. You can take the supplement orally or under the tongue (sublingually). You can also get injections to be administered by yourself or by a nurse.

Just So You Know

Methylcobalamin is the best form of the supplement. This is also called the *methylated form* of B$_{12}$. It's the active form that makes its way into the brain and nervous system, so it helps all kinds of neurological conditions.

Many people looking for B_{12} make the mistake of buying cyanoco-balamin, which is not natural. It's a semisynthetic version of the real deal. It's generally considered to be safe, and it's found in hundreds of supplements worldwide. As its name suggests, cyanocobalamin has a water-soluble cyanide group attached to its chemical structure, whereas methylcobalamin carries a methyl group. This is a very important distinc-tion. The body's natural stash of B_{12} is in the adenosylcobalamin form, not the methyl or cyano forms. The methyl in methyl B_{12} helps lower homocys-teine, an inflammatory chemical in the body that raises your risk of heart disease. Also, methyl B_{12} is the only form that can help you generate an important antidepressant and pain-relieving chemical called SAMe (S-adenosyl-L-methionine).

Remember I told you that people with low B_{12} look like they have Alzheimer's? Well, a study published in January 2010 found that people with Alzheimer's have low levels of SAMe in their brains. You can buy supple-ments of SAMe at any pharmacy or health food store, but you can also make this incredible substance yourself when you have methyl B_{12} on board, not cyano. Indeed, the ability of B_{12} to protect nerve cells may also be thanks to the increased SAMe in the body.

Cyanocobalamin is extremely popular and sold nationwide. But since you are reading my book and want my opinion, I am gently pushing you (okay, maybe I'm shoving a little, but I really care) toward methyl B_{12}. Methyl B_{12} is better absorbed, and tissues retain it better. I want you to break out your magnifying glass and make sure your product says methyl-cobalamin on the label, not cyanocobalamin. I'm suggesting that you do this because your liver has to spin cartwheels in order to process the cyano type. Your liver and kidneys have to go through a time-consuming and taxing chemical reaction to jettison the cyanide molecule and convert the cyanocobalamin into methylcobalamin. Don't freak out, though. You're not going to die from cyanide poisoning if you take the inferior version; there's not enough of it.

The absorption of vitamin B_{12} depends on the presence of intrinsic factor, which is made in the GI tract. Many people do not have enough intrinsic factor to absorb B$_{12}$ from their food or supplements. That's one reason why maintaining gastrointestinal health is important. (For more on this, read Chapter 17 on probiotics.) People who opt for injections of B$_{12}$ almost exclusively get cyanocobalamin, not methylcobalamin. I don't recommend the cyano form for injections either. To get the methylcobalamin in an injectable form, you'll have to ask your doctor. (Okay, you'll actually have to nag!) And he or she will have to phone the local compounding pharmacy and ask them to make it.

Compounding pharmacies have the formula and make excellent, pure versions of injectable methylcobalamin all the time for the holistic-minded physicians in the area. Honestly, they know what they're doing. To find a compounding pharmacy, look in your Yellow Pages. If you can't find one there, contact the International Academy of Compounding Pharmacists at 800-927-4227 or www.iacprx.org. You can also try the Professional Compounding Centers of America at 800-331-2498 or www.pccarx.com.

If needles bother you or you just don't want to deal with the hassle of a prescription injectable form, then get an oral version of methylcobalamin; these supplements are sold at all health food stores. My point is: Get the methyl B$_{12}$ in any dosage form before you take cyano B$_{12}$. Studies have compared the two versions, and the methyl version always comes out on top. The studies are clear and undebatable. Individuals who took the natural methylcobalamin form of B$_{12}$ showed better concentration, exhibited more alertness, and experienced sleep that left them more refreshed.

You can expect to pay more for methylcobalamin, but in my opinion it's totally worth it. For the injectable version, we're talking something that costs $45 versus $15. So it's not a mortgage payment or anything. Oral supplements are $10 to $20 a bottle.

There is a low incidence of toxicity associated with methyl B$_{12}$, even at very high doses. With cyanocobalamin, on the other hand, it's easier to get excessive amounts and experience side effects. That's because your body has to do more processing with cyanocobalamin, and tiny amounts of cyanide molecules may accumulate over time and cause subtle vision damage.

For whatever reason, if you have to take the cyano form of B_{12}, my best advice is to take it for only a few months or less, especially if you are taking relatively high dosages. Taking large doses of any form of B_{12} (methyl or cyano) will tilt all your vitamin Bs out of ratio. Some people just naturally have a lot of B_{12} to begin with. Very often, people with mitral valve prolapse or rheumatoid arthritis have higher levels of B_{12} and/or cobalt levels, so taking high supplemental doses could be harmful. It may not be wise for people with schizophrenia to take high doses of B_{12} either, except on the advice of their doctors.

Installing a Nutrient Security System

Medical experts maintain that no amount of B_{12} will help you if you take the supplement by mouth and happen to lack intrinsic factor in your digestive tract. This substance is a protein secreted by certain cells in the stomach. In humans, it aids in the absorption of vitamin B_{12} from your intestine. If you can't make or use intrinsic factor properly, the condition of B_{12} deficiency (pernicious anemia) results. So one way to install a foolproof security system and be 100 percent sure you're getting methyl B_{12} is to bypass your digestive tract. There are three ways to do that:

1. Take methyl B_{12} tablets sublingually (so it goes from your mouth to your bloodstream).

2. Take methyl B_{12} shots intramuscularly (so it goes from muscle into your bloodstream).

3. Take methyl B_{12} formulas that are combined with intrinsic factor (which gives you a better chance of absorbing B_{12} if you don't make it yourself).

What's in My Cupboard?

The B vitamins are interdependent. In other words, it's very easy to tilt your Bs out of their perfect balance. If you take B_{12} chronically, you may become deficient in another B vitamin. So whenever you take high doses of a single B vitamin, take a B complex as well so that the other Bs are on board. If you take high doses of B$_{12}$ only occasionally or daily, but for less than a month or two, then you don't need the B complex.

Preferred Sublingual Methyl-B12 by Applied Health: These tablets give you B$_{12}$ in the proper methyl form, providing 5,000 mcg (5 mg) in one naturally sweetened cherry tablet. Many people require large doses of B$_{12}$, and this product provides just that. Speak to your doctor about substituting this formula for prescribed injections of B$_{12}$. (Hey, who likes needles, anyway?)

Methylcobalamin by Life Extension: Each dissolvable lozenge contains 5,000 mcg. The formula does not contain any artificial sweeteners, colorants, gluten, or milk. This is another strong version of B$_{12}$ that could be taken if you're needle shy.

Sublingual B$_{12}$ by ProThera: Each chewable tablet contains 5,000 mcg methyl B$_{12}$.

B$_{12}$ Infusion by Enzymatic Therapy: This product contains pure methylcobalamin in a chewable tablet offering 1,000 mcg per dose. It is free of yeast, dairy, and gluten. Because it is all natural, color variations may occur in the rapidly absorbed tablets.

Methyl B-12 1000 by Jarrow Formulas: These lozenges taste really good and are free of all allergenic ingredients. I often carry some of these in a little pill case in my purse for a quick pick-me-up. They also come in a 5,000 mcg strength.

Methylcobalamin lozenges by KAL: Each lozenge contains 1,000 mcg methyl B$_{12}$ in a natural berry flavor.

Advanced B-12 Complex by Source Naturals: This formula contains both methyl B$_{12}$ and another active form of B$_{12}$ called adenosylcobalamin, providing B$_{12}$ in two highly usable forms. It also contains some folic acid since B$_{12}$ works better when its partner folic acid is hanging around.

B-Complex #12 by Thorne Research: I like this formula because it contains two active forms of B$_{12}$ as well as all the active versions of the other B vitamins. So it's a full B complex with lots of B$_{12}$.

Niacin (Vitamin B₃)

Niacin was the third B vitamin to be discovered, so it's often referred to as vitamin B_3. It is best known for its ability to open blood vessels and capillaries wider. Capillaries are the tiniest blood vessels in your body; they supply your skin and hard-to-reach areas. Some capillaries are so narrow that blood cells have to flow through them in single file, like a procession. If they get clogged up over the years, they can completely close off. When niacin comes along and widens them, more blood flows. Health nerds like me call this process vasodilation. When it occurs, you turn pink, get a heat sensation everywhere, and feel all tingly. It's a good thing if you have Reynaud's disease, because niacin sends blood flowing to your hands and feet.

The fact that niacin can widen arteries and increase blood circulation to such an extent means that it helps lower blood pressure and cholesterol while supplying more blood to the heart. In fact, studies confirm that niacin can help with all of these conditions and more.

The first statin cholesterol-lowering drug, lovastatin (Mevacor), was introduced to the American market in 1986. It made millions for its makers, of course, but the simple nutrient niacin has the ability to do the job at least as well and maybe better. And now I'm going to tell you something that just annoys the heck out of me, and I'm sure it's going to upset you, too, especially if you have high cholesterol. As far back as 1994, doctors knew that niacin performed better than statin cholesterol drugs. They knew it!

In a small, head-to-head study published in the *Archives of Internal Medicine* that compared niacin with lovastatin, niacin outperformed the drug. In the randomized, placebo-controlled 26-week study, niacin raised the level of good cholesterol (HDL) by 33 percent compared to lovastatin's measly 7 percent. What's more, niacin was also shown to simultaneously lower levels of lipoprotein(a)—or Lp(a)—and fibrinogen, two substances that are strong risk factors for a heart attack. It lowered LDL (the bad kind of cholesterol) a little bit too. Lp(a) is really important. You won't hear doctors talking about it much, but elevated Lp(a) can make you 10 times more likely to develop heart disease than high LDL, which everyone seems to obsess over.

So it looks like niacin actually does work harder than statins to protect your heart and circulatory system. That's hard to believe, and I'm betting that most folks reading this book have never been told that niacin just might work better than a statin drug.

Niacin has the added benefit of reducing fibrinogen levels. Fibrinogen is a substance that makes blood thick and clotty, and high levels contribute to strokes. Best of all, niacin has the HDL-raising capabilities that statins can only dream of having.

So why isn't niacin suggested more often for lowering cholesterol? For one thing, this nutrient can't be patented in its natural form, so drug companies can't make tons of money from it. Some smart cookies in the pharmaceutical world found a way to patent an extended-release formula that is sold by prescription. This drug is very effective and fairly affordable, too, but it is not the same as natural niacin, the way it's found in nature.

As I mentioned, there is one pesky side effect of niacin. When the nutrient is taken in the therapeutic doses necessary for lowering cholesterol, it undergoes conversion in the body to form the active compound niacinamide. During this conversion, your blood vessels widen (which is a good thing), but as they do, you experience flushing—heat and redness.

Within an hour of taking a large dose of plain niacin (not extended release), your face might turn beet red. This response is known as a niacin flush. If you're supersensitive, you'll feel like a firecracker! Menopausal women can sympathize here because they deal with hot flashes (ahem, power surges) all the time. Some people find that taking one aspirin (81 to 325 mg) or ibuprofen (Advil, Motrin) is enough to curtail the prickly, hot effect induced by niacin. You should take the aspirin about 30 minutes before you take the niacin in order to minimize (or hopefully eliminate) the heat!

Because of these naughty side effects, I always recommend that people taking niacin be supervised by their doctors, even though the supplement is inexpensive and widely available in health food stores. Nevertheless, niacin is still commonly used for heart disease and is often suggested by physicians in the know. Taking the correct form of niacin (nicotinic acid) is an established natural treatment for high cholesterol.

If you'd like to try niacin as a cholesterol-lowering treatment (or as an alternative to statin medications, or as an add-on with your statin), please discuss it with your doctor. Unless your doctor has asked you to do so, you should not be using large doses of niacin to lower your cholesterol at the same time you're taking statins because cholesterol is actually important to the body. Surprise! We need it to stay healthy, happy, and strong, and yet it feels to me that many health professionals are on a mission to lower your cholesterol to the point of unwellness.

I'm pointing out that niacin works! So do the drugs, and the combination of your OTC supplement with your prescribed medication is going to do an outstanding job of driving your numbers down. It is well known today that niacin enhances the effect of statins, and the two are commonly prescribed together. I just don't want you to take this combination without consulting with your doctor. You need to be under a doctor's supervision for either form of treatment. Some drugmakers are combining niacin with statins. Two medications on the market that combine niacin with a statin are Simcor and Advicor. That's how good the combination of niacin plus statin works; it's so good that pharmaceutical companies are cashing in on it! But maybe you could get by on just the vitamin?

Niacin can help with many other conditions related to blood circulation. In one study published in the *British Journal of Clinical Practice* in 1988, niacin was shown to help with intermittent claudication, a condition that involves heaviness, achiness, burning, or cramping in the legs that happens while walking and goes away when resting. It's a result of poor blood flow, and niacin helps because it makes the blood flow better. The dosage in the study was very high, 2,000 mg twice daily, much higher than I would recommend. After 3 months, patients in the treated group were able to walk with more comfort and had larger changes in claudication times when compared with patients who received placebo. If you have this condition, feel free to ask your doctor if you should slowly work your way up to a high dosage like this, based upon the findings of the study. Your physician will know what's right for you.

The therapeutic benefits of niacin are by no means limited to the heart and circulatory system. Studies show that this B vitamin is helpful for many other conditions. In one small but important study of 80 women who were experiencing heavy menstrual cramps, niacin appeared to help. The women took 100 mg twice daily starting 7 to 10 days before menses was to begin, and the same dose several times a day during heavy cramping. Some 90 percent of the women in the study reported significant benefit.

In this study, researchers used a special form of niacin that requires you to learn a new big name—inositol hexaniacinate (IHN). You don't have to pronounce that, just commit it to memory so that you can read labels at the health food store and find it. This form of niacin won't make you turn beet red. It's not found in nature. It's made chemically by attaching six molecules of niacin to one large molecule of inositol, hence the name inositol hexaniacinate. Your body requires time to break this tight molecule apart, so it's considered slow release for all practical purposes. To give you an idea, it takes about 6 to 10 hours to unlatch all the niacin molecules with this form, whereas with plain niacin (the flushing kind) your body can utilize it within 30 minutes to an hour.

Niacin also seems to work a little bit like a tranquilizer, but milder. Some studies show that niacin's effect on the body is similar to antianxiety drugs in the benzodiazepine class, such as Valium (diazepam), Xanax (alprazolam), Ativan (lorazepam), and others. Doctors in Italy have even used niacin to help people get off these addictive drugs. Since niacin mildly mimics the medication, it helps curtail the effects of withdrawal. If you are prone to anxiety or depression, you might want to add a niacin supplement in a low dose to your regimen. Now don't get too excited. Niacin's calming effect is not going to solve marital problems or disagreements with your teenager, but it could help bring a little peace of mind if you're a worrywart.

⚠ Niacin, Nutrient of Many Names

I wish scientific people would simply call niacin vitamin B_3 to keep life simple, but B_3 is anything but. It's known by all sorts of names. Let me briefly try to help you understand what you might see on product labels so that you know what you're getting and what symptoms it might help you overcome. Vitamin B_3 comes in two basic forms:

1. Niacin, also called nicotinic acid.

2. Niacinamide, the amide form of niacin. "Amide" is simply a chemistry term that recognizes that the molecule is metabolized differently. This compound is biologically active. In a perfect world, your body converts niacin to niacinamide.

Now think this out slowly with me. It's clear from number one above that niacin is also called nicotinic acid. So it makes sense to learn that the amide form of niacin (niacinamide) can also be called nicotinamide. And that compound, in fact, is the body-ready activated version your cells utilize. And therein lies the confusion. You can see either niacinamide or nicotinamide on product labels.

Now listen carefully. When nicotinamide undergoes a chemical reaction in your body, it forms an important by-product (metabolite) called nicotinamide adenine dinucleotide, which is thankfully abbreviated as NAD on product labels. You also see it abbreviated as NADP;

Because it increases blood flow to the eyes and the brain by widening those tiny capillaries, this powerful B vitamin also seems to help people with the common vision disorder macular degeneration. It also helps at the beginning stages of Alzheimer's disease.

There is also evidence to show that nicotinamide helps with arthritis. This form is involved in preserving and improving beta cell function, too. Beta cells are the ones that reside in your pancreas and produce your insulin. This means nicotinamide enhances insulin secretion and improves the

the "P" stands for phosphate. Sometimes you see it as NADH. (Don't ask me why they put an "H" on it, because I already have a headache from all this.) And are you sitting down? Sometimes you see this NAD or NADP or NADH as "coenzyme 1" on product labels!

I told you they should just call it B_3, didn't I?

I'm not kidding when I tell you that you can see vitamin B_3 labeled in all these different ways, depending on what type of B_3 it is and who the manufacturer is.

Now stick with me because the plot thickens even more. There is a variation on B_3 called inositol hexaniacinate that is also commercially available! The advantage of inositol hexaniacinate is that inositol itself is an essential compound, and some people are deficient in it. Taking it in this form is advantageous because inositol (also known as vitamin B_8) is a good antidepressant! I think researchers have nothing better to do than confuse the public like this, but it's true, so if you do the math, you'll see that good ole B_3 might be called nine different names!

Certain forms of B_3 only do so much in the body. For example, niacinamide or nicotinamide does not generally cause the infamous hot flash, nor does it lower cholesterol as well as niacin. Niacinamide or nicotinamide does, however, make energy for you and protect your gastrointestinal tract, especially your pancreas. Niacinamide jumps into your energy-producing pathways to help make ATP, which helps with cellular respiration and energy metabolism throughout the human body. This is a very important role.

sensitivity of your cells to insulin (it makes the insulin you have more effective). To make a long story short, nicotinamide protects you from pancreatic insufficiency and diabetes, so it's helpful for both treatment and prevention of this disease. FYI, it is helpful for both type 1 and type 2 diabetes. You will find studies on the Internet that say that niacin can raise blood sugar, but this is controversial and I think that you're fine taking this supplement at low doses and with adequate monitoring. For more on diabetes, read my book *Diabetes without Drugs*.

Niacin is often found in supplements used to detoxify the body. Because it improves blood flow to capillaries, this nutrient apparently helps pull toxic buildup from fatty cells and tissues. Releasing toxins like this could make you feel itchy, and that's normal. (Of course, if you're looking to detoxify your cells and dump all that waste, your best bet is to focus on your diet and make sure you get lots of fresh produce, fruits, and home-made juices, because eating better makes your biochemical system run more efficiently. Most importantly, you should reduce your trans fat intake. Yes, that means saying no to fried chicken and potato chips.)

A serious niacin deficiency, a condition known as pellagra, involves diar-rhea, poor appetite, muscle weakness, fatigue, irritability, rough or cracked skin, sore red eyes, eye pain, headache, mood swings, inflamed tongue, depression, anxiety, and memory loss. After some time, niacin deficiency may lead to chronic diarrhea, dehydration, dementia, Alzheimer's disease, derma-titis, and other skin problems. Any of these symptoms can develop in people who routinely drink alcohol or those who take drug muggers of niacin.

When niacin runs low, so does riboflavin, and possibly B_6 and other B vitamins. The B family sticks together and its members work in conjunc-tion with one another. That's why it's always good to take a well-rounded B complex even while supplementing with one B vitamin in particular.

As I mentioned, niacin is also known as nicotinic acid. When some people hear that term, they are leery of taking it because they think it could hurt them the way nicotine in cigarettes does, but this is not true. Nicotinic acid does not pose the same danger as the nicotine in cigarettes. In fact, niacin used to be widely known as nicotinic acid; the term was changed to help allay these concerns.

The nicotine in cigarettes is actually a drug mugger of niacin. One of the ways that smoking causes such catastrophic effects in the human body is by competing with niacin for your cells' love and affection. More specifi-cally, nicotine looks so incredibly similar to nicotinamide (niacin's active form) that it fakes your cells out and interferes with the absorption and utilization of nicotinamide. From the starving cells' point of view, smoking causes nicotinamide deficiency.

Most experts feel that it's rather hard to become deficient in niacin, but I don't think it's that rare. In my book, deficiencies are common in people who routinely drink alcohol, eat processed foods, take high dosages of other B vitamins (causing a relative deficiency in niacin), are genetically stumped when it comes to activating B_3 to its body-ready form, or take drug muggers of niacin. So you see that quite a lot of people are probably niacin deficient. And if you are wondering what type of B_3 I suggest out of all those crazy names, I think that nicotinamide or its metabolite NADH are the better forms for drug mugging replenishment. If you are simply trying to lower your cholesterol, I recommend taking plain niacin (nicotinic acid) and working the dose up slowly to get used to the flush effect, which will subside over time.

Too much niacin in supplemental form (and what's too much for you may not be enough for someone else) may interfere with blood sugar control (as we've seen, some studies show that it can raise blood sugar), increase gout episodes, damage the liver, and increase the homocysteine level. Homocysteine is an inflammatory chemical that contributes to heart disease. To be clear: If you take the right dose of niacin, it can help prevent and treat heart disease, but if you take too much, you could actually contribute to the problem. That was what researchers discussed in a 1996 study published in *Coronary Artery Disease*. So it's a really good idea to discuss the therapeutic use of niacin with your health-care provider.

Drug Muggers of Niacin (Vitamin B₃)

Acid Blockers

Cimetidine (Tagamet)

Esomeprazole (Nexium)

Famotidine (Pepcid and Pepcid Complete)

Lansoprazole (Prevacid 24HR)

Nizatidine (Axid)

Omeprazole (Prilosec OTC)

Pantoprazole (Protonix)

Rabeprazole (Aciphex)

Ranitidine (Zantac)

Antacids (all of them because they change the pH in the gut)

Antibiotics (just a few examples)

Amoxicillin (Amoxil)

Azithromycin (Z-Pak)

Cefaclor (Ceclor)

Cefdinir (Omnicef)

Cephalexin (Keflex)

Ciprofloxacin (Cipro)

Clarithromycin (Biaxin)

Doxycycline (Doryx)

Erythromycin (E.E.S.)

Isoniazid (INH)

Levofloxacin (Levaquin)

Minocycline (Minocin)

Penicillin (Pen VK)

Sulfamethoxazole and
trimethoprim (Bactrim Septra)

Tetracycline (Sumycin)

Trimethoprim (Proloprim)

Antigout

Probenecid (Benemid, Col-
Benemid)

Anti-Inflammatory Drugs
(NSAIDs)

Celecoxib (Celebrex)

Diclofenac (Voltaren)

Etodolac (Lodine)

Ibuprofen (Advil, Motrin)

Indomethacin (Indocin)

Ketoprofen (Orudis)

Naproxen (Aleve, Anaprox,
Naprosyn)

Sulindac (Clinoril)

Antituberculosis Agents

Ethambutol (Myambutol)

Isoniazid (INH)

Rifampin (Rifadin)

Aromatase Inhibitors for breast
cancer

Anastrozole (Arimidex)

Cholesterol Agents

Cholestyramine (Questran)

Colestipol (Colestid)

Blood Pressure Drugs

Diuretics, loop:

Bumetanide (Bumex)

Ethacrynic acid (Edecrin)

Furosemide (Lasix)

Diuretics, thiazide:

Any combination drug that
contains HCTZ or
hydrochlorothiazide (dozens of
drugs contain this)

Chlorothiazide (Diuril)

Chlorthalidone (Hygroton)

Hydrochlorothiazide or HCTZ
(Hydrodiuril)

Methyclothiazide (Enduron)

Metolazone (Zaroxolyn)

Diuretics, sulfonamide:

Indapamide (Lozol)

Triamterene/HCTZ (Dyazide,
Dyrenium, Maxzide)

Hormone Replacement
Therapy/Oral Contraceptives

Estradiol (Activella, Climara,
CombiPatch, Estraderm,
EstroGel, Menostar)

Estrogen-containing drugs
(Estrace, Estring, Femring, and
many others—there are dozens!)

Estrogens, conjugated (Prempro,
Premphase)

Ethinyl estradiol (found in many
birth control pills)

Laxatives

SERMs (Selective Estrogen Receptor
Modulators—used for breast cancer)

Raloxifene (Evista)

Tamoxifen (Nolvadex)

Toremifene (Fareston)

Sulfonamides (Sulfa antibiotics, some diabetes medications)

Miscellaneous

Alcohol

Anything that mugs vitamin B$_6$ (because B$_6$ converts niacin to nicotinamide, so without B$_6$ you could run low)

Estrogen dominance

Low-protein diets

Nicotine (smoking)

Niacin: Put This on Your Plate

Mushrooms, lean beef, liver, eggs, dairy products, chicken and other poultry, wild salmon, yellowfin tuna, corn grits, any kind of nut, peanut butter, and enriched cereals. Fermented foods (sauerkraut) and kefir improve probiotic status, and that increases B$_3$. True—your beneficial bacteria help make this important nutrient!

Also note that your body naturally produces niacin from tryptophan-rich food and that the niacin made in your own cells won't make you flush the way dietary supplements of niacin can. Tryptophan is found in small amounts in oats, chocolate, bananas, dairy products, meat, turkey, fish, chickpeas, sunflower seeds, pumpkin seeds, nuts, and spirulina.

An Absurdly Inexpensive Way to Feel Better

If you take too much niacin, you may become deficient in your other B vitamins. So whenever you take a single B vitamin, it may be wise to take a B complex also so the other Bs are on board.

For general health: 50–100 mg per day

Drug mugger dose: 100–1,000 mg per day

Therapeutic dose: 1,000–2,000 mg per day (But ask your doctor first.)

Just So You Know

The word *niacin* actually comes from the combination of NIcotinic ACid vitamIN. (I've capitalized the letters NIACIN so you can see this clearly.)

The special flush-free form of niacin, inositol hexaniacinate, is widely available in health food stores. Many people say that this type is less irritating to the stomach, too. There are also prescription versions of niacin available, and your doctor may order one of them for you if you have high cholesterol. Just be aware that prescription versions of extended-release niacin have been associated with liver damage, so if you take one, have your doctor order liver function tests about every 6 months. It's best to take niacin in smaller doses at first and then work your way up. If you gradually increase the dosage, you are less likely to experience the skin sensations that are so common with niacin. Therapeutic dosages vary widely, from 100 to 2,000 mg, but usually are between 1,000 and 2,000 mg. You can take aspirin or ibuprofen a half hour before taking your niacin (prescription version or OTC). Since niacin increases blood flow, it makes sense that you should avoid hot drinks and even alcohol around the time you take your supplement. This will help reduce the amount of facial flushing. If you are prescribed bile acid resin drugs (i.e., colestipol, cholestyramine), which are also used to lower cholesterol, separate the dose from niacin by 6 hours or more.

Caution: Because niacin widens arteries and increases blood flow, it will naturally reduce blood pressure. If you take therapeutic doses of niacin, please be careful when you get up from a lying or sitting position. Your supplement or medication may cause you to feel dizzy or faint. Getting up slowly may help until this effect lessens after a week or two as your body gets accustomed to the niacin on board.

If you have gout, do not take niacin without your physician's consent because it competes for elimination with uric acid. If your body is busy clearing niacin, then your uric acid might build up, triggering a gout attack. It's rare, but I want you to be aware of it. One more thing: Do not take niacin (especially the extended-release form) if you have liver problems, unless your doctor approves and monitors your liver function. People with liver dysfunction are better off with plain niacin or niacinamide (not extended release).

Install a Nutrient Security System

Assuming you have no malabsorption issues and you have sufficient acid in your stomach, niacin is absorbed from your gastrointestinal tract with ease. One way to help improve GI health and therefore niacin production and uptake is to make sure that you have a healthy supply of natural beneficial bacteria (probiotics) as well as digestive acid. Betaine supplements increase digestive acid and are sold at health food stores.

What's in My Cupboard?

Niacin (B-3) Caps by Twinlab: Each capsule contains 1,000 mg plain niacin (vitamin B₃) and is free of corn, soy, yeast, rice, barley, wheat, dairy products, citrus, fish, egg, and artificial flavors and colors.

Niacinamide Flush Free 250mg by Jarrow Formulas: Each capsule contains 250 mg niacinamide.

B-Complex #3 by Thorne Research: This product contains 20 mg plain niacin along with 275 mg niacinamide. The best thing about this brand is that it also contains niacin's sisters and brothers (the other B vitamins that are naturally found in a B complex—methylcobalamin, pyridoxine, thiamine, pantothenic acid, biotin, and the rest).

Kyolic Kyo-Chrome by Wakunaga: This multitasking formula contains aged garlic (odorless), which has been shown to lower cholesterol in numerous studies, along with niacin and chromium to help stabilize cholesterol and blood sugar. It is made with the utmost attention to quality. The garlic is grown organically.

HDL Booster by Enzymatic Therapy: These capsules contain the perfect combination of niacinamide, vitamin C, folic acid, natural vitamin E, and some arginine (which widens arteries and improves blood flow). In addition, they have a blend of helpful herbs, including hawthorn, garlic, and grape seed. This product is specifically geared to improve heart health and help normalize cholesterol.

Slo-Niacin and Niaspan: These are two different slow-release niacin preparations available only by prescription from your doctor, so they are FDA approved to treat high cholesterol. Never break, crush, or chew slow-release formulas unless they are scored and you are told that it is safe to do so by your pharmacist. In my opinion, these prescription versions don't have any tremendous advantage over OTC versions, but you may have insurance that allows you to pay a small co-pay for a prescription, whereas the OTC version would be completely out-of-pocket. Be sure to monitor liver enzymes routinely through your doctor's office if you take extended-release formulas (prescription or over the counter). It's a simple blood test.

Potassium

You never want to run low on potassium. If you do, you could develop problems all over your body, especially in your muscles and nerves. Unfortunately, it's all too easy to experience a shortfall of this important mineral, especially if you have diarrhea or if you get mugged by a drug. Potassium deficiency can come on slowly, either from taking drug muggers or from poor nutrition, chronic illness, or pain. Symptoms usually include muscle weakness, fatigue, drowsiness, poor reflexes, muscle spasms, leg cramps, heart arrhythmias, and nerve excitability. Potassium deficiency can come on very quickly in certain cases, and result in all of the above symptoms as well as severe irregular or rapid heartbeat, confusion, high or low blood pressure, vomiting, abdominal distension, paralysis, sensations of pins and needles, and fainting.

Many scientific studies have been done on this important mineral. It's now well established that low potassium can cause increased risk of high blood pressure and death from heart attack and stroke. It's ironic that many blood pressure medications make the potassium drug mugger list, because potassium is needed for healthy blood pressure! Other signs and symptoms of too little potassium include constipation, osteoporosis, constant thirst, and heart disease.

Potassium is very important to your heart and blood pressure. It ensures a regular heartbeat. This mineral is called an electrolyte because it helps with water balance and electrical circuitry in the body. It helps fire nerve impulses, aiding in muscle contraction. Without that electrolyte assist from potassium, muscles couldn't work properly.

Some people claim that potassium supplementation can help cure alcoholism, but this is simply not true. People who are withdrawing from alcohol may become deficient in potassium during this debilitating stage, so adequate supplementation may be necessary under the care of a physician. But potassium supplements do not stop the craving for alcohol, nor do they ease symptoms of withdrawal.

In addition to blood pressure medications, the long list of drug muggers of potassium includes medications that improve breathing, reduce pain, and promote regularity.

Some of you may underestimate the power of an allergy or asthma nasal spray such as Flonase, but it is a corticosteroid. Even though it goes through your nose and not through your mouth (orally) or through your skin (injection), a steroid is a steroid and chronic use can impact your health to some degree. In fact, chronic, long-term use of Flonase may be causing you to lose potassium—and zinc—much faster than a person who does not take steroid drug muggers. There are numerous studies, one dating back as far as 1975, that suggest corticosteroids can result in reduced minerals. Yes, we've known about it this long. Has your physician told you yet? Basically, in that early study, eight patients with lung disease who were taking prednisone were evaluated. Higher dosages of the drug were associated with more excretion of potassium (so less was left in the body). Patients who were treated for a long time (several years) retained less of their potassium supplement, suggesting that levels of potassium will go down the longer you take the drug.

Most adults get enough potassium in their diets. If, for some reason, you do need to take a potassium supplement, be careful not to overdo a good thing, because this mineral affects the heart and interacts with many prescribed drugs. For example, potassium may cause a dangerous rise in the level of amiloride, a drug used to treat water retention and fluid buildup. In OTC dosages, problems like this are extremely rare. It's most likely to occur with prescribed potassium because the dosages are exponentially higher.

Doctors sometimes prescribe fairly high dosages of potassium and then carefully monitor their patients' blood levels every few months. Certain patients, like those with chronic kidney disease, will more than likely require higher dosages.

Potassium is irritating to the delicate mucosal lining of the digestive tract and so could increase the risk of ulcers if taken along with other medications that are hard on the stomach, like atropine, belladonna, or the bone-building drugs used for osteoporosis. If you take digoxin, make sure that your potassium level is measured routinely and that you don't run low on it, a condition called hypokalemia. Developing low potassium while taking digoxin can be fatal. Having too little potassium is much worse for you than having too much because hypokalemia causes dangerous cardiac arrhythmias. Did you catch that? Low potassium is far more dangerous than a high level. It's usually the other way around.

People who sweat a lot or exercise vigorously have an increased need for potassium. This is the basis of those sports drinks on the market (like Gatorade) that replenish lost potassium. Potassium is also available at the pharmacy in prescribed strengths of up to 20 mEq (milliequivalents), which is about 1,500 mg. Potassium is often measured in milliequivalents in laboratory tests, although the supplements are converted to milligrams. Most supplements sold at health food stores come in dosages of 99 mg. Why not a hundred? Go figure.

Various types of potassium drugs are sold by prescription. The brand names include Micro-K Extencaps, Klor-Con, Slow-K, and K-Dur. These forms should be taken with a meal and a full glass of water. But whether you take high dosages or low dosages of potassium, the mineral is very hard on the stomach and often creates stomach upset when taken orally. It can seriously increase the risk of gastric and esophageal irritation. There's even a possibility that it may poke microscopic holes in the delicate mucosal lining of the esophagus, stomach, or intestines. This seems to occur more often if the potassium is taken in liquid form without enough water to chase it down. Extended-release formulations, usually taken by prescription, have been associated with ulcers, too.

One way to get around the gastric issue caused by oral potassium is to buy the OTC form in powder and put a little in your bathwater. Potassium goes right through your skin exactly the same way magnesium does. But be careful and use only small dosages as directed on the label.

Potassium powder is not dosed like Epsom salts, which you can dump plenty of into the bathtub and just relax. You only need a teaspoon or capful of potassium, depending on what your product's label directions say. Consult your doctor to find out what dosage is right for you.

Drug Muggers of Potassium

Acid Blockers

Cimetidine (Tagamet)

Esomeprazole (Nexium)

Famotidine (Pepcid and Pepcid Complete)

Lansoprazole (Prevacid 24HR)

Nizatidine (Axid)

Omeprazole (Prilosec OTC)

Pantoprazole (Protonix)

Rabeprazole (Aciphex)

Ranitidine (Zantac)

Analgesics

Aspirin (Bayer, Ecotrin, St. Joseph)

Butalbital compound and aspirin (Fiorinal)

Carisoprodal and aspirin (Soma Compound)

Hydrocodone and acetaminophen (Lorcet, Lortab, Norco, Vicodin)

Ketoprofen (Orudis)

Oxycodone and aspirin (Percodan)

Salicylate drugs or herbs

Antibiotics (just a few examples)

Amoxicillin (Amoxil, Augmentin)

Azithromycin (Z-Pak)

Cefaclor (Ceclor)

Cefdinir (Omnicef)

Cephalexin (Keflex)

Ciprofloxacin (Cipro)

Clarithromycin (Biaxin)

Doxycycline (Doryx)

Erythromycin (E.E.S.)

Isoniazid (INH)

Levofloxacin (Levaquin)

Lomefloxacin (Maxaquin)

Minocycline (Minocin)

Moxifloxacin (Avelox, Vigamox)

Tetracycline (Sumycin)

Anticonvulsants

Pregabalin (Lyrica) (Not a drug mugger; this boosts potassium levels.)

Antacids

Aluminum and magnesium hydroxide (Maalox, Mylanta)

Aluminum carbonate gel (Basaljel)

Aluminum hydroxide (Amphojel, AlternaGEL)

Calcium carbonate (Tums, Titralac, Rolaids)

Magnesium hydroxide (Phillips' Milk of Magnesia)

Sodium bicarbonate (Alka-Seltzer, baking soda)

Antigout

Colchicine (Colcrys)

Antivirals

Delavirdine (Rescriptor)

Foscarnet (Foscavir)

Lamivudine (Epivir)

Nevirapine (Viramune)

Zidovudine, AZT (Retrovir)

Zidovudine and lamivudine (Combivir)

Blood Pressure Drugs

Hydralazine (Apresoline)

ACE inhibitors:

Enalapril and HCTZ (Vaseretic)

Angiotensin II receptor blockers:

Telmisartan and HCTZ (Micardis HCT)

Valsartan (Diovan)

Valsartan and HCTZ (Diovan HCT)

Calcium-channel blockers:

Nifedipine (Procardia)

Verapamil (Calan, Verelan)

Diuretics, loop:

Bumetanide (Bumex)

Ethacrynic acid (Edecrin)

Furosemide (Lasix)

Torsemide (Demadex)

Diuretics, thiazide:

Any combination drug that contains HCTZ or

hydrochlorothiazide (dozens of drugs contain this)

Atenolol and chlorthalidone (Hygroton)

Chlorothiazide (Diuril)

Chlorthalidone (Hygroton)

Hydrochlorothiazide or HCTZ (Hydrodiuril)

Methyclothiazide (Enduron)

Metolazone (Zaroxolyn)

Diuretics, sulfonamide:

Indapamide (Lozol)

Diuretics, potassium-sparing diuretics (Possibly; however, this is not conclusive.)

Bronchodilators

Albuterol (syrup, tablets, nebulizer solution and inhalers like Ventolin, ProAir, and Proventil)

Corticosteroids

Dexamethasone (Decadron)

Hydrocortisone (Cortef)

Methylprednisolone (Medrol)

Prednisolone (Pediapred liquid)

Prednisone (Sterapred)

Inhaled corticosteroids:

Budesonide (Rhinocort)

Fluticasone (Flonase)

Glaucoma

Acetazolamide (Diamox)

Hormone Replacement Therapy/ Oral Contraceptives

Estrogen-containing drugs

Estrogens, conjugated (Premarin, Premphase, Prempro)

Immunosuppressants

Cyclosporine (Sandimmune)

Tacrolimus (Prograf)

Laxatives

Bisacodyl (Dulcolax)

Long-Acting Beta Agonists (LABAs)

Salmeterol (Serevent inhaler and Advair diskus)

Parkinson's Drugs

Levodopa and carbidopa (Sinemet)

Stool Softeners

Docusate and casanthranol (Peri-Colace)

Miscellaneous

Alcohol

Cesium supplements

Coffee, tea, and soda (caffeinated)

Excessive salt intake

Insulin

Stinging nettle herb

White willow bark

Potassium: Put This on Your Plate

Swiss chard, tomato puree, figs, currants, seeds, mushrooms, spinach, romaine lettuce, celery, beets (boiled), beet greens, mustard greens, fennel, broccoli, winter squash, blackstrap molasses, grilled snapper, mackerel, eggplant, kale, brussels sprouts, turmeric, asparagus, cauliflower, apricots, potatoes, raisins, ginger, yams, kiwifruits, chile peppers (dried), adzuki beans, cabbage, barley, bananas, oranges, avocados, watermelon, kidney beans, pistachios, prunes, and salt substitutes.

An Absurdly Inexpensive Way to Feel Better

Even though hypokalemia (low potassium) is far more dangerous to your heart than hyperkalemia, it's all too easy to get yourself in trouble with potassium supplements if you also take prescribed medications or have a chronic illness. In these situations, it's best to concentrate on food sources if you feel you need an additional supply of this mineral or to consult with your doctor before taking large doses of potassium.

For general health: 200–400 mg per day with food and plenty of water

Drug mugger dose: 300–1,000 mg per day (Consult your physician for proper dosage.)

1 cup acorn squash: 900 mg

1 banana: 450 mg

1 cup watermelon: 550 mg

½ cup raisins: 550 mg

8 ounces Gatorade: 30–40 mg

Just So You Know

Do not crush or chew tablets that are extended-release supplements, such as Slow-K or Klor-Con. Take all doses of potassium with a full glass of water or juice. It's better to take small doses throughout the day rather than one big dose. Always follow the label directions on your formula regardless of the dosages that are provided here. The dosages in this book are provided as general information, but individual needs vary widely.

You know you are getting too much potassium if you develop diarrhea, nausea, stomach pain, or confusion. Some people who exceed normal doses or have poor gut integrity experience darkened, tarry stools—a sign that GI bleeding has occurred. You should stop taking potassium immediately and call your doctor if this happens. Other warning signs that you are getting too much potassium include slow heartbeat; numbness; anxiety; fatigue; heaviness of the legs; and tingling in the hands, feet, or lips. Another word of caution: Some drugs, such as ACE inhibitors, heparin, beta-blockers, and NSAIDs, increase potassium.

Install a Nutrient Security System

When you lose potassium, you often lose protein in the body as well. One way to improve these simultaneous losses is to make a smoothie that contains both. It's yummy and good for you! Just put all of these ingredients in your blender and give it a whirl:

1 banana (or 5 pitted apricots)

1 cup orange juice (fresh squeezed if possible)

½ cup fresh or frozen strawberries (or raspberries)

**1 scoop whey protein powder (hemp or rice protein powder if you
prefer vegan)**

What's in My Cupboard?

Potassium Amino Acid Complex by Solgar: These veggie caps are kosher and contain 99 mg of potassium in a bioavailable amino acid complex. This product is sugar free, gluten free, and dairy free.

Potassium Gluconate 99 by GNC: These are vegetarian caps and are kosher. They contain 99 mg of potassium per capsule. GNC also makes an intelligent formula that contains potassium and magnesium in a 1:1 ratio. It's called **Potassium and Magnesium Aspartate 250.**

Potassium Gluconate by NOW: Each teaspoonful (3.48 grams) of this powder contains 540 mg of potassium, which can be taken once daily with food. You can add a little to your bathwater for additional absorption through your skin. Check with your doctor about dosage.

Potassium Plus by Enzymatic Therapy: This innovative blend provides food-grade potassium from the juices of oranges and sugarcane. It also provides a wonderful combination of trace minerals, including selenium, silicon, boron, nickel, and tin. You need these minerals for healthy blood pressure as well as bone health. If that isn't good enough, it also contains B_6 and pantothenic acid (vitamin B_5), which help reduce cholesterol and homocysteine while raising your energy level. This blend is perfect for blood pressure and heart health!

Probiotics

You've probably heard the word *probiotic* or seen the words *live active cultures* on yogurt containers. These are popular terms found on food and supplement labels to describe living bacteria that your digestive tract needs for good health.

Let's back up. You may not have even realized that you have good bacteria in your intestinal tract. You weren't born with them. In fact, at birth you had a weak immune system and no bacteria at all living inside you. When you started to consume food for the first time—mother's milk and other foods introduced later—you also ingested beneficial bacteria that attached themselves to your gut wall and started to grow. They helped you build a strong immune system.

During your childhood, a healthy camp of good bacteria naturally took up residence in your gut. As a young adult, you are supposed to have trillions of these helpful microorganisms living in your gut. Your camp of intestinal flora is like a fingerprint. No other human on Earth has the same exact camp of microorganisms. Good bacteria protect you from bad bacteria. It's shocking, but a healthy gut should have about 3 pounds of normal intestinal flora. A 2009 study published in the *Journal of Evolutionary Biology* and conducted at the University of Arizona College of Medicine found that some of the healthy flora is stored in the appendix, which had long been thought to be useless. People without an appendix need to be vigilant about creating and maintaining a constant camp of flora because they have lost their storage unit.

The good bacteria colonize the entire surface of our intestinal tracts and affect every single aspect of our health. In fact, people with enough healthy bacteria in their guts are less likely to develop heartburn, gas, diarrhea, and constipation. The good news is that if for some reason you don't have this colony of happy campers in your gut, if something has happened to wipe them out—more on this in a moment—you can introduce them with a probiotic supplement. This supplement is helpful for anyone with any type of gastrointestinal complaint. In fact, I think everyone should take probiotics if they are willing to take one supplement a day.

Probiotic supplements contain many different strains of bacteria, but they all generally come from two genuses, either *Lactobacillus* or *Bifidobacterium*. These two groups are known to regulate the immune response by increasing secretory immunoglobulin A (IgA), which means that they strengthen your ability to fight off germs. They also reduce dangerous inflammatory chemicals in your body, produce antimicrobial substances, improve the gut's mucosal lining (which may prevent food allergies), modulate gene expression, and, in a process known as decreasing pathogen adhesion, prevent pathogens from infecting the gut.

Why do I tell you all this scientific stuff when we are just talking about gut bugs? Because I want you to have enough information to inform your health-care practitioners of your desire to supplement with probiotics, and why. These bacteria are very, very important to people with chronic illnesses, but virtually everything you put in your mouth, from foods to drugs, will mug beneficial bacteria. In my book, restoring these friendly organisms is key to optimal health. Getting your individual camp to flourish is better than taking doses of probiotics into your system that your body may not even recognize.

If you want to learn more about this important topic, follow the work of Doug Kaufmann, the host of the *Know the Cause* television program (www.knowthecause.com) and the author of numerous books on the subject, including *The Fungus Link to Health Problems* and *Infectious Diabetes*. His books offer life-changing information that can help you restore good health. Within a minute of meeting Doug, you know you are in the presence of someone special who genuinely cares about your health and wants to make your life better. Watch him on TV and you'll see exactly what I mean. Some of our TV shows together are posted at his Web site, and I do a medical minute on his show now, too.

When I interviewed Doug Kaufmann for this book, he talked about fires, as in the kind that burn down forests! Just go with him on this, as it's a fantastic way to look at your gut:

"Reforestation is the necessary process of landscape restoration that occurs when fire burns through the natural terrain of a forest. Soon thereafter, in an effort to save not only the terrain of the forest itself, but the wildlife, forest keepers quickly plant new fledgling indigenous trees and plants. Disease in the forest and the animals will be successfully abated by this process.

"Why hasn't anyone thought of restoring the terrain of the intestines after a similar 'fire'? Antibiotics are analogous to the forest fire because life-forms (bacteria) are destroyed. Unbeknownst to many physicians, antibiotics are most often poisonous fungal by-products called mycotoxins. I have long contended that intestinal damage caused by antibiotics often comes back to haunt a patient long after the antibiotic therapy has stopped.

"I suspect that serious systemic diseases known to be caused by mycotoxins could be averted if doctors would understand the importance of mandating *pro*biotics with each and every *anti*biotic prescribed. If you have ever taken antibiotics and now suffer from any number of symptoms and/or diseases, a 30-day trial run of probiotics and a grain-free diet should be instituted. It seems that even the human body needs to 'go green' with regard to reforestation!"

Antibiotics save lives and I like them as a class of drugs, but they are the worst drug muggers of beneficial bacteria. If you've ever taken an antibiotic, you've decimated your healthy camp of bacteria; the antibiotic goes off like a shotgun in your gut. That's not an excuse to stop taking your antibiotic, though. Naturally, you need them if you can't fight off dangerous infections yourself. But I personally think the entire category of antibiotics should be renamed *Normalfloricus stupidicus*. They are stupid because they can't distinguish the good guys from the bad guys, so they kill everything in sight, normal flora included. That's why you end up with diarrhea, cramps, vaginal yeast infections, or jock itch every time you take an antibiotic.

When you need to take an antibiotic, you should supplement with a probiotic to replenish what the drug mugger steals. While I realize that antibiotics destroy the beneficial bacteria—including a probiotic supplement—I still recommend that you take a supplement even while you're on your course of antibiotics. By doing this, you reseed the gut with healthy flora and can significantly reduce the gastrointestinal side effects of the drug therapy. Basically, you are just running damage control. It may translate into getting softer stools on day 10, rather than terrible cramps and diarrhea on day 4.

I recommend that you take probiotics at least twice a day, but more often if you want to. If you can get only two doses in, take the first one 4 to 6 hours after your morning antibiotic dose, and again at night 2 hours after your last antibiotic dose (if you take the antibiotic at night, that is).

Studies conducted on lactobacillus GG, a special strain of bacterium, showed that the supplement reduced antibiotic-induced diarrhea. However, I recommend probiotic supplements every day, not just during antibiotic usage.

You need to have normal flora to help you digest and absorb your food. A person with a lot of beneficial bacteria has a stronger immune system because these small friends neutralize many dangerous and cancer-causing substances. When you have a healthy camp of bacteria in your gut, dangerous organisms can't take over so easily. Without enough beneficial flora, you wind up with an overgrowth of *Candida albicans* yeast, gut dysbiosis, *Escherichia coli,* parasites, and other bad bugs. People who lack beneficial flora frequently experience yeast infections, urinary tract infections, skin problems, fatigue, jock itch, irritable bowel syndrome, belching, diarrhea, heartburn, and chronic fatigue.

Most people who don't have enough good bacteria inside them experience a lot of gas, bloating, or cramps after eating. Did I say gas? Yes, a lot of that! People tend to get used to these symptoms and chalk them up to irritable bowel syndrome, or perhaps bad genetics, so I want to emphasize the importance of probiotics. Having healthy levels of intestinal flora can help you feel better and may, in some cases, relieve bowel conditions like those I mentioned above as well as constipation.

Remember, it's not just the following list of drug muggers that can create an imbalance in your intestinal tract. Stress, illness, junk foods, sugary foods, alcohol, and coffee also tilt your gut flora in the wrong direction.

The lactobacillus and bifidobacterium strains are the most popular of the probiotic supplements you find in health food stores. They help your body make B vitamins such as biotin, folic acid, B_6, B_{12}, and niacin, among others. They also can increase the bioavailability of minerals such as magnesium, iron, copper, and manganese. The added minerals are important and help boost mood, improve immunity, increase energy, stabilize blood pressure, and regulate heart rhythm. Beneficial bacteria also help maintain a healthy pH, which is slightly acidic, between 5.5 and 6.5. The slightly acidic environment is conducive for the friendly microorganisms and helps to drive out the harmful ones. This means a healthy environment for your beneficial bacteria to grow and thrive. Good bacteria help process estrogen and thyroid hormones, so indirectly they can help ease menopausal symptoms and protect against breast cancer.

When it comes to picking a supplement, you need to understand the terms on product labels. Living bacteria in supplements are often measured in CFUs, or colony-forming units. Taking 10 billion to 40 billion CFUs per day is not uncommon, but 1 billion to 5 billion units is more typical. More is not better, because you don't want an unfavorable reaction. Supplements commonly contain 5 to 15 different strains of friendly bacteria, but even though they are considered harmless, you may be allergic to them because they are not part of your flora fingerprint. You may find some of the following names on your product: *Lactobacillus acidophilus, L. paracasei, L. rhamnosus, Bifidobacterium lactis, B. bifidum,* and many others. CFU is a bit of a marketing concept. The CFU doesn't matter to me as much as that you take a probiotic that is alive and viable.

Drug Muggers of Beneficial Bacteria

This list could fill a book. Pretty much anything that goes into your mouth (meaning processed foods, alcohol, and medications) can destroy the gut flora so to save space I am just summarizing. Consider probiotic replenishment the foundation of getting better. Take a high-quality brand to strengthen your immune system and to help you digest all the other foods and vitamins that you take each day.

Acid Blockers
  All

Antacids
  All

Antibiotics
  All

Antivirals
  All

Hormone Replacement Therapy/ Oral Contraceptives
  All estrogen-containing drugs

OTC Medicines
  Virtually all

Prescription Medicines
  *Virtually all

SERMs (Selective Estrogen Receptor Modulators—used for breast cancer)

Sulfonamides (Sulfa antibiotics, some diabetes medications)

Miscellaneous
  Estrogen dominance
  Many herbal products that disrupt integrity in the GI tract
  Nutrients like prescription-strength folic acid, Lovaza, Nephro-vite, and prenatals
  Vitamin K (phylloquinone) found in some multivitamins

*The drug muggers list would take a hundred pages if I were to list all of them.

Probiotics: Put This on Your Plate

In most chapters so far I have offered a list of foods, but with probiotics it's a little more complicated. Allow me to share with you a couple of the most important foods to add to your diet—kombucha tea and kefir.

   Drinking kombucha (kombu) tea is a new health craze. Some health food stores carry it or can order it for you. It's almost like drinking vinegar or sparkling apple cider to me. You get used to the taste, and some brands taste really good. It's fermented tea (*Camellia sinensis*), and it's superpacked with probiotics. I think kombucha is a notch up from kefir because it also contains some healthy organic acids, vitamins, minerals, and enzymes and there is no dairy. It contains all the B vitamins, which give you energy and help you process fats and carbs. It also contains vitamin C, a strong immune system booster.

Research has shown that kombucha may have antibiotic-like effects against harmful bacteria (like *E. coli*) and dangerous fungi. If you have *C. albicans* or multiple allergies, I would pass on this drink because we can't predict how you will react to the multitude of various bacteria and yeasts in kombucha. Others can drink it anytime, but be warned, it can spark energy. That's a good thing.

Kefir is a sort of fermented milk. As you just saw with kombucha, fermented foods can be good for us. Think of it as liquid yogurt. It contains enzymes and lots of friendly microorganisms to help the ecosystem of your gut thrive. Drink kefir on an empty stomach any time of day.

Speaking of yogurt, you probably already know that the right kind of yogurt is replete with healthy, friendly bacteria. What's the right kind? Preferably one that's homemade or from the farmers' market. Store-bought yogurt sometimes contains beneficial bacteria, but it also may contain additives or colorants. Many of these products are laden with sugar and candylike toppings. That very likely means that the probiotics inside will be rendered useless. That's because fruit additives and sweeteners may kill off the bacteria after the product has been on the shelf. If you want fruit on your yogurt, it's better to wash fresh organic blueberries or strawberries and put them there yourself.

Store-bought yogurt is okay as long as it says "live active cultures" and is plain—no artificial sweeteners, sugar, colors, candy, or added fruits. I really hesitate to recommend manufactured yogurt because I know that you will go straight to the store and buy yourself a great big tub of Double Dutch Brownie Caramel Fudge Banana Split Yogurt with sprinkles on top. I really want you to buy it plain, which is important because you want your yogurt to contain living cultures of probiotic strains, not dead bacteria that have been killed off by all the sugar and flavorings, not to mention pasteurization, which also kills off those live active cultures. Let's not go there today. Trust me on this. Plain yogurt is better than processed kinds, and supplements are a step up from that. I'd prefer that you buy plain yogurt or kefir since these are sure to contain live active cultures that actually are alive. Sauerkraut, preferably organic and raw, is another healthy choice.

An Absurdly Inexpensive Way to Feel Better

For general health: 10–40 billion CFU per day, on an empty stomach. Take it 4 hours away from medicine and 2 hours away from food if possible. Many people find that taking it at bedtime works best.

Drug mugger dose: Take probiotics one to three times daily on an empty stomach.

Just So You Know

It's virtually impossible to overdose on probiotics, but you may be getting too much if you start to develop gas or other intestinal symptoms. Remember, these supplements are supposed to relieve intestinal problems, not cause them. If you experience any discomfort at all, it may be related to a die-off reaction of the bad bugs. It shouldn't last more than 3 days. Not all brands are created equal, and some contain starch, gluten, fillers, and prebiotics, which may be upsetting to a few sensitive people. Prebiotics are different from probiotics. They are basically just food for the probiotics, or beneficial bacteria. Prebiotics are nondigestible substances that stimulate the growth of certain bacterial flora species such as bifidobacteria and lactobacilli. Probiotics flourish in the presence of prebiotics, so some supplements combine the two. That said, some people are sensitive to this additive and get sicker from the combo. This discomfort is the result of your taking a probiotic that contains microorganisms that are not natural to your own camp. If you recall, at the outset of this chapter, I said that each human has a unique fingerprint of flora. So when you take a probiotic that is perceived as foreign to your own individual camp, your immune system wakes up and starts attacking your body to get rid of these new and "dangerous" gut bugs. This is why it's best to take probiotics (and prebiotics) that allow your own camp to flourish. It's better than taking a smorgasbord of foreign gut bugs. Dr. Ohhira's Probiotics is a good choice if this is a concern for you. (See "What's in My Cupboard?" below.) Some examples of prebiotics you might see on a formula label include: lactulose, lactitol oligo-fructose (and sc-FOS), inulin, galactooligosaccharides (GOS), tagatose, iso-maltooligosaccharides, polydextrose, and digestion-resistant maltodextrin.

Install a Nutrient Security System

Most consumers think that taking a probiotic is all they need to do, and they just randomly pick any one of dozens on the store shelf. But the bacterial strain matters because you have a flora fingerprint. Certain strains are more helpful than others at beating particular issues, so learn to be choosier if you want to install a good security system for your body. More specifically, if you are trying to prevent allergic responses and asthma attacks, then *L. reuteri* has been shown to help. If you are riddled with *C. albicans* or gut dysbiosis and get yeast infections all the time, then perhaps the friendly yeast *Saccharomyces boulardii* is your best bet. *S. boulardii* is also strongly recommended for preventing antibiotic-associated diarrhea and traveler's diarrhea, according to a review article published in the *World Journal of Gastroenterology* in 2010. This meta-analysis of 27 trials including 5,029 patients showed that *S. boulardii* was significantly effective (and safe) in 84 percent of the randomized, placebo-controlled treatments. You can buy *S. boulardii* by that name or as the brand Florastor. And if *Helicobacter pylori* (known to cause ulcers) is your problem bug, then products containing *L. salivarius* could help. And if you have an autoimmune disorder, your best supplements might be Nutrex Hawaii's Spirulina Pacifica, Dr. Ohhira's brand, vitamin B_{12}, and low doses of melatonin.

What's in My Cupboard?

Probiotic supplements should be purchased with care because if you're not taking live active cultures, you may not be getting the very best effect, although some Israeli research suggests that even carcasses of dead lactic acid bacteria are beneficial in certain persons. Probiotic supplements are very fussy. They're sort of fragile because they are so sensitive to heat, light, oxygen level, and loud noise.

So Delicious Coconut Milk Yogurt by Turtle Mountain: It's in my fridge because it's dairy free and soy free and really yummy. The company does not use artificial sweeteners or artificial colors. It contains six live and active cultures including *L. bulgaricus, S. thermophilus, L. plantarum,* and others. I don't rely on this for my probiotic supplementation, though.

Pro-Bio by Enzymedica: I often recommend the Enzymedica line because they are high-quality supplements with no fillers. This enteric-coated product contains various strains of probiotics that are guaranteed potent at room temperature (many supplements require refrigeration). The capsules are small and easy to swallow. One of the strains in Pro-Bio is *Bacillus subtilis,* which is the source of an enzyme, nattokinase, that supports heart health and circulation. It is one of the most useful heart-healthy strains in the world and can also improve intestinal flora. The other living strains in this brand improve immune function, digestion, and detoxification, and help you manufacture essential enzymes and vitamins. It is sold at health food stores nationwide, or visit www.enzymedica.com.

Dr. Ohhira's Probiotics by Essential Formulas: This product was developed by a Japanese microbiologist and his team. It contains a synergistic blend of living beneficial bacteria along with amino acids, vitamins, minerals, organic acids, and bacteriocins. The beneficial bacteria remain with their original food source to stimulate growth and create the perfect environment for your own beneficial bacteria—what I call your flora fingerprint. Dr. Ohhira's probiotics are safe for the entire family, although the dosage changes from children to adults. The product is vegetarian and never genetically modified. It is free of gluten, soy, and dairy.

Primal Defense HSO Probiotic Formula by Garden of Life: This is Jordan Rubin's whole food blend of probiotics. He is the author of *The Maker's Diet.* This brand contains the nutrients and beneficial bacteria that you would normally get from healthy soils, those that are untouched by pesticides, herbicides, and other chemicals. The product contains 14 species of hardy, nondairy organisms that survive stomach acid and bile.

Saccharomyces boulardii by NutriCology: This particular brand of *S. boulardii* is found in the fridge in most health food stores. This company has a lot of integrity. Its product is very pure and may be an excellent addition to any probiotic supplementation because it is a yeast and we need friendly yeast, too. *S. boulardii* has nothing to do with *C. albicans* strains. In fact, this dietary supplement can help you beat *C. albicans* infections by running them out of the house. It has been extensively studied and found to support gastrointestinal health and to increase secretory IgA, which improves immunity. There are no preservatives or diluents in this brand, and it's hypoallergenic.

Probiotic All-Flora by New Chapter: This product is organic and contains nine strains of live probiotics cultured together on a nondairy, whole food base. The makers combine the live bacteria with growth-promoting prebiotics to feed the probiotics so they work better. The prebiotics come from organic apples and organic inulin sourced from Jerusalem artichokes. The bacteria strains in this blend provide billions of units per dosage; the strains used are *Streptococcus thermophilus*, *Lactobacillus rhamnosus*, *Bacillus breve*, *L. acidophilus*, *B. infantis*, *B. longum*, *L. plantarum*, *L. salivarius*, and *L. helveticus*. The product is gluten free, but it does contain fermented soy and fish.

Kyo-Dophilus Probiotics Plus Enzymes by Kyolic: This product is used in thousands of hospitals and university research centers. Kyolic manufactures this high-quality product from three specially cultured, nondairy, heat-stable strains of friendly bacteria. The trio survives stomach acid. I really like the fact that this product does not require refrigeration for stability, as many probiotics do. This supplement provides digestive enzymes to help you break down your meals, in addition to the probiotics. It could be helpful for people with nonspecific digestive problems. It contains *L. acidophilus*, *Bifidobacterium bifidum*, and *B. longum*.

Spirulina Pacifica by Nutrex Hawaii: Spirulina contains a host of naturally occurring probiotics that will also help you manufacture your own.

Pyridoxine (Vitamin B$_6$)

Pyridoxine makes us happy! Also known as vitamin B$_6$, this nutrient is really important when it comes to boosting your mood, improving your sleep, and nourishing your entire nervous system. It accomplishes all this because it boosts levels of serotonin, GABA, and dopamine, all three of which are happy brain chemicals that support healthy mood, relaxation, and sleep. In fact, pyridoxine is one of the most important B vitamins in the body because it also helps you make red blood cells and create energy. If you've been diagnosed with iron deficiency anemia, there's a good chance that your anemia could be related to a vitamin B$_6$ deficiency, not a true iron deficiency, as is sometimes mistakenly thought.

Vitamin B$_6$ also nourishes your nerves. Ironically, too much of it can damage the nerves. This nutrient is often recommended for peripheral neuropathy, the nerve damage associated with diabetes and shingles. Sometimes it is recommended (along with physical therapy) for carpal tunnel syndrome, the painful wrist condition that can develop in people doing jobs that require repetitive motion.

Pyridoxine's therapeutic benefits do not stop there. Vitamin B$_6$ is so good at soothing the nerves and the entire central nervous system that some physicians recommend it for women with strong PMS symptoms and tearfulness around the time of their periods. I often recommend it for PMS, and many of my clients report that their breast tenderness is relieved and their mood improved.

If you would like to give pyridoxine's PMS-relieving benefits a try, research suggests taking a dose of about 50 to 100 mg of vitamin B$_6$ per day for 2 weeks before your menses is to begin. If fibrocystic breast pain is an issue for you, I can't help but mention that both natural progesterone cream and iodine supplements are used to relieve that. These supplements may reduce your risk for breast cancer if they are dosed properly and good-quality supplements are used. These are sold over the counter at health food stores.

Scientific studies support pyridoxine's role in breast health. There are several reasons that I've reached that conclusion. The most obvious is that vitamin B$_6$ helps reduce homocysteine, a known cancer-causing chemical in the body. High homocysteine is known to contribute to the formation of estrogen-induced breast cancer and most other cancers, if not all. In 2003, Harvard researchers published a study in the *Journal of the National Cancer Institute* that concluded that a diet high in vitamin B$_6$ (and folate) could offer some protection against breast cancer. This didn't surprise me. After all, these B vitamins help make DNA, your basic genetic code. The study followed 121,700 females (nurses, actually) and looked at lifestyle risk factors from 1976 to 2003. Of the 712 nurses who developed breast cancer, researchers found that they had lower levels of folic acid in their blood. They also found that women with a higher intake of vitamin B$_6$ and higher blood levels of this vitamin had a lower incidence of breast cancer.

Our sex hormones estrogen, progesterone, and testosterone are kept in check by vitamin B$_6$ (and folate). This means that they are less likely to exert excessive or toxic effects in the presence of sufficient vitamin B$_6$. Your vitamin B$_6$ status plays an important role in preventing diseases driven by these hormones, such as breast and prostate cancer. If you want to learn how to protect yourself from these conditions, please refer to my e-book *Breast Cancer Protection* available on my Web site, www.dearpharmacist.com. It is only about 50 pages long, but it's extremely comprehensive. Taking vitamin B$_6$ is just one of many ways you can reduce risk.

Vitamin B$_6$ also protects the heart by lowering the homocysteine level. Homocysteine damages arteries feeding the heart, making it easier for blood to clump together into clots and clog up the arteries. Vitamin B$_6$ is critical for anyone facing heart disease or atherosclerosis.

Drug muggers that rob this nutrient leave you more susceptible to heart disease. Love a good steak several times a week? Listen up, because vitamin B$_6$ is needed to break down protein found in meats and dairy products. The more animal protein you consume, the more vitamin B$_6$ you should take.

Pyridoxine is water soluble, so it gets into many water-based cells in your body, but not into the fatty tissues. Like other B vitamins, it cannot be stored, so you will need to make sure that you get enough vitamin B_6 on a daily basis whether through foods, supplements, or both.

If you become deficient in this vital nutrient, you could experience weakness, mental confusion, depression, insomnia, or PMS. Pregnant women may experience more nausea as a result of being shy on vitamin B_6.

Like niacin, pyridoxine is a mild tranquilizer, so if you run low, you may feel irritable and nervous or you may not sleep well at night. All this makes you feel even more tired the next day, and of course the insomnia persists. It becomes a vicious cycle.

You may also become anemic if you don't get enough pyridoxine. Remember, vitamin B_6 helps you make red blood cells. Some people who are deficient notice problems with their skin and develop lesions or seborrheic dermatitis. Some also experience mouth pain, tongue sores, or tongue discoloration.

Since B_6 helps you make red blood cells, it makes sense that running low on B_6 could lead to iron deficiency anemia, and that, my friends, is a leading cause of hypothyroidism. Hypothyroidism is a factor in the development of diabetes. So now you may understand why I wrote this book. Replenishing one nutrient can spare you years of suffering and a medication merry-go-round.

Drug Muggers of Pyridoxine (Vitamin B_6)

Acid Blockers

Cimetidine (Tagamet)

Esomeprazole (Nexium)

Famotidine (Pepcid and Pepcid Complete)

Lansoprazole (Prevacid 24HR)

Nizatidine (Axid)

Omeprazole (Prilosec OTC)

Pantoprazole (Protonix)

Rabeprazole (Aciphex)

Ranitidine (Zantac)

Antacids

Aluminum and magnesium hydroxide (Maalox, Mylanta)

Aluminum carbonate gel (Basaljel)

Aluminum hydroxide (Amphojel, AlternaGEL)

Calcium carbonate (Tums, Titralac, Rolaids)

Magnesium hydroxide (Phillips' Milk of Magnesia)

Sodium bicarbonate (Alka-Seltzer, baking soda)

Antibiotics (just a few examples)

Amoxicillin (Amoxil, Augmentin)

Azithromycin (Z-Pak)

Cefaclor (Ceclor)

Cefdinir (Omnicef)

Cephalexin (Keflex)

Ciprofloxacin (Cipro)

Clarithromycin (Biaxin)

Doxycycline (Doryx)

Erythromycin (E.E.S.)

Isoniazid (INH)

Levofloxacin (Levaquin)

Lomefloxacin (Maxaquin)

Minocycline (Minocin)

Moxifloxacin (Avelox, Vigamox)

Sulfamethoxazole and trimethoprim (Bactrim Septra)

Tetracycline (Sumycin)

Anticonvulsants

Phenytoin (Phenytek)

Aromatase Inhibitors for breast cancer

Anastrozole (Arimidex)

Barbiturates

Blood Pressure Drugs

Hydralazine (Apresoline)

ACE inhibitors:

Enalapril and HCTZ (Vaseretic)

Diuretics, loop:

Bumetanide (Bumex)

Ethacrynic acid (Edecrin)

Furosemide (Lasix)

Torsemide (Demadex)

Diuretics, sulfonamide:

Indapamide (Lozol)

Diuretics, thiazide:

Any combination drug that contains HCTZ or hydrochlorothiazide (dozens of drugs contain this)

Chlorothiazide (Diuril)

Chlorthalidone (Hygroton)

Hydrochlorothiazide or HCTZ (Hydrodiuril)

Methyclothiazide (Enduron)

Metolazone (Zaroxolyn)

Bronchodilators

Albuterol (Proventil, Ventolin, ProAir HFA)

Albuterol and ipratropium (Combivent)

Cycloserine (Seromycin)

Theophylline (Uniphyl, Slo-bid, Theo-24, or Theo-Dur)

Cardiac Glycoside

Digoxin (Lanoxin, Lanoxicaps, Digitek)

Chelating Agent

Penicillamine (Cuprimine)

Cholesterol Agents

Cholestyramine (Questran)

Colesevelam (Welchol)

Colestipol (Colestid)

Corticosteroids (all of them)

Betamethasone (Diprolene, Luxiq)

Cortisone (Cortone Acetate)

Dexamethasone (Decadron)

Fluocinolone (Synalar topical)

Halobetasol (Ultravate topical)

Mometasone (Elocon)

Methylprednisolone (Medrol)

Prednisolone (Pediapred and
    Orapred liquid)

Triamcinolone (Aristocort)

Inhaled corticosteroids:

Budesonide (Rhinocort)

Flunisolide (Nasacort, Nasalide,
    Nasarel)

Fluticasone (Flonase)

Fluticasone and salmeterol (Advair)

Diabetes Medications

Metformin (Fortamet, Glucophage,
    Glucophage XR, Glumetza,
    Riomet)

Metformin and sitagliptin (Janumet)

**Hormone Replacement Therapy/
Oral Contraceptives**

Estradiol (Activella, Climara,
    CombiPatch, Estraderm,
    EstroGel, Menostar, and many
    others)

Esterified estrogens (Estratab)

Estrogen-containing drugs (Estrace,
    Estring, Femring, Menest)

Estrogens, conjugated (Premphase,
    Prempro)

Ethinyl estradiol (Ortho-Novum,
    Triphasil, among others)

Levonorgestrel (found in many
    birth control pills)

MAO Inhibitor Drugs (See
    complete list on page 50.)

**Nonsteroidal Anti-Inflammatory
Drugs, or NSAIDs** (They deplete
other nutrients that are required to
convert B_6 to P5P, such as zinc, and
they deplete other sister B vitamins
like B_{12} and folic acid, as well as C.)

Aspirin (Bayer, Bufferin)

Diclofenac (Voltaren)

Ibuprofen (Advil, Motrin)

Nabumetone (Relafen)

Naproxen (Aleve, Anaprox,
    Naprosyn)

Parkinson's Drugs

Levodopa and carbidopa (Sinemet)
    (Separate from B_6 by 4 to 6 hours
    or ask the doctor about taking a
    supplement.)

SERMs (Selective Estrogen Receptor
Modulators—used for breast
cancer)

Raloxifene (Evista)

Tamoxifen (Nolvadex)

Toremifene (Fareston)

Miscellaneous

Alcohol

Aluminum poisoning

Candida albicans overgrowth

Chelation therapy

Estrogen dominance

Excessive protein intake

Riboflavin drug muggers (since
    riboflavin is needed to activate B_6)

Zinc deficiency

Zinc drug muggers (since zinc is
    needed to activate B_6)

Vitamin B$_6$: Put This on Your Plate

Sprouts, spinach, bell peppers, turnip greens, garlic, yellowfin tuna (baked), cauliflower, mustard greens, beans, bananas, raw celery, cabbage, asparagus, steamed broccoli, turmeric, kale, collard greens, brussels sprouts, watermelon, cod (baked), Swiss chard, and nuts.

An Absurdly Inexpensive Way to Feel Better

The B vitamins are interdependent. In other words, it's very easy to tilt your Bs out of balance. If you take too much pyridoxine, you may become deficient in your other B vitamins. So whenever you take a single B vitamin, it may be wise to take a B complex also so that the other Bs are on board.

For general health: 10–25 mg daily (if you are taking active P5P, then the dose is 5–15 mg daily)

Drug mugger dose: 50 mg once or twice daily (with P5P, the dose is 15–30 mg once or twice daily)

Just So You Know

Because vitamin B$_6$ is so energizing, I suggest taking it in the morning rather than at night. When a food product at the grocery store says that it's been fortified with vitamin B$_6$, they have used pyridoxine hydrochloride, the principal type of B$_6$ found in most supplements. The active, body-ready version is pyridoxal 5'-phosphate (P5P), which is what you get from eating plant-based foods and from converting B$_6$ in your gut with the help of other micronutrients and minerals.

Taking just a plain vitamin B$_6$ supplement is fine for most people. The body goes on to activate the nutrient to its usable form, P5P. For that reason, you will not see brands of vitamin B$_6$ included in my recommended products list. It's widely available and costs pennies per day. The body-ready form of P5P is a smidgen tougher to find, so I've included only those in my list. I have found you brands that are already activated so you can fully and readily absorb them.

Vitamin B_6 is eliminated through the urine (like the other B vitamins), but it is possible to get too much. Having vivid dreams or nightmares is one sign of excessive vitamin B_6. Other signs include numbness, tingling, and other nerve-related problems in the hands, arms, or legs. Any kind of new neurological symptom could mean you are ingesting too much. You may want to switch brands or back off the dosage if you notice these types of side effects. The best way to supplement with vitamin B_6 is to take little doses throughout the day along with a B complex so you have the full spectrum of Bs on board.

Install a Nutrient Security System

One of the most important things you can do to improve your vitamin B_6 security system is to control yeast production in your gut. I'm thinking mainly of *C. albicans*, but there are dozens of other yeasts that could flourish if your GI tract isn't functioning well. What do yeasts have to do with vitamin B_6? They produce a neurotoxin called acetaldehyde that not only wipes out your vitamin B_6, but also depletes another substance (alpha-ketoglutaric acid) that you need to activate vitamin B_6 to its body-ready form, P5P. To control the yeast beast, minimize sugar consumption, and take healthy probiotics and a friendly yeast called *Saccharomyces boulardii* and, if your doctor approves, a little zinc (2 to 5 mg daily). Careful, though, because too much zinc will mug copper.

What's in My Cupboard?

Pyridoxal 5-Phosphate by Metabolic Maintenance: This brand delivers B_6 to you in its active, body-ready form so you can readily absorb the nutrient and put it to work. The capsules are free of fillers, preservatives, and allergens.

Pyridoxal 5-Phosphate by Food Science of Vermont: This is pure P5P. It does not require any activation by the liver and is fully bioavailable in this form. The company offers vegetarian caps with no artificial colors, fillers, or gluten.

B-Complex #6 by Thorne Research: This product contains a full range of B vitamins with higher amounts of P5P. All are also in their active, body-ready forms.

Pyridoxine P5P by Allergy Research Group: This is an allergen-free combination of pyridoxine hydrochloride and P5P (the active form) in case you have trouble activating the pyridoxine. This company specializes in formulating high-quality, allergen-free supplements at affordable prices.

Coenzymated B-6 by Source Naturals: These are sublingual tablets with natural peppermint flavor. This brand allows you to bypass your gut and liver, thereby improving absorption. This product contains the active P5P version of B_6, so it really takes a load off your system in terms of absorbing and activating it. I would suggest this form to recovering alcoholics and to people with yeast issues, liver or pancreatic problems, intestinal malabsorption issues such as celiac or Crohn's disease, or genetic flaws in their ability to activate B_6 to P5P. This is also a good choice for anyone who wants to guarantee better absorption and utilization. It does contain tiny amounts of sorbitol, which some people are sensitive to.

Coenzyme Active B-6 Caps by Country Life: Here's a B_6 product that I'm in love with because each capsule contains 25 mg of active P5P along with 25 mg pyridoxine alpha-ketoglutarate. That last ingredient is a combination of vitamin B_6 and an important biological compound involved in energy production. It's great because your body puts the coenzyme complex to work immediately, directly at the sites of action. Your liver doesn't have to think.

Pyridoxine P5P by NutriCology: This brand offers a high dose of 275 mg per capsule. They split up the contents of the B_6, providing plain pyridoxine hydrochloride and P5P. The advantage to this is that you get a sustained action of sorts because the P5P goes to work right away while your body converts the plain pyridoxine to P5P over the course of a few hours. The dose is rather large, and in my opinion this high-quality product might best be used short-term to build up levels quickly. Take it for a month unless your doctor says otherwise, or take it several times a week (not daily). And, of course, any time you drive one B vitamin very high, it's best to take it along with a B complex.

Riboflavin (Vitamin B₂)

Have you ever taken a multivitamin and then noticed that your urine was fluorescent yellow a few hours later? It's from the riboflavin (or vitamin B₂). The effect is harmless but makes for interesting conversation for 12-year-olds. This phenomenon happens because riboflavin is actually a dye. Its Latin-based name is derived from *ribose,* which means sugar, and *flavus,* which means yellow. In fact, it's used as a colorant in some foods, including baby food, cheese, and cereal. When used this way, it is called E101; the "E" stands for Europe. Because riboflavin really is fluorescent (!) under ultraviolet light, engineers in various industries use it to detect leaks. Don't worry, though, you won't glow in the dark if it's in your system. In fact, it's vital.

As a B vitamin, riboflavin works in concert with the other Bs. It plays a role in your body's creation of energy. Riboflavin supports mitochondrial function. Remember that mitochondria are the tiny powerhouses in each of your cells that create energy from the ATP molecule. Riboflavin also works hard to improve thyroid hormone levels, and that in turn affects metabolism, helping you burn calories. If you already have hypothyroidism (low thyroid hormone), you have a problem converting your riboflavin into a usable form that works for you, so talk to your doctor about taking more of this important B vitamin.

This nutrient also protects your nerves and helps you cope with life if you eat stress for breakfast, lunch, and dinner. It's also helpful if you grind your teeth. Seriously, tooth grinding can occur in people who are stressed out and riboflavin deficient. The reason it works so effectively in this case is because this B vitamin makes your adrenal glands function better and produce anti-stress hormones that help you cope with whatever is going on in your life.

Riboflavin is needed to make the nutrient glutathione, a powerful free radical scavenger. In fact, a doctor can measure glutathione reductase activity in your red blood cells to assess your riboflavin nutritional status. Another way to do this is by testing micronutrients. Women are especially at risk of running low because the many drug muggers of riboflavin include estrogen-containing drugs such as oral contraceptives and hormone replacement therapy.

Riboflavin is great for tired or overweight women, especially those who have migraines, too. This is incredible because millions of dollars are spent on migraine medications that only help temporarily and never solve the problem. One way we think riboflavin works is by supporting mitochondrial function in the brain. Your mitochondria can also be called your powerhouses because they generate energy and burn fat and sugar. Riboflavin is the precursor to two important coenzymes—FAD (flavin adenine dinucleotide) and FMN (flavin mononucleotide). When shopping for riboflavin, you often see references to these two compounds, so get familiar with them. They are life sustaining and absolutely essential in powering the energy-producing mitochondrial chain of events, or what is called the electron transport chain. In other words, the party can't get started producing energy unless enough riboflavin is present and can morph into FAD and FMN. A deficiency of riboflavin starves the brain of oxygen and energy. That's when the migraine pain sets in and you have to call your boss and tell him or her you're down for the count.

Medical science has known about the potential benefits of riboflavin as a treatment for migraines for quite some time. Back in 1998 a randomized, placebo-controlled trial looked at the B vitamin's effect on 55 patients who frequently suffered with migraines. Researchers gave the participants 400 mg of riboflavin every day for 3 months. In terms of headache days, 59 percent of patients improved by at least 50 percent as compared with 15 percent of those taking placebo. The scientists concluded that riboflavin was significantly better than placebo in reducing the number of headaches, though it took almost 3 months for optimal benefits.

Another study of 23 people ages 20 to 65 and published in the 2004 issue of the *European Journal of Neurology* also found that riboflavin helped decrease the frequency of migraines. The aim of this study was to investigate riboflavin's preventive powers. Participants were given 400 mg of riboflavin per day for 3 months, and researchers evaluated headache frequency, duration, and intensity and the need for antimigraine drugs. After 6 months, headache frequency was cut in half and the need for drugs also decreased from 7 pills to an average of 4.5 pills per month. Researchers concluded that "riboflavin is a safe and well-tolerated alternative in migraine prophylaxis."

There are few things worse than chronic head pain. After all, your head is your motherboard, so if this little tidbit of information helps you get your life back, then I'm totally tickled! Riboflavin is cheap and easy to find anywhere. The only thing to remember is that if you take too much of one B vitamin, you tilt your Bs out of balance and can develop a relative deficiency of the others. Taking a B complex may be necessary while you drive up your level of riboflavin. Be sure to read the other chapters about the rest of the B vitamins, too, because you want to be aware of the symptoms of any vitamin deficiency, just in case it happens.

Migraines do seem to occur more frequently in people who are deficient in riboflavin. I recall telling this little secret to a woman named Alice at the pharmacy one evening as I was filling her prescription for Imitrex (sumatriptan), a medication that helps relieve migraines. I suggested riboflavin. Alice took my advice and immediately purchased a bottle. I also told her to stop drinking diet sodas because they contain artificial sweeteners, some of which have been associated with headaches in some people.

Soon after, I received an e-mail from Alice expressing gratitude. For the first time in 7 years, she had gone 6 days in a row without a headache, and she felt more energetic. In her words: "I can now fully enjoy my life again. I feel like I am getting to know my children again after all these years. I can focus on them and play with them, and it is all because of you."

It is really gratifying to help people, and it is wonderful to know that this woman no longer needs to fill her Imitrex prescription every month.

The benefits of riboflavin do not stop there, however. Riboflavin (and biotin) help create luxurious hair, pretty skin, and strong nails. Pregnant women may derive benefit from added riboflavin because it helps the developing fetus grow properly and it prevents pregnancy cramps. A deficiency of riboflavin during pregnancy can increase the risk of pre-eclampsia fivefold. Preeclampsia occurs in 5 to 8 percent of pregnant women and causes high blood pressure in both mom and baby. Riboflavin is found in prenatal vitamins because it may help prevent the condition. Make sure your formula contains it; you can ask your pharmacist. You can also ask your obstetrician-gynecologist whether you need additional ribo-flavin, more than is already in your prescribed formula.

Your body needs riboflavin to help digest foods and activate other B vitamins, such as B_6 and niacin. If you're a big meat eater, you need extra riboflavin to digest the fat and protein in your meals. Riboflavin helps make red blood cells, so if you run out of riboflavin, you may subsequently develop iron deficiency anemia and become fatigued. This is superbly interesting to me because I have known so many people who are iron deficient and can't get better even after taking iron supplements for months and months. I've learned that they either have leaky guts (and can't absorb the supplements from the gut) or, and this is the biggie, they are riboflavin deficient! So listen carefully if you find that you are the poster child for iron deficiency or you know for sure that you have trouble absorbing iron. You should ask your doctor if you can take the higher dosage (like the drug mugger dose) of riboflavin I recommend below, along with your iron supplement.

You don't often hear of riboflavin deficiency because the symptoms are hard to pin down and easy to cover up with medication. For example, some people have a decreased sensitivity to touch, temperature, vibration, or position that may occur in the hands, legs, or feet. It may be very subtle and fly under the radar because they just accept their bizarre circum-stances (which cause no pain). Riboflavin deficiency is fairly common in elderly people and in those with anorexia, bulimia, HIV, inflammatory bowel disorders, chronic diarrhea, celiac disease, diabetes, and heart disease. And, of course, if you push other B vitamins, then you can get a relative deficiency of riboflavin (which can also go unnoticed for months or years).

If you have watery, fatigued, or bloodshot eyes (and it's not because you're up late writing books!), it's possible that you are just short on riboflavin. Riboflavin deficiency can cause tearing, itching, or burning in or around the eyes; blurred vision; and sensitivity to light. If you have a deficiency, people might assume you are hung over or exhausted because your eyes look so bloodshot.

The skin is also affected by riboflavin deficiency. People with a deficiency can develop sores on the tongue or the corners of their lips, which could crack. Their skin may start to dry out or peel, and this can occur anywhere. Redness and rash are very common with a riboflavin deficiency. A rash can sometimes occur in the most unfortunate places, like the groin. Some people use riboflavin supplements to ease rosacea, as it helps prevent pustule formation by improving the skin's tone and secretions.

Drug Muggers of Riboflavin (Vitamin B₂)

Acid Blockers

Cimetidine (Tagamet)

Esomeprazole (Nexium)

Famotidine (Pepcid and Pepcid Complete)

Nizatidine (Axid)

Omeprazole (Prilosec OTC)

Pantoprazole (Protonix)

Ranitidine (Zantac)

Rabeprazole (Aciphex)

Ranitidine (Zantac)

Antacids

Aluminum and magnesium hydroxide (Maalox, Mylanta)

Aluminum carbonate gel (Basaljel)

Aluminum hydroxide (Amphojel, AlternaGEL)

Calcium carbonate (Tums, Titralac, Rolaids)

Magnesium hydroxide (Phillips' Milk of Magnesia)

Sodium bicarbonate (Alka-Seltzer, baking soda)

Antibiotics (all of them, just a few examples here)

Amoxicillin (Amoxil)

Azithromycin (Z-Pak)

Cefaclor (Ceclor)

Cefdinir (Omnicef)

Cephalexin (Keflex)

Ciprofloxacin (Cipro)

Clarithromycin (Biaxin)

Doxycycline (Doryx)

Erythromycin (E.E.S.)

Levofloxacin (Levaquin)

Minocycline (Minocin)

Sulfamethoxazole and trimethoprim (Bactrim Septra)

Anticonvulsants

Phenobarbital (Solfoton)

Antidepressants, Tricyclic

Amitriptyline (Elavil)

Desipramine (Norpramin)

Doxepin (Sinequan)

Imipramine (Tofranil)

Nortriptyline (Pamelor)

Antimetabolites

Methotrexate (Rheumatrex, Trexall)

Antinausea Drugs

Promethazine (Phenergan)

Antivirals

Delavirdine (Rescriptor)

Foscarnet (Foscavir)

Lamivudine (Epivir)

Nevirapine (Viramune)

Zidovudine, AZT (Retrovir)

Zidovudine and lamivudine (Combivir)

Aromatase Inhibitors for breast cancer

Anastrozole (Arimidex)

Blood Pressure Drugs

Diuretics, loop:

Bumetanide (Bumex)

Ethacrynic acid (Edecrin)

Furosemide (Lasix)

Torsemide (Demadex)

Diuretics, potassium-sparing: diuretics (Possibly; however, this is not conclusive.)

Diuretics, sulfonamide:

Indapamide (Lozol)

Diuretics, thiazide:

Any combination drug that contains HCTZ or hydrochlorothiazide (dozens of drugs contain this)

Chlorothiazide (Diuril)

Chlorthalidone (Hygroton)

Hydrochlorothiazide or HCTZ (Hydrodiuril)

Methyclothiazide (Enduron)

Metolazone (Zaroxolyn)

Cancer Drugs

Doxorubicin (Adriamycin)

Hormone Replacement Therapy/ Oral Contraceptives

Estradiol (Estrace, Climara, Estraderm, Estring, Activella, Femring, CombiPatch, EstroGel, Menostar, and many others)

Estradiol and testosterone (Estratest, Depo-Testadiol)

Estrogen-containing drugs, such as oral contraceptives

Estrogens, conjugated (Premphase, Prempro)

Ethinyl estradiol (found in many birth control pills)

Levonorgestrel (found in many birth control pills and Plan B)

Norethindrone (found in many birth control pills)

Psychiatric Drugs

  Chlorpromazine (Thorazine)

  Fluphenazine (Prolixin)

  Haloperidol (Haldol)

  Thioridazine (Mellaril)

  Trifluoperazine (Stelazine)

SERMs (Selective Estrogen Receptor Modulators—used for breast cancer)

  Raloxifene (Evista)

  Tamoxifen (Nolvadex)

  Toremifene (Fareston)

Sulfonamides (Sulfa antibiotics, some diabetes medications)

Miscellaneous

  Alcohol

  Anorexia

  Estrogen dominance

  High dosages of any other B vitamins

Riboflavin: Put This on Your Plate

Dairy products, lean meats, beef liver, crimini mushrooms, spinach, asparagus, Swiss chard, mustard greens, broccoli, collard greens, turnip greens, eggs, whole grains, yogurt, green beans, cabbage, strawberries, cauliflower, goat's milk, raspberries, brussels sprouts, summer squash, tempeh, plums, soybeans (cooked), and almonds.

An Absurdly Inexpensive Way to Feel Better

Unless advised otherwise by your health-care provider, you'll want to get the following doses as part of a B complex supplement. B vitamins work together, and it's easy to tip them out of balance by taking supplements of individual Bs.

  For general health: R5P (riboflavin 5'-phosphate): 50–200 mg per day

  Drug mugger dose: 200–400 mg per day

  Migraines: Usually 200 mg twice daily for 60 days, then reduce to maintenance level of 25–50 mg daily

Just So You Know

Riboflavin may be taken without regard to meals, but most people take their B vitamins with food to maximize absorption and minimize tummy upset. If you enjoy strenuous exercise or have a lot of stress in your life, you will probably need a higher amount than the average person. If you have a genetic polymorphism (a defect of sorts) that prevents you from activating riboflavin to its bioavailable form (R5P), then you'll need to take the active form of this nutrient. You can get genetically tested if you suspect you have this genetic defect. Vitamins you buy in the store aren't active until your body carries out a few chemical reactions on them. Polymorphism prevents this simple process. I'm telling you this because when you buy riboflavin (or CoQ10, pyridoxine, or folic acid), you have two choices. You can buy these nutrients and have your body convert them for you, or you can buy the body-ready form (usually at a lower dose than the precursor). You saw an example of this in Chapter 8 on CoQ10. CoQ10 is widely available, and so is its active body-ready version, ubiquinol. Similarly, when riboflavin is activated in your body, it becomes R5P; you can buy supplements in this activated form, although they are a little harder to find. See my list on page 256.

Riboflavin also helps vision, but taking too much of it could backfire and cause cataracts or poor nighttime vision. Other possible reactions to high doses of riboflavin may include itching, numbness, burning, prickly sensations, and sensitivity to light.

Install a Nutrient Security System

Riboflavin is activated to R5P in the intestines, where it is then absorbed, so having a healthy gut goes a long way toward improving and maintaining your level of this important B vitamin. Probiotic supplements can help keep your gut in a healthy state. In addition, you can't activate riboflavin to R5P without sufficient amounts of digestive acid, which is sold in supplemental form at health food stores (look for betaine hydrochloride or trimethylglycine). You can find out if you make enough stomach acid with a gastrin test, which is a blood test. For more information, see Chapter 17, Probiotics.

What's in My Cupboard?

The B vitamins are interdependent, and it's very easy to tilt your Bs out of balance. If you take too much riboflavin, you may become deficient, so to speak, in your other B vitamins. So whenever you take a single B vitamin, it's wise to also take a B complex so that the other Bs are on board.

B-2 by Source Naturals: These hypoallergenic tablets contain 100 mg of riboflavin. The product is easy to find at health food stores.

B-2 by NOW: This formula offers 100 mg riboflavin in an easy-to-swallow capsule. It is also easy to find at health food stores.

Riboflavin 5' Phosphate by Thorne Research: This is activated riboflavin! If you take this product, your body doesn't have to expend energy to convert plain riboflavin into R5P. The nutrient is instantly bioavailable. This matters for many people who have digestive disorders, take a lot of medicine, or don't have enough acid or normal flora in their intestinal tracts.

Riboflavin-5-Phosphate by Douglas Labs: This, too, is activated riboflavin. This product is sold through your health-care practitioner; it is not found in health food stores or pharmacies. You can search online or have your doctor fax his or her license to Douglas Labs to order it for you.

B-2 by Bluebonnet: This products offers 100 mg riboflavin. It is kosher and free of sugar and allergens such as milk, eggs, fish, wheat, soy, corn, and gluten.

Vitamin B2 by Solgar: These vegicaps contain 100 mg per capsule and are kosher and free of all allergens. This brand is widely available.

Migra-Eeze by Life Extension: This multitasking formula contains a powerful blend of herbs and vitamins designed to help with headaches. Two softgels contain 400 mg riboflavin (some of which is in the body-ready R5P form), along with butterbur and ginger, two herbs known to help reduce the frequency and pain of migraine headaches. This product is free of milk, egg, fish, peanuts, crustaceans, shellfish (lobster, crab, shrimp), tree nuts, wheat, yeast, gluten, corn, rice, and artificial sweeteners, flavors, colors, and preservatives. It is sold online at www.vitacost.com and www.lef.org.

Selenium

Selenium is a trace mineral most commonly known for its role in the thyroid gland. As you probably know, thyroid hormone helps regulate your metabolism, which means it has a great impact on your weight, your energy level, and your mood. A happy thyroid equals a happy person. And a skinny person, too. But the role of selenium does not stop there. A selenium deficiency can lead to heart disease, macular degeneration, cataracts, exhaustion, poor immune function, and frequent infections. A selenium deficiency can also make for a poor ratio of HDL to LDL cholesterol. It protects and boosts your immune system by increasing the number of helpful cells that fight off pathogens while suppressing inflammatory, pain-causing chemicals. And just like its cousin zinc, selenium protects the prostate gland, improves sperm count, and helps men with fertility problems.

The recommended daily amount set by the FDA is 40 to 70 mcg per day for adult males and 45 to 55 mcg for adult females, but based on numerous studies, I feel that a little bit more might be beneficial, especially for people with thyroid problems or poor immune function. Some studies show lower rates of cancer, heart disease, and thyroid disease in people who have healthy levels of selenium. It also appears that people with rheumatoid arthritis who have lower selenium levels tend to experience more pain, stiffness, inflammation, swelling, and loss of mobility in their joints. People with digestive tract problems such as celiac or Crohn's disease or irritable bowel syndrome tend to run out of this mineral quickly.

A number of studies have pointed to the role of selenium in thyroid disease. No surprise there, as the human thyroid gland has the highest concentration of selenium per gram of tissue of all the organs. Most people don't realize this, but our bodies require selenium to produce the powerful antioxidant glutathione. The body has trouble making the enzyme glutathione peroxidase without selenium on board, and this enzyme protects your body from harm by neutralizing dangerous inflammatory and cancer-causing chemicals that act like bullets in the body. This explains why selenium is so helpful to the immune system. It nourishes your thyroid gland and produces chemicals that do good housekeeping on your cells.

Many autoimmune thyroid disorders worsen in the presence of low selenium. When the immune system mistakenly attacks the thyroid gland, a condition known as Hashimoto's disease may result. In this autoimmune form of hypothyroidism, the thyroid gland is slowly destroyed by a person's own immune system. Your doctor will measure your thyroid peroxidase (TPO) antibodies; the higher they are, the more destruction is occurring. Studies show that people with Hashimoto's, who have high TPO antibodies, can benefit from selenium (as well as a gluten-free diet). Supplementing with about 200 mcg of selenium each morning for 3 months could significantly lower antibodies that attack the thyroid gland. One study published in the *Journal of Clinical Endocrinology and Metabolism* in 2002 followed 70 women for 3 months. Nine of the patients in the selenium-treated group had completely normalized antibodies compared with only two patients in the placebo group. Researchers found that in regions with higher incidences of selenium deficiency, more thyroiditis was occurring. This is because less selenium in the body translated into less glutathione peroxidase (the cleanup crew). The researchers said: "Even mild selenium deficiency may contribute to the development and maintenance of autoimmune thyroid diseases."

Selenium is a strong antioxidant that is often employed in treating cancer. Some studies indicate that death rates from lung, colon, rectal, and prostate cancers are lower among people with higher selenium intake. But not all studies regarding selenium and cancer are positive. In January 2009 in the *Journal of the American Medical Association*, for example, researchers published their data on a high-profile cancer study called SELECT, which stands for Selenium and Vitamin E Cancer Prevention Trial. They found no apparent difference in prostate cancer risk between groups of people who supplemented daily either with selenium, vitamin E, both, or placebo. But how strong a conclusion can one draw when this research had so many limitations? For example, they could have used a better form of selenium that had shown clinical benefit in prior trials. They also could have enrolled subjects who were relatively deficient in selenium rather than subjects with normal or higher baseline values. The conclusion is fuzzy from where I sit.

The bottom line is that if you want to take selenium, follow the directions on the label, which usually call for 100 to 200 mcg per day, and if you are dealing with something serious like Hashimoto's, a drug mugging effect, or even pain from pancreatitis, ask your doctor about taking higher dosages, about 400 to 600 mcg per day for a short while (a few months). Selenium seems to be able to block the growth of blood vessels that tumors need for their food supply. So it is able to starve a tumor to death. If you're being treated for cancer, you should discuss selenium supplements with your physician.

It's worth emphasizing that selenium is a powerful immune system booster. People who become deficient in selenium have lower resistance to infections, including viruses. This was shown in a small study done at the University of Liverpool in 2004 that concluded that increased selenium intake helped people clear poliovirus from their systems. I realize that polio and swine flu are completely different infections, but my point is that selenium can increase production of infection-fighting cells (like natural killer cells, which attack cancer, and infection-fighting T cells) and help people fight infections that cause shingles, cold sores, and other types of herpesvirus symptoms, so why not the flu?

A study published in the *Journal of Infectious Diseases* in 2000 looked at selenium's role in people with HIV and concluded that the trace mineral could increase useful immune system chemicals like interleukin-2 while down-regulating (or calming down) the production of neurotoxic chemicals like interleukin-8 and tumor necrosis factor-alpha. In other words, selenium can provide significant protection for people with HIV. Pretty major stuff for one little micronutrient! Bottom line: If you have HIV, it's worth asking your doctor about taking a selenium supplement.

What's important here is that selenium appears to help your body defend itself rather well no matter what kind of challenges your immune system faces.

A more recent article elaborated on the use of selenium and other anti-oxidant supplements (such as resveratrol, vitamin E, and NAC/glutathione) and their effect on the pandemic virus H5N1, also called bird or avian flu. The authors, who published their findings in 2006 in *Medical Hypotheses*, concluded:

> Key mediators in these processes include selenium, vitamin E, NAC/glutathione, resveratrol, and quercetin. Taken prophylactically, and throughout the duration and recovery of an H5N1 infection, the nutritional supplement formula may aid humans infected with H5N1 influenza to survive with a reduced likelihood of major complications, and may provide a relatively low-cost strategy for individuals as well as government, public-health, medical, health-insurance, and corporate organizations to prepare more prudently for an H5N1 pandemic. Some evidence also indicates that the supplement formulation [the authors describe] may be effective as an adjunctive to H5N1 vaccine and anti-viral treatments, and should be tested as such.

These authors are suggesting that a handful of inexpensive nutrients, including selenium, might help some people fend off a pandemic virus. Since swine flu contains some genetic material derived from the bird flu, it stands to reason that selenium could play a role in helping protect people from that virus as well should it ever be revived. Thankfully, by spring 2010, the swine flu blew over, and we apparently won't have to worry too much about that anymore, but other infectious organisms abound. I'm certainly not going to wait for yet another study to tell me that selenium is helpful to my immune system. I'm just going to go ahead and take it. Because I'm relatively healthy and I don't take medications, I take only one bottle of selenium supplements a year, starting in the fall. I don't take the whole bottle at once, of course. I take 1 capsule (200 mcg) daily until the bottle is empty.

Protection against infectious agents is just the tip of the iceberg in what taking a selenium supplement might offer you. If you run low on selenium, you will have more fatigue; a higher level of LDL cholesterol; sticky, thick blood; and mental fatigue, anxiety, and depression. Because it is such a strong antioxidant and can sweep up free radicals, selenium is recommended for people with any kind of cell damage.

I read a National Health and Nutrition Examination Survey that concluded that most Americans obtain adequate selenium from their diets. I disagree. You may not realize this, but we used to get a lot more selenium in our diets than we do now. That's because selenium (and many other important minerals) used to be found in plentiful supply in the soils used to grow our foods. But as a result of industrialization, the use of chemicals and pesticides, and other factors, our soils have become virtually barren of many life-sustaining minerals, including selenium. Because of this, it's possible to run low even if you don't take a drug mugger on the list below.

Steroids deplete minerals, including selenium, magnesium, and zinc. In a 1987 study published in the *Journal of Rheumatology*, patients with rheumatoid arthritis had selenium levels measured, including in the plasma and red blood cells. They were compared to a control group of similar age and sex. High doses of corticosteroid treatment (about 20 to 60 mg of prednisolone per day) correlated to reduced selenium levels in the patients. The reason for this is not entirely clear, but what is clear is that something bad is happening to selenium levels in patients, and selenium is needed for a healthy immune system.

Drug Muggers of Selenium

Acid Blockers

Cimetidine (Tagamet)

Esomeprazole (Nexium)

Famotidine (Pepcid and Pepcid Complete)

Lansoprazole (Prevacid 24HR)

Nizatidine (Axid)

Omeprazole (Prilosec OTC)

Pantoprazole (Protonix)

Rabeprazole (Aciphex)

Ranitidine (Zantac)

Antacids

Aluminum and magnesium hydroxide (Maalox, Mylanta)

Aluminum carbonate gel (Basaljel)

Aluminum hydroxide (Amphojel, AlternaGEL)

Calcium carbonate (Tums, Titralac, Rolaids)

Magnesium hydroxide (Phillips' Milk of Magnesia)

Sodium bicarbonate (Alka-Seltzer, baking soda)

Antidepressants, including Tricyclic and SSRI Medicines

(a few examples)

Amitriptyline (Elavil)

Desipramine (Norpramin)

Fluoxetine (Prozac)

Nortriptyline (Pamelor)

Paroxetine (Paxil)

Sertraline (Zoloft)

Trazodone (Desyrel)

Aromatase Inhibitors for breast cancer

Anastrozole (Arimidex)

Corticosteroids (all of them)

Betamethasone (Diprolene, Luxiq)

Cortisone (Cortone Acetate)

Dexamethasone (Decadron)

Fluocinolone (Synalar topical)

Halobetasol (Ultravate topical)

Mometasone (Elocon)

Methylprednisolone (Medrol)

Prednisolone (Pediapred and Orapred liquid)

Triamcinolone (Aristocort)

Inhaled corticosteroids:

Budesonide (Rhinocort)

Flunisolide (Nasacort, Nasalide, Nasarel)

Fluticasone (Flonase)

Fluticasone and salmeterol (Advair)

Hormone Replacement Therapy/ Oral Contraceptives

Estradiol (Estrace, Climara, Estraderm, Estring, Activella, Femring, CombiPatch, EstroGel, Menostar, and many others)

Estrogen-containing drugs (hormone replacement therapy and birth control)

Estrogens, conjugated (Prempro, Premphase)

Ethinyl estradiol (found in many birth control pills)

SERMs (Selective Estrogen Receptor Modulators—used for breast cancer)

Raloxifene (Evista)

Tamoxifen (Nolvadex)

Toremifene (Fareston)

Sulfonamides (Sulfa antibiotics, indapamide, and some diabetes medications, but this is just a hunch since this class of drugs is known to deplete many other minerals.)

Miscellaneous

Alcohol

Burn victims are at risk for selenium (and vitamin E) depletions

Celiac or Crohn's disease or IBS

Estrogen dominance

Gastric bypass

Gluten-free diet

Heavy metal toxicity (Likely all heavy metals but these for sure)

Cadmium burden (which occurs from smoking)

Mercury burden (which occurs from certain seafood, environmental chemicals, and amalgams)

Selenium: Put This on Your Plate

Food sources include walnuts, tuna, swordfish, herring, shrimp, mollusks, soybeans, corn, wheat, rice, chicken, eggs, cheese, turkey, beef, oatmeal, and vegetables. Brazil nuts have the highest concentration of selenium per gram, so eat a small handful each day.

An Absurdly Inexpensive Way to Feel Better

For general health: Selenium citrate or picolinate, 100 mcg once daily

Drug mugger dose: 100–200 mcg one to three times daily

Just So You Know

Selenium may be taken throughout the day, but if you take it once a day (rather than two or three times), then go ahead and take it in the morning so it can get to work and make some energizing thyroid hormone for you. The forms above are just fine, though some experts feel that when selenium is bound to an amino acid, it has a slight edge in terms of absorption. If you want that form, look for either selenomethionine or selenocysteine. Selenomethionine is an organic form of selenium and is easier to absorb than inorganic selenite forms. In fact, a clinical trial found that selenomethionine is absorbed almost 20 percent better than selenite.

Selenomethionine is the natural way selenium exists in food, so it is my preference. Another version, which is bound to a yeast, is also highly bioavailable. You'll find it listed on labels as "high selenium yeast" or "SelenoExcell." Bear in mind that selenized yeast is really just brewer's yeast that has been grown in selenium-rich broth and then turned into a selenium supplement. It's fine to take, but it probably has gluten in it no matter what the label states. That's because gluten is found in virtually all forms of brewer's yeast.

Selenium doses of greater than 300 to 500 mcg daily can be harmful for some people because they spark production of too much thyroid hormone. You know you are getting too much selenium if you start to lose your hair, become nauseated, vomit, or get abdominal cramps or a racing heart. It's rare, but in some people excessive amounts of selenium (selenosis) manifest as nerve damage, spots on the nails, nausea, and vomiting.

Install a Nutrient Security System

To ensure that you are getting selenium from your foods, it's important to have enough vitamin B_6 on board, specifically pyridoxal 5'-phosphate, the active form of B_6. Whenever you take vitamin B_6, your body converts it to P5P. You can simply purchase P5P in certain proprietary blends. You need to have P5P on board as a cofactor (an assistant) to help get the selenium out of your food. It's sort of like a shuttle. The B_6 also helps make the selenium work better in your body.

Vitamin E also works hand in hand with selenium. So to install the tightest security system, make sure you are getting enough natural vitamins E and B_6. You can eat a lot of leafy greens for the vitamin B_6 and nuts for the vitamin E, or just take supplements labeled "natural vitamin E."

What's in My Cupboard?

Selenium Picolinate by Thorne Research: These capsules deliver 200 mcg per dose in a form of selenium readily absorbed by the body.

Selenium by Nutraceutical Sciences Institute (NSI): This product gives you selenium in the bioavailable amino acid chelated form, selenomethionine, so it's easier on the stomach. Each kosher capsule provides 200 mcg selenium.

E and Selenium Food Complex by New Chapter: This company manufactures a whole food supplement line. Since selenium and vitamin E work better together, this combination is perfect. The formula is easy to digest because it's natural. It's basically food so usually it does not irritate the stomach lining. This particular blend contains turmeric and ginger, two powerful anti-inflammatories, along with spinach extract, blueberry, fenugreek, and other herbs to support health and wellness. Each vegetarian capsule contains 100 mcg of natural selenium and 50 IU of natural vitamin E, which includes the entire family of eight molecules of vitamin E, rather than an isolated form like most other supplements.

SelenoExcell Selenium Yeast 200 mcg by Natural Factors: Each capsule contains 200 mcg in a bioavailable form of organically bound selenium yeast. SelenoExcell is actually the trademarked name for this patented selenium yeast complex, so you may see that name on the labels of other products sold at health food stores. This product contains no artificial preservatives, colors, sweeteners, dairy products, soy, corn, starch, or wheat.

Selenium by Futurebiotics: Each capsule provides 200 mcg of selenium as amino acid chelate. The label states that this product is free of yeast, starch, sugar, salt, wheat, gluten, soy, corn, dairy products, and artificial colors and preservatives.

Selenium 200 by GNC: These tablets contain 200 mcg of Seleno-Excell and are vegetarian friendly and kosher.

Yeast-Free Selenium by Solaray: This is 100 percent organically bound (to methionine) selenium, so it's a highly absorbable chelated version. It is yeast free. I like this brand because you can find it practically anywhere, it's very affordable, and it's easy to digest.

Thiamine (Vitamin B₁)

Thiamine is known as B₁ because it was the first of the B vitamins to be identified by scientists. Like all the other Bs, thiamine works better in concert with its cousins than it does by itself. It's water soluble, which means that you have to take it daily since it is not stored in your cells. A true deficiency of thiamine causes beriberi, a condition that's rare in the United States except in people with alcoholism or chronic diarrhea. More often, people who develop thiamine deficiency fly under the radar with symptoms chalked up to aging rather than to nutritional deficits.

Thiamine is important to the digestive process of breaking down carbohydrates, fats, and protein, so it plays a role in maintaining weight, lowering blood sugar, and reducing cholesterol. This makes it incredibly important to people of all ages.

Although this vital nutrient can be helpful in preventing and treating a whole host of conditions, let's start by dispelling a couple of myths. Some people think that thiamine can repel insects. Some thiamine does get excreted through the skin, and insects are apparently put off by this residue. The theory is that if you have a good enough supply on board, you might be less likely to get bitten. Hmm. If I ever travel to the Amazon River Basin, where insects are the size of small VWs, I won't be counting on thiamine. But I will keep this information in my back pocket, right next to a big flyswatter.

Some misguided people also think that thiamine can prevent motion sickness, for example on a cruise. This reminds me of the last Caribbean cruise I went on. A guest at my table kept saying how dizzy she was from the swaying of the ship (which was not moving one iota). She asked for health advice while I was eating dinner. Finally, over the cheesecake, I suggested that the next night she should skip the 2½ glasses of cabernet sauvignon before dinner and the Frangelico for dessert, as these sorts of things tend to make the boat sway. In her case, thiamine would have been helpful only to replenish what the drug mugger alcohol stole. But it doesn't relieve motion sickness.

So what does thiamine do? To begin with, a deficiency of thiamine can cause macular degeneration, reduced appetite, fatigue, weakness, poor digestion, chronic constipation, an inability to gain weight, paresthesia (pins and needles or a sensation that someone is poking you with toothpicks all over the place), and mental fatigue. It can also lead to depression, nervousness, mental exhaustion, and insomnia. If the deficiency persists, the muscles become affected, which could cause leg cramps and general muscle weakness.

That last symptom is a big concern because your heart is a muscle and it's not supposed to be weakened. In a state of thiamine deficiency, the heart muscle gets a tad lazy and stops pumping properly. This leads to hypertrophy (enlargement) of the heart. Then, because circulation slows down, even the scalp loses blood flow, causing the hair to fall out and new hair growth to slow down.

Even though thiamine deficiency is fairly rare, it is getting more common thanks to processed foods and sweets made with refined white sugar, neither of which supplies adequate amounts of the nutrient. Alcohol, though, is the biggest drug mugger of thiamine, so imagine all those people who enjoy wine with dinner. They are more than likely deficient in B₁.

People with diabetes can greatly benefit from taking a thiamine supplement because it can help prevent diabetic retinopathy, blurry vision, atherosclerosis, and the plaque buildup that especially affects diabetics. All this gunk is what squeezes off arteries to the heart, limbs, and eyes.

Naturally, people with heart disease could also benefit because thiamine not only helps normalize cholesterol, but also has a mild diuretic effect, both of which are helpful. If you take this supplement, be sure to take it in the morning so you're not running to the bathroom during the wee hours.

You'll soon see from my drug mugger list that some heart medications are drug muggers of thiamine. Obviously, anyone who takes a drug mugger is at higher risk for thiamine deficiency. One study found that 98 percent of people with congestive heart failure who took the loop diuretic furosemide (approximately 80 mg daily) were deficient in thiamine. Furosemide is a drug mugger of many nutrients; imagine it making you spill out all the goodies that you need, as well as that excess fluid that is causing your blood pressure to rise. If you have to take a diuretic such as furosemide, consider replenishing what this mugger is stealing. In this chapter, it's clear that a deficiency of thiamine can make you lose your mind! In 2003, in a study published in the *Canadian Journal of Clinical Pharmacology*, 32 patients with congestive heart failure were evaluated. The study took place at the University of Ottawa Heart Institute. The patients were all being treated with at least 40 mg per day of furosemide. The patients were split into two groups, depending on the dosage of furosemide received. Their levels of thiamine were measured, and the results astonished me. Evidence of thiamine deficiency was found in 98 percent of folks who took at least 80 mg of furosemide per day. Thiamine deficiency was also found in more than half (57 percent) of patients taking just 40 mg per day. Just so you know, 40 mg is the most commonly dispensed dose at the pharmacy, so this is what most people take! My conclusion is that most people who take furosemide are walking around with thiamine deficiency and don't even know it (until now). Aren't you glad you're reading this? Based on this study, it looks like taking a thiamine supplement is a must for any heart failure patient on a loop diuretic.

All the B vitamins play a role in protecting the nerves and improving nervous system function. Thiamine can help improve numbness and tingling (peripheral neuropathy), burning sensations, painful and tender feelings in the limbs, and headache. If you run low on thiamine, you can develop all of these problems along with fatigue, depression, and memory loss.

If you drink alcohol, you must take a thiamine supplement because alcohol is a huge drug mugger of this nutrient. Longtime alcoholics are prone to malnutrition, causing more pronounced thiamine deficiency. This is the part that sounds crazy: Chronic drinkers frequently develop mental confusion, staggering gait, and visual disturbances. Doesn't that sound like what happens after a few beers? But they experience all these neurologic disturbances (called Wernicke's encephalopathy) even while sober. Thiamine can help relieve these symptoms. It's simple but true. If you are deficient in B_1, then your body has a much more difficult time breaking down the alcohol and clearing it out of your body. So B_1 deficiency is a risk factor for hellish hangovers.

You are probably wondering if thiamine can be used as a hangover remedy. Sure it can. It is much better than other hangover helpers such as orange juice and raw eggs. The study I'm going to share with you was published in *Inflammation Research*, was supported by the US Veterans Administration, and is nothing short of remarkable. Laboratory rats were given enough acetaldehyde to kill them (acetaldehyde is one of the metabolic by-products of alcohol and cigarettes). Then some of them were given the antioxidant nutrients vitamin B_1, vitamin C, and L-cysteine. Guess what? The rats that were given the antioxidant cocktail did not die. I have a family member who struggles with alcohol, and it's challenging for all of us who love him, so I strongly urge you not to drink. Realistically, I know that some people will ignore this advice. If you choose to drink anyway, you can take 200 or 250 mg thiamine before you get the party started, then take 100 mg more before bed along with 1,000 mg vitamin C and 600 mg NAC (cysteine), which scavenges the acetaldehyde. Be aware that acetaldehyde can cause pancreatitis.

Do problems with your memory have you concerned that you might be developing Alzheimer's disease? Then a thiamine supplement is a good choice for you. Thiamine helps improve memory by mimicking acetylcholine, a crucial memory molecule in your brain cells. It sharpens both memory and focus, and apparently also reduces your risk of developing Alzheimer's. Thiamine helps make acetylcholine through the production of acetyl coenzyme A, which feeds directly into your Krebs cycle, the metabolic pathway that gives you energy. In other words, thiamine deficiency can cause mitochondrial dysfunction. This all translates into being exhausted all the time!

Thiamine plays a big role in the digestive process, so people with gastrointestinal disease (who don't absorb the nutrient properly) can often benefit from taking a supplement. Among them are people with poor liver function, irritable bowel syndrome, Crohn's disease, or celiac disease. People who have had gastric bypass surgery often run out of thiamine because they have poor absorption in their gastrointestinal tracts.

Dieting can also cause an individual to run low on thiamine. A woman who goes on a crash diet and practically starves herself for several weeks in order to look thinner at her 10th high school reunion is likely going to that event with a thiamine deficiency. Chronic dieting or simply not eating (if you have chronic pancreatitis pain, for instance, and can't eat much at all) can also be a problem. Low levels of acetylcholine have been tied to anorexia, so taking thiamine may help people with this condition. (Remember, thiamine mimics acetylcholine in the body.) Thiamine overdose is rare, even in high dosages, but it is possible. You're getting too much if you develop headaches, tremors, irritability, rapid pulse, or insomnia, or if a blood test shows that your level of thyroid hormone has fallen below normal. By thyroid hormone I mean free T_3 specifically, not T_4 (the inactive form).

Drug Muggers of Thiamine (Vitamin B₁)

Acid Blockers

Cimetidine (Tagamet)

Esomeprazole (Nexium)

Famotidine (Pepcid and Pepcid Complete)

Lansoprazole (Prevacid 24HR)

Nizatidine (Axid)

Omeprazole (Prilosec OTC)

Pantoprazole (Protonix)

Rabeprazole (Aciphex)

Ranitidine (Zantac)

Antacids

Aluminum and magnesium hydroxide (Maalox, Mylanta)

Aluminum carbonate gel (Basaljel)

Aluminum hydroxide (Amphojel, AlternaGEL)

Calcium carbonate (Rolaids, Titralac, Tums)

Magnesium hydroxide (Phillips' Milk of Magnesia)

Sodium bicarbonate (Alka-Seltzer, baking soda)

Antibiotics (Just a few here, but all of them are drug muggers.)

Aminoglycosides

Amoxicillin (Amoxil)

Azithromycin (Z-pak)

Cefaclor (Ceclor)

Cefdinir (Omnicef)

Cephalexin (Keflex)

Ciprofloxacin (Cipro)

Clarithromycin (Biaxin)

Doxycycline (Doryx)

Erythromycin (E.E.S.)

Levofloxacin (Levaquin)

Minocycline (Minocin)

Penicillin (Pen VK)

Sulfamethoxazole and trimethoprim (Bactrim Septra)

Tetracycline (Sumycin)

Anticonvulsants

Phenytoin (dilantin) (Space supplement at least 4 hours away from the medication.)

Zonisamide (Zonegran)

Antivirals

Delavirdine (Rescriptor)

Lamivudine (Epivir)

Nevirapine (Viramune)

Foscarnet (Foscavir)

Zidovudine, AZT (Retrovir)

Zidovudine and lamivudine (Combivir)

Aromatase Inhibitors for breast cancer

Anastrozole (Arimidex)

Cardiac Glycoside

Digoxin (Lanoxin, Lanoxicaps, Digitek)

Blood Pressure Drugs

Diuretics, loop:

Bumetanide (Bumex)

Ethacrynic acid (Edecrin)

Furosemide (Lasix)

Torsemide (Demadex)

Diuretics, potassium-sparing: (Possibly; however, this is not conclusive.)

Diuretics, sulfonamide:

Indapamide (Lozol)

Diuretics, thiazide:

Any combination drug that contains HCTZ or hydrochlorothiazide (Dozens of drugs contain this.)

Chlorothiazide (Diuril)

Chlorthalidone (Hygroton)

Hydrochlorothiazide or HCTZ (Hydrodiuril)

Methyclothiazide (Enduron)

Metolazone (Zaroxolyn)

Bronchodilators

Theophylline (Uniphyl, Theo-24, or Theo-Dur)

Hormone Replacement Therapy/ Oral Contraceptives

Estradiol (Estrace, Climara, Estraderm, Estring, Activella,

Femring, Combipatch, EstroGel, Menostar, and many others)

Estrogen-containing drugs (hormone replacement therapy and birth control)

Estrogens, conjugated (Premphase, Prempro)

Ethinyl estradiol (found in many birth control pills)

SERMs (Selective Estrogen Receptor Modulators—used for breast cancer)

Raloxifene (Evista)

Tamoxifen (Nolvadex)

Toremifene (Fareston)

Sulfonamides (Sulfa antibiotics, some diabetes medications)

Miscellaneous

Alcohol

Betel nuts (also called bettlenuts or areca nuts, these are popular in Taiwan)

Coffee

Estrogen dominance

Genetic problems that prevent you from activating B_1

Quercetin and rutin (two popular dietary supplements)

Raw shellfish or raw seafood (such as sushi, oysters, or mussels)

Sulfites found in foods as a preservative

Tea (because of the tannins in tea, so even decaf)

Tobacco (nicotine)

Thiamine: Put This on Your Plate

Romaine lettuce, asparagus, spinach, sunflower seeds, yellowfin tuna, celery, green peas, tomatoes, eggplant, mustard greens, brussels sprouts, cabbage, watermelon, carrots, squash, broccoli, corn, kale, pineapple, oats, oranges, split peas, peanuts, lentils, and whole wheat.

An Absurdly Inexpensive Way to Feel Better

If you take too much thiamine, you may become deficient in your other B vitamins. Remember that whenever you take a single B vitamin, it is wise to take a B complex, too, so that the other Bs are in your system.

For general health: 5–10 mg per day

Drug mugger dose: 20–50 mg per day

Heart disease, alcoholism, or diabetes: 50–250 mg per day (Ask your doctor for his or her input on this.)

Just So You Know

People who have cancer or are undergoing chemotherapy should stick to very low dosages. Thiamine is sometimes given to combat the B_1 deficiency associated with fast-growing cancers like leukemia, but low doses are used because some studies have found that doses of more than 3 mg per day could backfire and increase the growth of the tumor. It's not completely clear, because chemotherapy itself can cause thiamine deficiency, but supplementing with too much can spark faster tumor growth in certain people. So my advice is to ask your doctor if thiamine is right for you, and if so, stick to what he or she advises.

Also, you will find lots of B_1 supplements with something called benfotiamine. This is a patented, fat-soluble, synthetic version of thiamine also called S-benzoylthiamine-O-monophosphate. This molecule is a precursor to thiamine and appears to be very effective in replenishing nutritional deficiencies. There is clinical research suggesting that benfotiamine offers protection against advanced glycation end products, or AGEs, which are typically associated with age-related diseases such as diabetes, Alzheimer's, cataracts, heart attack, and stroke. Reducing AGEs is one of the best things you can do if you want to reverse diabetes or blood sugar abnormalities. Simply put, thiamine, and more specifically benfotiamine, appears to have antiaging benefits. But remember that this is not a natural form of thiamine. Ask your doctor if it's right for you.

Install a Nutrient Security System

The more refined the food, the less thiamine you get. If you eat the typical American diet, you will become thiamine-depleted in about 3 to 4 weeks. It doesn't take long! Remember, this is a water-soluble vitamin, so it's not stored in your body. You have to constantly replenish this nutrient. It's always better to get your nutrients from foods rather than supplements, but I feel that supplementation is necessary for some people.

To install the tightest security system and get the highest content of thiamine from your foods, always choose brown rice (not white rice), whole grain bread (not white bread), and so forth. When supplementing, it's better to take smaller doses throughout the day than to take one large dose. Your body just takes what it needs and excretes the rest.

Thiamine is also a must for anyone taking high dosages of any other B vitamin since that can cause a relative deficiency of thiamine. Bs exist as a family (called B complex), so if you take one in a high dose, your body is tilted in the direction of the B you're taking. You won't even realize a deficiency is in the making because it could take weeks or months to develop, and all the while you think you're losing your mind, forgetting stuff all the time, and maybe even developing paresthesia, that prickly feeling all over. It's really not that uncommon, because many people take high doses of methyl B_{12} for demyelination disorders or fatigue. Other people commonly take high dosages of folic acid (or 5-MTHF, the active form) to improve estrogen metabolism or protect against heart disease. Some people take high dosages of B_6 for carpal tunnel. My point is that if you drive up the level of a particular B vitamin, you are very likely going to suffer a relative deficiency of thiamine, and it's superuncomfortable.

What's in My Cupboard?

Vitamin B-1 by Solaray: This product contains pure thiamine in a whole food base. Solaray uses natural sweeteners and flavors in all of its products, as well as natural preservatives such as vitamin E and rosemary extract.

Vitamin B-1 by Swanson: These small capsules provide 100 mg thiamine hydrochloride in rice flour, so it's gluten free. This company also offers the synthetic version of B_1 I mentioned that is considered to be more easily absorbed because it's fat soluble so it gets into the cells faster and easier. It's called benfotiamine. Contact information: www.swansonvitamins.com.

B-Complex #1 by Thorne Research: I like this brand for people who are in good general health because it contains a full range of all the B vitamins including pantothenic acid, riboflavin, folic acid, niacin, B_6, and others. It also has a good amount of B_1 (200 mg per capsule). It is yeast free, magnesium stearate free, and free of all diluents, flowing agents, and allergens. It doesn't get any purer than that!

B1 Caps by Twinlab: These hard gelatin capsules contain 100 mg pure crystalline thiamine that is yeast free and free of other allergens. It does not have any coatings, bindings, or colorings and is gluten free.

B-1 by Nature Made: This product contains 100 mg of thiamine with no artificial colors, flavors, or preservatives. It's also gluten free and USP certified for purity and potency.

High Potency B-1 by Source Naturals: This product is strong, offering 500 mg per tablet. The company also produces 100 mg tablets.

Benfotiamine by Nutraceutical Sciences Institute (NSI): This product, sold at www.vitacost.com, is the fat-soluble precursor to thiamine. It is kosher.

Mega Benfotiamine by Life Extension: This is a pure, high-potency specialty product (250 mg) free of all allergens.

Thiamine by injection: This is given by your doctor, particularly holistic MDs, but they will usually test your blood first to see if you're deficient (since they feel it's rare). I don't think blood level is as important as the clinical picture, though. I've seen people get remarkably better on thiamine injections or oral supplements despite their so-called normal blood levels.

One of the most effective ways to get thiamine (and other Bs) into your system is with an IV drip in a mixture called a Myers cocktail. I've tried this and found it to be just amazing because it created so much energy for me and it lasted for days.

Vitamin C

Vitamin C is a powerful antioxidant that is best known for protecting you against a cough or cold. Linus Pauling, the two-time Nobel Prize winner, made this nutrient famous in the 1970s. Does it really work? Many experts still think so. I'm one of them.

When it comes to the benefits of vitamin C, helping to prevent and heal colds is just the tip of the iceberg. It is great for sweeping away free radicals, those naturally occurring molecules that damage the body's cells. Studies have shown that it does boost your immunity to infections and cancer. But it gets better. Vitamin C (also called ascorbic acid) is good for so much more than just your immune system.

Vitamin C is crucial for your heart because it protects your heart valves, arteries, and capillaries, ensuring adequate blood supply to and away from your heart.

Believe me when I tell you that vitamin C can act as a natural cholesterol reducer, behaving just like a weak statin drug. In 2008, a researcher published a review in the *Journal of Chiropractic Medicine* that analyzed data pooled from 13 different studies. He concluded that: "Supplementation with at least 500 mg [daily] of vitamin C, for a minimum of 4 weeks, can result in a significant decrease in serum LDL cholesterol and triglyceride concentrations." This meta-analysis of 13 trials found an 8.8 percent decrease in triglycerides in 405 patients with high cholesterol. Both LDL (low-density lipoprotein) cholesterol and triglycerides are blood fats that contribute to heart disease. Another study from 2008 concluded that vitamin C lowers CRP—which stands for C-reactive protein—just as well as statins in those with high CRP levels. CRP is a strong marker for cardiovascular risk—think heart attack. This study followed 396 healthy nonsmokers for 2 months. The participants were divided into three groups and given either 1,000 mg of vitamin C daily,

800 mg of vitamin E daily, or placebo. In the vitamin C group, there was a 25 percent reduction in CRP and no effect with the vitamin E group. So if vitamin C can reduce CRP, I'd recommend this nutrient to everyone who is overweight, diabetic, or at risk for heart disease.

Just two more comments on heart disease since it's the number one killer in the United States. First, another relatively new antioxidant called astaxanthin (BioAstin) can also reduce CRP. (See page 285 for more on this.) Even though drug companies are aware of the studies showing how well natural vitamin C lowers cholesterol, you only see advertisements for the drugs, don't you? One doctor who pays special attention to the role of vitamin C in supporting heart health is Matthias Rath, MD. It's worth spending some time on his Web site: www.drrathresearch.org.

Second, millions of you are taking baby aspirin once daily in order to keep your blood flowing smoothly. Aspirin is one of those drugs that people pop without giving it a second thought, and it's been around for decades. But aspirin just so happens to make you urinate more vitamin C than is good for you! True story—your levels of vitamin C are lowered with chronic intake of aspirin, and it happens due to increased urinary excretion of vitamin C. What does that mean exactly? A lot! For example, vitamin C is needed to help make connective tissue and collagen in your body. Maybe this is why NSAID therapy is associated with osteoporosis, increased joint destruction, and poor cartilage formation. People with rheumatoid arthritis are often deficient in vitamin C, and not surprisingly, they are often taking aspirin or NSAID-type drugs for pain.

Vitamin C also has anticancer properties. There's another good reason to enjoy citrus fruits, which are high in this important nutrient. Isaac Eliaz, MD, knows a lot about this. He is a pioneer in the field of integrative medicine, a researcher, a clinician, and the author of dozens of research studies, which you can read about on his Web site, www.dreliaz.org.

Dr. Eliaz has dedicated his life to conquering cancer and other supposedly incurable diseases. You might call him the Sherlock Holmes of health—just replace the magnifying glass with a microscope. Dr. Eliaz is the mastermind behind an innovative product called PectaSol-C Modified

Citrus Pectin. It's like citrus rind in a capsule. Citrus rind is brimming with various polysaccharides, but don't let the big word scare you. They are just long chains of sugar, and they confer important health benefits such as protecting you from cancer, detoxifying your body, and snatching up heavy metals that harm you.

I interviewed Dr. Eliaz about the importance of vitamin C and cancer-fighting supplements such as MCP. He said, "As frightening as a cancer diagnosis is, I assure you that you need not battle it alone. There are safe, highly effective natural therapies that can augment and support your other treatment strategies." He should know. He formulated one of them.

Vitamin C also promotes healthy gums and teeth and helps you heal wounds, burns, and scars. This vitamin is also helpful when you indulge in foods that are probably best avoided. For example, it's a good idea to beef up your vitamin C intake—say, with fresh-squeezed orange juice, camu camu berries, or even a squeeze of lemon—if you are planning to eat a hot dog, bacon, or a bologna sandwich. I'd prefer you skip these foods, of course, but if you insist, at least get some C into your belly a few minutes before eating processed meats. The vitamin C helps neutralize the nitrites and nitrates in these foods before they latch onto your healthy cells and potentially damage the DNA (possibly contributing to cancer). You get only a little help from the C when you eat these foods, but it's better than nothing.

I learned this trick from my friend Health Ranger Mike Adams, the founder of www.naturalnews.com. He encourages people to get healthy with natural foods, phytochemicals, and high-quality supplements, and he posts informative articles and podcasts to really motivate you. Recently, he launched a comprehensive, easy-to-use database that helps people find interesting books by the most knowledgeable health-care authors of our time.

Speaking of unhealthy indulgences, you should also know that smokers need more vitamin C because nicotine is a drug mugger of C (as well as niacin).

Studies have shown that vitamin C protects against cataracts. It's also a great beauty supplement because it helps you make collagen and seems to reduce the occurrence of brown age spots.

Vitamin C enhances the amount of iron you absorb, and it keeps it hanging around a little longer. You might say that foods rich in vitamin C can protect against iron deficiency anemia in susceptible people such as women who have heavy menses or those who have slow, chronic blood loss. If you have iron deficiency anemia, drink one of my amazing juices—Juice C Juice (rich in vitamin C) or Iron Bonanza (see pages 364 or 368). Women who have preeclampsia during pregnancy have been found to have low levels of vitamin C. And because C concentrates in the adrenal glands, it's crucial for your energy levels. This is why people who run low on vitamin C feel weak and tired and get frequent infections. Vitamin C has also been shown to reduce lead, a heavy metal toxin, in the body.

This nutrient also helps put you in a good mood because it activates brain chemicals that support positive feelings—for example, serotonin and dopamine. When people run low on vitamin C, they often feel depressed and tired, so be sure to take C when you are dealing with a lot of stress.

A deficiency may also lead to easy bruising, bleeding gums, nosebleeds, and dark circles under the eyes from all those broken capillaries leaking blood. People with severe vitamin C deficiency develop a disorder called scurvy. They can also develop gallstones more frequently, but too much vitamin C increases your risk for kidney stones. It's a catch-22.

Many medications rob your body of C, most notably aspirin, as well as oral contraceptives, steroids, analgesics, and antidepressants.

And this is neat: People who have higher histamine levels—for example, those with allergies—might enjoy the antihistamine effect that vitamin C in high dosages offers. These people seem to have trouble falling asleep because of congestion, so it may not be a bad idea to boost vitamin C intake in the evening. Ask your doctor if a higher dose of 1,000 to 2,000 mg at bedtime would be a good alternative to all those nasal sprays, inhalers, and pills. This won't work overnight, but after a few weeks, you may notice fewer sniffles. Another option, perhaps even more beneficial, is C's cousin, quercetin. Try 2,000 to 3,000 mg three times daily. Think of it as Mother Nature's Claritin.

Drug Muggers of Vitamin C

Acid Blockers

Cimetidine (Tagamet)

Esomeprazole (Nexium)

Famotidine (Pepcid and Pepcid Complete)

Lansoprazole (Prevacid 24HR)

Nizatidine (Axid)

Omeprazole (Prilosec OTC)

Pantoprazole (Protonix)

Rabeprazole (Aciphex)

Ranitidine (Zantac)

Analgesics

Aspirin (Bayer, Ecotrin, St. Joseph)

Carisoprodol with aspirin (Soma Compound)

Hydrocodone and acetaminophen (Lortab, Norco, Vicodin, Lorcet)

Methocarbamol and aspirin (Robaxisal)

Oxycodone and aspirin (Percodan)

Antacids

Aluminum and magnesium hydroxide (Maalox, Mylanta)

Aluminum carbonate gel (Basaljel)

Aluminum hydroxide (Amphojel, AlternaGEL)

Calcium carbonate (Rolaids, Titralac, Tums)

Magnesium hydroxide (Phillips' Milk of Magnesia)

Sodium bicarbonate (Alka-Seltzer, baking soda)

Antibiotics (a few examples)

Amoxicillin (Amoxil)

Azithromycin (Z-Pak)

Cefaclor (Ceclor)

Cefdinir (Omnicef)

Cephalexin (Keflex)

Ciprofloxacin (Cipro)

Clarithromycin (Biaxin)

Doxycycline (Doryx)

Erythromycin (E.E.S.)

Levofloxacin (Levaquin)

Minocycline (Minocin)

Sulfamethoxazole and trimethoprim (Bactrim Septra)

Tetracycline (Sumycin)

Anti-Inflammatory Drugs (most)

Diclofenac (Voltaren)

Etodolac (Lodine)

Ibuprofen (Advil, Motrin)

Indomethacin (Indocin)

Ketoprofen (Orudis)

Naproxen (Aleve, Anaprox, Naprosyn)

Sulindac (Clinoril)

Antivirals

Delavirdine (Rescriptor)

Foscarnet (Foscavir)

Lamivudine (Epivir)

Nevirapine (Viramune)

Zidovudine, AZT (Retrovir)

Zidovudine and lamivudine (Combivir)

Aromatase Inhibitors for breast cancer

Anastrozole (Arimidex)

Barbiturates

Pentobarbital (Nembutal)

Phenobarbital (Donnatal, Luminal)

Secobarbital (Seconal)

Blood Pressure Drugs

Diuretics, loop:

Bumetanide (Bumex)

Ethacrynic acid (Edecrin)

Furosemide (Lasix)

Torsemide (Demadex)

Diuretics, potassium-sparing:

Amiloride (Midamor)

Spironolactone (Aldactone)

Triamterene (Dyazide, Dyrenium, Maxzide)

Diuretics, sulfonamide:

Indapamide (Lozol)

Diuretics, thiazide:

Any combination drug that contains HCTZ or hydrochlorothiazide (dozens of drugs contain this)

Chlorothiazide (Diuril)

Chlorthalidone (Hygroton)

Hydrochlorothiazide or HCTZ (Hydrodiuril)

Methyclothiazide (Enduron)

Metolazone (Zaroxolyn)

Corticosteroids

Dexamethasone (Decadron)

Fluocinonide (Lidex)

Methylprednisolone (Medrol)

Prednisolone (Orapred liquid, Pediapred)

Prednisone (Deltasone)

Triamcinolone (Aristocort cream)

Inhaled corticosteroids:

Budesonide (Rhinocort)

Flunisolide (Nasacort, Nasarel, Nasilide)

Fluticasone (Flonase)

Triamcinolone (Azmacort inhaler)

Hormone Replacement Therapy/ Oral Contraceptives

Estradiol (Estrace, Climara, Estraderm, Estring, Activella, Femring, CombiPatch, EstroGel, Menostar, and many others)

Estrogen-containing drugs (hormone replacement therapy and birth control)

Estrogens, conjugated (Premphase, Prempro)

Ethinyl estradiol (found in many birth control pills)

Levonorgestrel (found in most birth control pills and Plan B)

SERMs (Selective Estrogen Receptor Modulators—used for breast cancer)

Raloxifene (Evista)

Tamoxifen (Nolvadex)

Toremifene (Fareston)

Miscellaneous

Alcohol

Nicotine products (cigarettes, cigars, chewing tobacco, nicotine patches)

Vitamin C: Put This on Your Plate

Camu camu berries, bell peppers (especially red), parsley, broccoli (steamed), cauliflower, strawberries, lemon juice, romaine lettuce, brussels sprouts, papaya, kale, turnip greens, kiwifruits, oranges, tomatoes, grapefruit, raspberries, asparagus, celery (raw), pineapple, watermelon, cranberries, summer squash, blueberries, carrots, garlic, apricots, beef liver, sweet potatoes, plums, onions, and baked potatoes (with skin).

An Absurdly Inexpensive Way to Feel Better

For general health: 100–300 mg divided into two or three doses throughout the day (rather than one big dose) so you have some vitamin C on board all day

Drug mugger dose: 300–2,000 mg divided into two or three doses throughout the day

Just So You Know

Vitamin C, or ascorbic acid, is a water-loving vitamin that all humans need and unfortunately are unable to manufacture. Surprisingly, humans don't make their own vitamin C, as some animals do. We have to ingest it in foods or supplements. The richest food sources are citrus fruits and other fruits and vegetables.

Dietary vitamin C supplements are sold in one of the following forms or a combination of them:

Ascorbic acid or ascorbate
Sodium ascorbate
Calcium ascorbate (Ester-C is the trade name of this patented form of vitamin C, which some believe to work faster than naturally occurring C.)

Some dietary vitamin C supplements are extracted from natural sources such as acerola, a cherrylike fruit, or rose hips (the seed pods of roses).

There are numerous forms of vitamin C on the market today, and each product claims to have some advantage over the others. The most common type is ascorbic acid. From that term alone you won't be able to tell if the product comes from a natural source or was made in a laboratory. Depending on what study you read, naturally derived C and synthetic versions confer similar positive benefits. Nevertheless, I feel that there are better forms of vitamin C out there, and on page 284 you will find the brands I recommend.

You are getting too much vitamin C if you start to develop stomach upset, diarrhea, gas and bloating, or kidney stones. The higher your level of copper, the greater your need for vitamin C. People with copper plumbing in their homes tend to accumulate the mineral in their bodies. People who have zinc deficiencies may have a relative increase in copper levels. Those two minerals should stay in balance. Read more about zinc in Chapter 24.

Very high doses of vitamin C (greater than 1,000 mg daily) should be avoided by pregnant women because it can increase the risk for preeclampsia.

Install a Nutrient Security System

Vitamin C is a powerful antioxidant. There's no doubt that it performs good housekeeping in your cells, sweeping up and eliminating free radicals. To install the tightest security system in your body, it's best to take vitamin C along with another natural nutrient called lipoic acid. You can buy alpha-lipoic acid (or R-lipoic acid) at health food stores. Why the dynamic duo? Vitamin C normally sweeps your body clean just one time before it exits the body with whatever it can latch onto. When lipoic acid is also on board, it regenerates vitamin C and gives it another go-round so it can scavenge additional dangerous toxins. This is true synergy and could bring incredible relief to people with painful neuropathy.

What's in My Cupboard?

Buffered Vitamin C 500 mg by Bluebonnet: These capsules are gluten free, sugar free, yeast free, and dairy free. They are kosher, too. They contain only pure vitamin C along with bioflavonoids from fresh oranges, tangerines, grapefruit, lemons, hesperidin, and rutin. Contact information: www.bluebonnetnutrition.com.

Citrus Bioflavonoid Complex 1,000 mg by Solgar: These vegetarian tablets are kosher, starch free, and gluten free, and contain a powerful blend of bioflavonoids derived from fresh fruits. Solgar products are sold at health food stores.

Buffered C Powder by Thorne Research: This product is pure crystalline vitamin C (calcium ascorbate) with no added fillers. It's a powder you mix with water or juice and drink. I put it in my smoothies or coconut water. It is hypoallergenic.

AdvanC Complex by Nutraceutical Sciences Institute (NSI): This product also combines vitamin C with citrus bioflavonoids. The advantage here is that the two work together, especially in their antioxidant activities and in strengthening blood vessels. This product is made in an exclusive process that combines ascorbic acid with a patent-pending mineral complex and C metabolites to produce an all-natural, pH-neutral formula. The nonacidic formula is gentler on the digestive system than plain vitamin C and easily absorbable. Contact information: www.gonsi.com or www.vitacost.com.

PectaSol-C Modified Citrus Pectin by EcoNugenics: This product provides the body with a multitude of compounds that have been studied and appear to have some anticancer effects. It can also bind heavy metals and remove them from the body, so you get a double whammy with one formula. There are many modified citrus pectin (MCP) formulas on the market, but this brand stands alone in terms of its high quality and published research that documents its benefits.

PectaSol-C is special because of the way it's formulated. The tiny particles are so small that they get into your hard-to-reach cells and create powerful healing changes in the body. In a study of individuals who had deadly forms of cancer (some in their final stages), MCP offered the participants better quality of life, reduced pain, improved clinical outcomes, and in one case of metastatic prostate cancer, a 50 percent reduction in PSA (prostate specific antigen). Could this product extend the lives of some men with prostate cancer?

It's a good idea to take a bottle of MCP (for this brand, 1 capsule twice daily on an empty stomach) each year just to be on the safe side. Why wait for a devastating diagnosis? Contact information: www.econugenics.com/mcp. You can read more about MCP and its developer, Dr. Eliaz, at www.dreliaz.org.

Emergen-C by Alacer: These are packets of tangerine- or raspberry-flavored powder that you mix with water. The supplement provides a whole host of vitamins, antioxidants, and minerals. Each packet delivers 1,000 mg vitamin C along with zinc, calcium, magnesium, quercetin, and B vitamins.

C-Plus Citrus Bioflavonoid Caps by Twinlab: This product is a powerhouse of vitamin C. Each dose (2 capsules) provides 1,000 mg of vitamin C and 650 mg of citrus bioflavonoids. It also contains 50 mg of rutin, which helps with capillary strength and vein insufficiency.

BioAstin Supreme by Nutrex Hawaii: One of nature's most powerful antioxidants, this product has been shown to reduce C-reactive protein by more than 20 percent in only 8 weeks. It can (and should) be taken with vitamin C for ultimate heart protection. Contact information: www.nutrex-hawaii.com, or ask your local health food store to get it.

Vitamin D

Vitamin D is one of the most fascinating and talked about nutrients today. I'm not trying to be morbid, but vitamin D is actually used in bait to kill rats. Don't be alarmed. You'd have to swallow the contents of 200 bottles of vitamin D before having a fatal reaction. Supplemental vitamin D is actually quite safe for humans even if it's bad for critters. And it's not just safe, it's vital to our survival.

Once ingested, vitamin D turns into a powerful hormone that targets more than 2,000 genes in the human body. Research has found that a vitamin D deficiency is a major factor in the development of at least 17 types of cancer, as well as stroke, heart attack, diabetes, and chronic pain.

Let There Be Light!

Sunlight spurs the production of vitamin D in our bodies. Without the sun, we would all die. So I'm wondering who went and made sunlight sound so bad? Maybe people who have something to sell you? Like sunscreen.

If you get 30 minutes of sunshine daily, you receive about 10,000 to 20,000 IU vitamin D. Plant that number in your brain because in a few minutes I'll tell you about supplementing with oral vitamin D. I'm not suggesting megadoses, but I want you to see how ridiculously low some of the guidelines are.

Sunshine makes vitamin D in your body, and D protects you from cancer. What is the sunscreen doing to you? According to a study published in *Environmental Health Perspectives* in 2008, low levels of sunscreen, less than swimmers typically apply, could kill coral in just 4 days. The popular brands tested had these four ingredients in common: paraben, cinnamate, benzophenone, and a camphor derivative. Certain sunscreens might even be killing coral reefs. People wearing sunscreen swim by the reefs, and the sunscreen releases dormant algae viruses into the water.

Some of the chemical ingredients used in popular sunscreen products have not even been tested for safety or approved by the FDA and now appear to be associated with cancer. They get absorbed right through the skin (which is very porous), and from there the chemicals go into the bloodstream. Do I sound a bit harsh? Sorry. Are you wondering what those fear-provoking ads about skin cancer have to do with getting adequate vitamins? By blocking the sun, certain sunscreens can lead to vitamin D deficiency, and this can increase your risk for skin cancer. In fact, we are now dealing with a national epidemic of vitamin D deficiency and an uncannily high rate of cancer. Could there be a connection?

We absolutely need this vitamin, which turns into a hormone in the body. It helps us stay healthy, prevents cancer, and improves insulin sensitivity (which means a lower risk of type 2 diabetes). I've hammered this issue in my column for a long time. Only recently has it made it to the mainstream media. Numerous well-designed clinical trials have shown that widespread vitamin D deficiency is real and very dangerous. I have no interest in the vitamin D industry. I want to protect you from cancer, and it just so happens that vitamin D is important for doing just that. The form of vitamin D we get is important as well.

It's alarming but true that rickets, the vitamin D deficiency disease, was once rare in the United States but is now once again of serious concern. In my opinion this has to be partly due to all the fear of sunshine and use of chemical-laden sunscreens.

So why is the recommended daily dose of vitamin D for adults only 600 IU? If we met 100 percent of the daily value for vitamin D, would it keep us from developing a deficiency and rickets? Possibly, but it certainly wouldn't help us promote good health. Earlier, you planted a number in your head. Do you recall how much vitamin D you get from being in the sun for 30 minutes? The answer is 10,000 to 20,000 IU vitamin D. So a daily value of even 600 IU falls sorely short of what most people can get from natural exposure. But since we are covered in sunscreen, working indoors, or living in regions where the sun doesn't shine for very long, it's safe to assume that we are all probably deficient.

I make it my job to research studies, and in recent years there were many alarming headlines in scientific journals. One of them, in the September 2009 issue of *Progress in Cardiovascular Nursing*, said: "Vitamin D Deficiency in the United States: A Growing Epidemic with Serious Health Consequences." Here's another one from the February 20, 2008, issue of the *Journal of the American Medical Association*: "Vitamin D Deficits May Affect Heart Health." The take-home point of this is that millions of people in the United States are deficient in vitamin D, and it can lead to many devastating consequences, including heart attack, poor immune function, and diabetic complications involving the heart. Furthermore, because vitamin D is an immune booster, I think it is extremely important if you are trying to ramp up immune function.

You're more likely to run out of D if you take a drug mugger of this important nutrient or if you're a vegetarian. Dark-skinned people can have less vitamin D stored in their bodies because it takes a lot more sunshine for dark skin to make the vitamin. Some people have a genetic issue that prevents them from fully utilizing the nutrient and need added vitamin D in their regimens. People with liver or kidney disease are unable to activate vitamin D properly to make it usable in the body.

Vitamin D undergoes some chemical reactions in the liver and kidneys in order to become activated. The active form is called 1,25-dihydroxy-cholecalciferol, which is usually shortened to *calcitriol*. People with normal kidney function continually convert vitamin D into calcitriol, which works as a hormone and a steroid, playing an enormous role in the hundreds of chemical reactions that keep us alive. One of its primary roles is in the immune system.

The rates of breast, prostate, and colon cancer as well as multiple myeloma cases are not decreasing. Studies now show that vitamin D plays a protective role against these cancers and many others.

Vitamin D helps you absorb calcium and phosphorus from your diet. If there is no vitamin D in your body, your bones don't get enough of these important minerals and you develop rickets. Vitamin D is essential for keeping bones strong. If you don't get enough, your risk for osteoporosis goes up because bones get softer. This is true because vitamin D works in tandem with calcium, so a deficiency in D could result in a deficiency in calcium. Browse through Chapter 7 on calcium for more on symptoms associated with low calcium.

In children, a deficiency causes knock-knee, bowed legs, spinal curvature, or dental problems. In adults, a deficiency could show up as osteoporosis, SAD (seasonal affective disorder, a form of depression), rheumatic pains, muscle weakness, gradual loss of hearing, and even a higher risk of cancer, particularly colon, prostate, and breast cancer, according to some cutting-edge research. In my previous book *Diabetes without Drugs*, I recommend vitamin D because it helps you cut cravings, reduce appetite, and improve insulin sensitivity. Vitamin D does the body good and does more than most people realize, even if you are not mugged by a drug.

Drug Muggers of Vitamin D

Acid Blockers

Cimetidine (Tagamet)

Esomeprazole (Nexium)

Famotidine (Pepcid and Pepcid Complete)

Lansoprazole (Prevacid 24HR)

Nizatidine (Axid)

Omeprazole (Prilosec OTC)

Pantoprazole (Protonix)

Rabeprazole (Aciphex)

Ranitidine (Zantac)

Antacids

Aluminum and magnesium hydroxide (Maalox, Mylanta)

Aluminum carbonate gel (Basaljel)

Aluminum hydroxide (Amphojel, AlternaGEL)

Calcium carbonate (Rolaids, Titralac, Tums)

Magnesium hydroxide (Phillips' Milk of Magnesia)

Sodium bicarbonate (Alka-Seltzer, baking soda)

Antibiotics (a few examples)

Amoxicillin (Amoxil)

Azithromycin (Z-Pak)

Cefaclor (Ceclor)

Cefdinir (Omnicef)

Cephalexin (Keflex)

Ciprofloxacin (Cipro)

Clarithromycin (Biaxin)

Doxycycline (Doryx)

Erythromycin (E.E.S.)

Levofloxacin (Levaquin)

Minocycline (Minocin)

Sulfamethoxazole and
trimethoprim (Bactrim, Septra)

Tetracycline (Sumycin)

Anticonvulsants

Carbamazepine (Tegretol, Carbatrol)

Ethosuximide (Zarontin)

Gabapentin (Neurontin)

Phenobarbital

Phenytoin (Dilantin)

Primidone (Mysoline)

Valproic acid (Depakote,
Depakene)

Antifungals

Ketoconazole (Feoris, Nizoral)

Antituberculosis Agents

Ethambutol (Myambutol)

Isoniazid (INH)

Rifampin (Rifadin)

Aromatase Inhibitors for breast cancer

Anastrozole (Arimidex)

Barbiturates

Butalbital-containing drugs
(Fiorinal, Fioricet, Zebutal)

Blood Pressure Drugs

Calcium channel blockers:

Diltiazem (Cardizem)

Felodipine (Plendil)

Isoptin amlodipine (Norvasc)

Nifedipine (Procardia, Adalat)

Verapamil (Calan)

Diuretics, potassium-sparing (these are
not drug muggers, see examples
here):

Triamterene (Maxzide, Dyazide,
Dyrenium) may increase
vitamin D levels

Cholesterol Agents

Cholestyramine (Questran)

Colestipol (Colestid)

Fibrates (These drugs deplete
CoQ10 and Vitamin E, which
are two other fat-soluble
vitamins, so I think it's likely that
they deplete vitamin D, too.)

Clofibrate (Atromid)

Gemfibrozil (Lopid)

Fenofibrate (Tricor)

Statins (Some studies suggest a
statin-induced vitamin D
deficiency, which causes
muscle pain and cramps.
Have your doctor monitor
your levels twice annually
if you take a statin.)

Atorvastatin (Advicor, Lipitor)

Fluvastatin (Lescol)

Lovastatin (Altocor, Altoprev,
Mevacor)

Pitavastatin (Livalo, Pitava)

Pravastatin (Lipostat, Pravachol,
Selektine)

Rosuvastatin (Crestor)

Simvastatin (Lipex, Zocor)

Simvastatin and ezetimibe (Vytorin)

Simvastatin and niacin (Simcor)

Corticosteroids

Dexamethasone (Decadron)

Hydrocortisone (Cortef)

Methylprednisolone (Medrol)

Prednisone (Deltasone, Sterapred, Liquid Pred)

Inhaled corticosteroids:

Budesonide (Rhinocort)

Flunisolide (Nasarel, Nasalide)

Fluticasone (Flonase)

Laxatives that contain magnesium (such as magnesium citrate or Milk of Magnesia and stimulant laxatives)

Lipase Inhibitors

Orlistat (Alli, Xenical)

SERMs (Selective Estrogen Receptor Modulators—used for breast cancer)

Raloxifene (Evista)

Tamoxifen (Nolvadex)

Toremifene (Fareston)

Miscellaneous

Alcohol

Lack of sunlight

Liver or kidney damage

Malabsorption as in Celiac, Crohn's, IBS, or pancreatic insufficiency

Mineral oil

Olestra (fat substitute often used in "light" potato chips)

OTC diet aids and fat blockers (kidney bean extract or starch neutralizer, for example)

Vitamin D: Put This on Your Plate

Wild cold-water seafood, including salmon, mackerel, tuna, sardines, cod, and halibut; milk; liver; egg yolks; and fortified cereal.

An Absurdly Inexpensive Way to Feel Better

Sunshine: Go out for 15–30 minutes every day without sunscreen (not at high noon). Be intelligent about the sun and enjoy it at safe hours during the early morning or late afternoon. Bare your belly and back.

If you avoid the sun, then take 4,000–5,000 IU daily. To get the equivalent in fortified milk, you'd have to drink 40–50 glasses of milk per day, and you don't want to do that. It's better to supplement with some cholecalciferol, vitamin D_3.

For general health: 1,000–5,000 IU per day

Drug mugger dose: 5,000–10,000 IU per day

Cancer or autoimmune disease: Speak to your doctor first, but I suggest
10,000–15,000 IU per day for 2 months, then reduce dosage.

Just So You Know

The name to look for on the label is vitamin D_3 or cholecalciferol. Avoid
vitamin D_2 or ergocalciferol, which is common in some supplements and
in prescription drugs containing vitamin D. This form comes from radiat-
ing fungus. It's a drug, not natural vitamin D, and it works only about half
as well. Your body won't fully recognize it or easily incorporate it.

A prescription version of vitamin D is Hectorol. It's a lab-created version whose chemical name is doxercalciferol. It annoys me that most of our
prescription versions of vitamin D are not natural forms of vitamin D_3, so
technically they are not even human forms of the nutrient. Vitamin D naturally occurs in seafood, such as salmon, cod, and halibut. In fact, cod liver
oil is your best source of vitamin D.

With many OTC brands, you get the real deal, D_3, and your body
understands and easily incorporates it since that's what's made in the
human body. In fact, according to a study in the *Journal of Clinical Endocrinology & Metabolism*, vitamin D_3 is 87 percent more potent at raising blood
levels than is vitamin D_2. It's fairly impossible to overdose on vitamin D if
you are getting it from sunlight, although you could wind up with a painful sunburn if you're not careful. It's also impossible to overdo vitamin D
by eating foods rich in it.

Some people take large supplemental doses all at once, and even this is
considered relatively safe for certain individuals. For example, people with
multiple sclerosis are often deficient in vitamin D, and in an effort to prevent
relapse and improve nerve health, some doctors recommend 50,000 IU per
week for these individuals. The type of vitamin D that most doctors prescribe comes from the pharmacy and is D_2, not natural D_3. I have to emphasize to you that D_2 is not what humans make from natural sunlight; we

make D_3. The prescription vitamin is much more expensive than D_3, which can be obtained in any health food store. By the time your body converts the D_2 into a usable form, you've lost about half of the dosage prescribed.

People with impaired kidney function may become deficient in vitamin D because they cannot effectively activate the nutrient to calcitriol, a powerful hormone. For these individuals, doctors sometimes prescribe high dosages of vitamin D in order to build levels back up. Depending on the problem, however, some patients with kidney disease need to avoid vitamin D supplements altogether. If you have kidney disease, the use of vitamin D is strictly up to your nephrologist, who knows your kidney function.

People with diabetes can benefit from vitamin D because it improves insulin sensitivity and reduces risk of pancreatic cancer.

If your health-care provider does a blood test and determines that you are low in this important nutrient, he or she may ask you to take a high dose of the vitamin for a limited amount of time. You should not be taking high-dose vitamin D on your own. It is stored in fatty cells and tissues, and cumulative dosing has the potential to cause problems over time.

Supplementing with doses between 2,000 and 5,000 IU per day is fine and indicated for many people. In fact, many doctors who stay up to date on nutritional research now recommend supplementing at this level. Once you get above 15,000 or 20,000 IU per day of supplemental vitamin D, I think you are teetering on the verge of too much—unless you are deficient as shown by a blood test and your doctor recommends you take this much for a limited time.

Do note that no matter what type of vitamin D supplement you take, it's best to take it with food. Actually, it's best to take it with breakfast. Why? Taking vitamin D in the morning puts the supplement in sync with your body's natural biorhythm. After all, it's already set up to take advantage of the morning sunshine, which triggers natural vitamin D production. It's hard to get too much vitamin D, but I would be remiss if I didn't at least give you the warning signs of excess. Too much vitamin D can cause excess calcium to build up in the bloodstream, which can cause weakness, confusion, headache, nausea and vomiting, constipation or diarrhea, dry mouth, or a metallic taste in your mouth. Other signs could be heart rhythm problems, increased thirst, and decreased appetite.

Special note: Some drugs actually increase the activity of vitamin D and can lead to overload. Estrogen-containing drugs and isoniazid or thiazide diuretics like hydrochlorothiazide, or HCTZ, are examples of these. Postmenopausal women who take both calcium (1,000 mg per day) and vitamin D (400 IU per day) appear to have a more significant risk of kidney stones over the course of several years. This was shown in the famous Women's Health Initiative study, but it was not clear whether the nutrients themselves or inferior brands of the nutrients may have caused the problem.

Install a Nutrient Security System

Some people who take vitamin D suddenly develop leg cramps and muscle pain. This happens most often because of an underlying magnesium deficiency that becomes evident as the level of vitamin D starts to climb. In other words, a vitamin D deficiency masks magnesium deficiency, so when D rises with supplementation, the magnesium deficiency rears its ugly head and causes symptoms—leg cramps, muscle pain, and possibly mild heart palpitations. Don't be discouraged and don't panic. Remember, you need vitamin D to slash your risk of cancer and other major diseases.

Vitamin D needs cofactors (think of them as assistants) to help the body utilize it properly. These include zinc, vitamin K_2, boron, vitamin A, and magnesium. Magnesium is absolutely the most important of all. What to do? If I were you, I'd increase my magnesium intake naturally through foods since magnesium from foods is absorbed very well. I wouldn't take a magnesium supplement, although I would recommend spirulina (because it's naturally high in magnesium; see Chapter 12). Magnesium is a key component of the chlorophyll molecule, and chlorophyll is found in green vegetables; this is why leafy greens are incredibly good sources of this mineral. Enjoy your green foods while supplementing with D to install the tightest security system possible. The cramping should stop with the magnesium-rich foods on board. Continue with the D.

What's in My Cupboard?

SuperEssentials Omega by Living Fuel: This product is an excellent combination of vitamin D_3 plus vitamin A in a perfect ratio, just as you would find them in cod liver oil. SuperEssentials also contains omega-3 fatty acids, vitamin E, and the impressive antioxidant astaxanthin, which helps unclog arteries, beautify the skin, and sweep away free radicals. Contact information: www.livingfuel.com.

Arctic-D Cod Liver Oil by Nordic Naturals: This doesn't taste like fish because it comes in flavors (lemon, peach, orange, spiced apple, and strawberry). A high-potency blend of essential fatty acids rich in pure DHA and EPA (two of the three main forms of omega-3s), this product contains low levels of natural, healthy forms of vitamin A, plus 400 IU of natural vitamin D (cholecalciferol). I like cod liver oil because it has important compounds, vitamins, and essential fatty acids that nourish the brain, joints, heart, arteries, and nervous system. This marine-derived formula is extremely pure and can improve vision, boost mood, ease menstrual discomfort, reduce joint pain, and cut down on your risk for heart disease. It is sold nationwide.

Super D3 by Allergy Research Group: This vitamin D comes from a natural source but not from the sea. It's from the lanolin of sheep wool. Lanolin, as you may know, is an oily substance that comes from the sebaceous glands of wool-bearing animals. It's often found in moisturizers and cosmetics. Each capsule contains 2,000 IU cholecalciferol along with a little bit of vitamins C and E for stability.

Vitamin D_3 by Country Life: This product is free of all common allergens, it's affordable, and it's easy to find in health food stores. It contains 5,000 IU vitamin D in the correct, natural form of cholecalciferol.

Vitamin D_3 Mixed Berry Flavor by ChildLife Essentials: This formula is made specifically for infants 6 to 12 months old, and children 1 to 12 years old. The liquid is alcohol free and contains all-natural ingredients. It has a natural berry flavor. Back in 2008, the American Academy of Pediatrics doubled its recommendation for vitamin D intake and suggested that children receive 400 IU per day. This could be particularly important for children with suppressed immune systems.

Liquid D$_3$ by LifeTime: This product, perfect for those who cannot take solid supplements or who have trouble with digestion, provides 4,000 IU per dose.

Full Spectrum Vitamin K by Allergy Research Group: This formula is named for its vitamin K content. It's a high-quality multitasking formula from a leading manufacturer of pure products. The ingredients in each softgel are intended to help with bone strength. They contain approximately 400–800 IU of D$_3$ derived from cod liver and tuna oils, along with vitamins A, K, and E.

Vitamin D$_3$ 5,000 IU Liquid Softgels by Nature Made: This is pure, natural vitamin D$_3$, and it's easy to find in health food stores and pharmacies nationwide. All vitamin D supplements created by Nature Made are in the form of D$_3$. There are no artificial colors, flavors, or preservatives. There are no allergens such as yeast or gluten. I think most people are deficient in natural vitamin D, and I like that this brand is easy to find, USP certified for purity, and very affordable.

Zinc

You need zinc in order to see, hear, taste food, and have sex. The mineral zinc participates in many life-sustaining biochemical reactions in your body by sparking activity in about 100 enzymes. Everyone needs this antioxidant for a strong, healthy immune system, and it helps wounds heal quickly. While researching this book, I learned how incredibly easy it is to lose this mineral, which is rarely talked about and almost taken for granted. It's lost through sweat, feces and urine, hair, skin, semen, and menstrual blood.

Zinc can help you if you are prone to digestive disorders. Typically, people with celiac or Crohn's disease, ulcerative colitis, or irritable bowel syndrome are deficient in zinc. Acid blockers make it to yet another drug mugger list. They zap your zinc supply. How ironic! You take an acid blocker because you're having issues with digestion, and you need zinc to help fend off infections of the gut and maintain a healthy lining.

Zinc is also important for helping men and women stay fertile. If you have fertility issues, this could be the supplement for you. You need zinc to make DNA. Adult men need about one-third more zinc than adult women because this mineral helps make testosterone. Sexually active men need a little more zinc than men who prefer to watch TV in bed. One article I read said that zinc is 100 times more concentrated in semen than in a man's bloodstream. There is also evidence to support zinc's protective effect on the prostate gland; it helps prevent and relieve symptoms of benign prostatic hypertrophy (often called BPH).

This important mineral also helps kill bacteria and viruses. It is a well-known immune protector that boosts the activity of various immune components—T cells, natural killer cells, and interleukin. Without enough zinc on board we get frequent colds and infections. This is a good reason to take it at the first sign of the sniffles. Zinc apparently can attach in the nose or mouth to the virus that causes the common cold and obliterate it before it can multiply. This keeps you from getting a full-blown infection and may shorten your misery time for a cold by up to 3 days. It could even help protect you from contracting swine flu (H1N1 virus).

An article published in the June 2009 issue of *Immunity and Ageing* stated:

> There are remarkable parallels in the immunological changes during aging and zinc deficiency, including a reduction in the activity of the thymus and thymic hormones, a shift of the T helper cell balance toward T helper type 2 cells, decreased response to vaccination, and impaired functions of innate immune cells. Many studies confirm a decline of zinc levels with age. Most of these studies do not classify the majority of elderly as zinc deficient, but even marginal zinc deprivation can affect immune function.

This is so important because many folks do not realize that zinc levels decline as we age, with or without drug muggers. It could explain in part why the frail and elderly are more susceptible to infections. Since zinc plays an important role in the prostate, it may be that zinc deficiency contributes to the prostate problems that affect so many elderly men. Another important paper published in *Molecular Medicine* in 2008 supports zinc's role in immune function. Researchers found that zinc was able to calm down the inflammatory response and boost immune cell response. It was also found to sweep away free radicals, meaning it has a powerful role in suppressing oxidative stress and pain-causing inflammatory chemicals.

Since zinc is needed to make both insulin and thyroid hormone, a deficiency could lead to diabetes and hypothyroidism, low production of thyroid hormone. It's important to note that people with diabetes often have this latter condition as well. In a 2009 study published in the *Review of Diabetic Studies*, researchers concluded, "Zinc supplementation reduced serum homocysteine and increased vitamin B_{12} and folate concentrations in type 2 diabetic patients with microalbuminuria." This means that people with diabetes, who often have microalbuminuria (a sign of kidney disease), can take zinc and improve their levels of B_{12} and folic acid. Not only that, but zinc also appears to reduce homocysteine, a dangerous chemical that promotes heart disease. Not too shabby for one little mineral that is considered "trace" because such tiny amounts impact health so greatly. Makes you want to eat oysters right now, doesn't it? Six oysters contain 77 mg of zinc.

Zinc works in tandem with vitamin A, so a deficiency in one could result in a deficiency in the other. Low zinc often means low vitamin A. This explains why some people deficient in zinc go on to develop visual problems, macular degeneration, and ultimately blindness. (See Chapter 5 for more symptoms of vitamin A deficiency.) Liver and pancreatic disorders are also associated with lower levels of zinc.

In summary, a zinc deficiency can have effects all over the body and may cause hearing loss, prostate problems, sexual difficulties, frequent infections, poor vision, night blindness, white spots under the fingernails, and muscle atrophy.

ACE inhibitors, which are blood pressure medications, may contribute to a deficiency in zinc, which could spark all kinds of problems. How do we know? Because in a 1998 study published in the *Journal of the American College of Nutrition*, a total of 34 patients with high blood pressure taking either Capoten (16 patients) or Vasotec (18) were followed for 6 months. There were 10 control subjects. Zinc levels were assessed at the beginning of drug treatment and after 6 months. The zinc was measured various ways, either in the serum, in the peripheral blood monocytes, or in the urine (collected over 24 hours). The researchers concluded that "treatment of hypertensive patients with captopril (Capoten) or enalapril (Vasotec) may result in zinc deficiency."

The soil has become depleted of important minerals like zinc in many parts of the world, which adds to the growing problem of mineral deficiency. It's actually quite common. Elderly people are usually deficient, as are alcoholics and people with kidney or liver disease. Vegetarians tend to run out of zinc more frequently than nonvegetarians, so I always recommend supplementation for anyone who is vegetarian or vegan. Also, people with malabsorption conditions such as candida overgrowth, celiac disease, Crohn's disease, and irritable bowel syndrome should supplement with zinc.

Drug Muggers of Zinc

Acid Blockers

Cimetidine (Tagamet)

Esomeprazole (Nexium)

Famotidine (Pepcid and Pepcid Complete)

Lansoprazole (Prevacid 24HR)

Nizatidine (Axid)

Omeprazole (Prilosec OTC)

Pantoprazole (Protonix)

Rabeprazole (Aciphex)

Ranitidine (Zantac)

Antacids

Aluminum and magnesium hydroxide (Maalox, Mylanta)

Aluminum carbonate gel (Basaljel)

Aluminum hydroxide (AlternaGEL, Amphojel)

Calcium carbonate (Rolaids, Titralac, Tums)

Magnesium hydroxide (Phillips' Milk of Magnesia)

Sodium bicarbonate (Alka-Seltzer, baking soda)

Antituberculosis Agents

Ethambutol (Myambutol)

Isoniazid (INH)

Rifampin (Rifadin)

Antivirals

Delavirdine (Rescriptor)

Etravirine (Intelence)

Foscarnet (Foscavir)

Lamivudine (Epivir)

Nevirapine (Viramune)

Zidovudine, AZT (Retrovir)

Zidovudine and lamivudine (Combivir)

Aromatase Inhibitors for breast cancer

Anastrozole (Arimidex)

Blood Pressure Drugs

Clonidine (Catapres)

Hydralazine (Apresoline)

Methyldopa (Aldomet)

Moexipril (Univasc)

ACE inhibitors:

Benazepril (Lotensin)

Captopril (Capoten)

Enalapril (Vasotec)

Enalapril and HCTZ (Vasotec HCT)

Fosinopril (Monopril)

Lisinopril (Prinivil, Zestril)

Moexipril (Univasc)

Quinapril (Accupril)

Ramipril (Altace)

Trandolapril (Mavik)

Angiotensin II receptor blockers:

Candesartan and HCTZ (Atacand
HCT)

Irbesartan and HCTZ (Avalide)

Valsartan and HCTZ (Diovan
HCT)

Diuretics, loop:

Bumetanide (Bumex)

Ethacrynic acid (Edecrin)

Furosemide (Lasix)

Torsemide (Demadex)

Diuretics, potassium-sparing:

Amiloride (Midamor) (This is not a
drug mugger; it may increase
levels.)

Triamterene/HCTZ (Maxzide,
Dyazide, Dyrenium)

Diuretics, sulfonamide:

Indapamide (Lozol)

Diuretics, thiazide:

Any combination drug that
contains HCTZ or
hydrochlorothiazide (dozens of
drugs contain this)

Chlorothiazide (Diuril)

Chlorthalidone (Hygroton)

Hydrochlorothiazide or HCTZ
(Hydrodiuril)

Losartan and HCTZ (Hyzaar)

Methyclothiazide (Enduron)

Metolazone (Zaroxolyn)

Chelating Agent

Penicillamine (Cuprimine)

Cholesterol Agents

Cholestyramine resin (Questran)

Ezetimibe (Zetia)

Fibrates:

Clofibrate (Atromid-S)

Fenofibrate (Tricor)

Gemfibrozil (Lopid)

Corticosteroids

Betamethasone (Diprolene, Luxiq)

Dexamethasone (Decadron) and
others

Methylprednisolone (Medrol)

Prednisolone (Pediapred Liquid)

Prednisone (Deltasone, Liquid
Pred, Sterapred)

Triamcinolone (Aristocort cream)

Inhaled corticosteroids:

Budesonide (Rhinocort,
Symbicort)

Flunisolide (Nasacort, Nasalide,
Nasarel)

Fluticasone (Flonase)

**Hormone Replacement Therapy/
Oral Contraceptives**

Estradiol (Estrace, Climara,
Estraderm, Estring, Activella,
Femring, CombiPatch, EstroGel,
Menostar, and many others)

Estradiol and testosterone
(EstraTest, Depo-Testadiol)

Estrogen-containing drugs
(hormone replacement therapy
and birth control)

Estrogens, conjugated (Premphase, Prempro)

Ethinyl estradiol (found in many birth control pills)

Levonorgestrel (in birth control and Plan B)

Norethindrone (found in many birth control pills)

SERMs (Selective Estrogen Receptor Modulators—used for breast cancer)

Raloxifene (Evista)

Tamoxifen (Nolvadex)

Toremifene (Fareston)

Miscellaneous

Calcium supplementation (in excess)

Casein (the protein in dairy)

Chelation therapy to remove heavy metals

Chocolate (because it's relatively high in copper)

Coffee, tea, and soda (caffeinated)

Copper supplementation (in excess)

Estrogen dominance

Food dyes rich in copper

Heavy metal toxicity (Likely all heavy metals but these for sure)

Cadmium burden (which occurs from smoking)

Mercury burden (which occurs from certain seafood, environmental chemicals and amalgams)

Smoking (because of the cadmium, a toxic heavy metal in cigarettes)

Zinc: Put This on Your Plate

Oysters, beef, lamb, crab, chicken, lobster, crimini mushrooms, spinach, summer squash, asparagus, Swiss chard, collard greens, milk, cheese, yeast, whole grains, miso, shrimp, maple syrup, broccoli, beans, green peas, yogurt, nuts, pumpkin seeds, and sesame seeds.

An Absurdly Inexpensive Way to Feel Better

To minimize stomach upset or diarrhea, take mineral supplements with food.

For general health: For women, 5–15 mg per day; for men, 10–25 mg per day

Drug mugger dose: 15–25 mg per day

Just So You Know

Zinc and a sister mineral, copper, are both neurotransmitters in the brain and have an impact on our moods. We have elaborate systems that regulate these trace minerals, and when they tilt out of balance, our health and mood pay the price. The ratio of copper to zinc is far more clinically valuable than the concentration of either one. Too much zinc and you have a relative deficiency of copper. Too much copper and your blood levels of zinc are diminished, which can spark severe PMS, panic attacks, anxiety, ADHD, autismlike syndrome, schizophrenia, hypomania, depression, personality changes, and even hallucinations.

Women at my lectures are always stunned when I tell them that the condition of estrogen dominance or the use of birth control pills can cause excessive copper (and zinc deficiency), leading to severe PMS and mood changes. It's a major "Aha!" I tell you this because many of these conditions are treated with psychoactive drugs. So many physicians never think to tease out a possible copper–zinc imbalance, which can be discovered with micronutrient testing. (See the Resources section on page 448 for information on nutritional testing.) When buying supplements, make sure you don't overdo zinc or copper. Sometimes you find supplements that combine these two important minerals in just the right ratio.

You know you're getting too much zinc if you develop nausea, stomach upset, joint pain, low blood pressure, urinary retention, diarrhea, or a metallic taste in your mouth.

Install a Nutrient Security System

I feel it's always best to absorb nutrients from our diets, and protein is important when it comes to zinc absorption. In particular, two amino acids, methionine and cysteine, improve the bioavailability of zinc. It's easy to get those if you eat animal proteins or make a protein supplement shake from whey, hemp, rice, or egg protein. Bread makes a difference, too. The zinc you get from whole grain products and plant proteins is less usable to you, thanks to their relatively high content of phytic acid, a substance that limits zinc absorption. Leavened whole grain breads have more bioavailable zinc than unleavened breads. And if you have a palate for oysters, by all means eat them! Oysters soar well above beef, which offers 6 mg an ounce to one oyster's 12 to 13 mg, and almonds, which offer about 1 mg an ounce.

What's in My Cupboard?

Pic-Mins by Thorne Research: This multimineral formula, made by a company known for its products' purity, contains minerals in their most highly absorbable forms. It features 15 mg zinc picolinate, along with selenium, chromium, molybdenum, boron, and vanadium.

Cold-EEZE by Quigley: These are lozenges containing 13.3 mg ionic zinc (zinc gluconate glycine), a form of zinc that starts to get absorbed right in your mouth. The gluten-free lozenges have clinical trials behind them, and they come in a variety of flavors that taste great compared to zinc's natural metallic flavor. This company's product line is free of dyes, preservatives, and artificial sweeteners, and some are even USDA-certified organic. I like this all-natural product line so much that I served as a clinical consultant for the company during cough and cold season several years ago.

L-OptiZinc by Nutraceutical Sciences Institute (NSI): These capsules provide zinc in the form of zinc methionine, which enhances absorption compared to many other zinc supplements with the zinc sulfate form. Methionine helps the body in other ways, too. As you know, when minerals are bound (chelated) to amino acids, as in this case, they become more immediately available and usable and are less upsetting to the stomach. Each capsule contains 30 mg of zinc.

Zinc Copper by Solaray: These capsules are impressive because they contain zinc and copper in the bioavailable amino acid chelate form, along with iodine. All three minerals support the pancreas, thyroid, and breast tissue. This product helps you make an important antioxidant, superoxide dismutase, which can help squash free radicals. It contains some pumpkin seed extract as well. What I like most is that this company gets its zinc and copper chelates from whole rice concentrate rather than the typical yeast, milk, or soy products.

Zinc Balance by Jarrow Formulas: This formula is nice because it contains 15 mg of zinc in the zinc methionine form and 1 mg of copper gluconate, preserving that important zinc-to-copper ratio.

Calcium Magnesium Plus Zinc by Solgar: This combination of minerals works better together than alone. Solgar has combined 1,000 mg calcium (a combination of calcium carbonate, calcium gluconate, and calcium citrate) with 400 mg of magnesium and 15 mg of zinc gluconate. I've included this one because it's a good trio and is easy to find.

Super Food by Bõku: This is a powerhouse green food supplement loaded with all the minerals you need, including zinc, enzymes, flaxseeds, probiotics, and powdered land and sea vegetables. It's a green drink, something I'm particularly fond of, as you know if you read my syndicated column. I mix a teaspoonful of it with a cup of natural organic apple juice each day to sweeten it a little. It is, in part, marine derived, so it contains many healthy ingredients to clear up all sorts of nagging symptoms. You might notice a difference in energy level after the first day or two, so it can be especially helpful if you take it right before athletic activity.

Spirulina Pacifica by Nutrex Hawaii: You can take this supplement by mouth as a tasteless tablet. It contains approximately 20 mg zinc in 3 tablets.

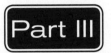

Part III

Getting the Most from Your Supplement

How to Pick a Great Supplement

My husband and I are both involved in health care. I am a writer and pharmacist who is passionate about natural medicine. Sam is a chiropractic physician. Between us, we have 40 years of clinical experience. We are both holistic practitioners and feel that drugs are overused and prescribed indiscriminately. Future generations may look back on this medicine-crazed time as barbaric.

As I was writing *Drug Muggers*, we both agreed that the number one health question we each receive in our respective professions is "How do I pick a great multivitamin?" Let's face it: The role of good nutrition and healthy supplements in health cannot be overemphasized, and the need for authentic and pure supplements is at an all-time high. So we decided to include a chapter that will help you navigate the aisles of pharmacies and health food stores and pick the best top-quality supplements for your needs.

Confronting the dizzying array of dietary supplements and vitamins is daunting and confusing to our patients and readers. Both my husband and I are Internet savvy and have seen a plethora of Web sites that propagate false information and sell supplements that are of poor quality. We've also examined Web sites that purport to do consumer testing and post reports deeming certain proprietary brands to be better than others. Then we've found out that these supposedly "better" companies have paid to have their brand-name products included on the lists. So how do you really know whom to trust and what companies are reliable?

I will help you sift through all the information and deception in the dietary supplement industry. In this chapter, you will become aware of the worst tricks in the industry so you can steer clear of—no, run from—poor-quality nutraceuticals. My goal is to teach you what to look for when you read vitamin labels.

Do You Need to Supplement?

Choices have consequences. For example, making the choice to smoke, drink, or lie on the couch watching TV every day rather than exercising eventually takes its toll. What about people who eat too many sweets, fried foods, and greasy burgers? An unhealthy diet does increase your need for supplementation. Let's get something clear, though. Even the best multivitamin supplement in the world can't make up for a lousy diet. It is a supplement, after all, not a remedy for bad habits. You have a choice, and you can choose to eat fewer processed and fattening foods and more "rabbit food."

Vitamins are present in fresh raw vegetables and fruits, to be sure. But in my opinion they aren't present in sufficient quantities to promote good health, reverse disease, or counteract all the toxins that surround us in the industrialized world we live in. Why is that? Our foods today are grown in mineral-devoid soils and riddled with pesticides and chemicals.

Many groups have special needs when it comes to nutrients. Women who are pregnant, nursing, or trying to conceive, for example, require larger amounts of certain nutrients to make sure their babies get the best start. And then there are senior citizens. Because levels of healthy nutrients and hormones decline in the elderly, they especially require added nutritional supplementation.

We all get vaccinated at birth and then take a slew of drugs throughout our lives, exposing ourselves to a continuous onslaught of unnatural chemicals. Many medications are drug muggers, often with the potential to slowly steal the life out of us. So the question isn't "Should I supplement?" Of course you should! The real question is "What are the best supplements to take to meet my individual needs?"

Why Do We Need Vitamins Anyway?

A common myth has it that if you eat well, you will automatically get all the vitamins and minerals you need solely from your food. Naturally I think you should eat a healthy diet. But even if you eat fresh fruits and vegetables every hour, you still get only a fraction of the essential nutrients you need from those foods. Remember, those "fresh" fruits and veggies are often grown in mineral-deficient soils that contain a lot of pesticides. Then the produce sits for days at the grocery store. Then more time passes while it sits in your fridge. Then you microwave it or boil it too long. The bottom line is that the vitamins and minerals in today's food supply have been greatly diminished by the time you eat them.

And let's not forget the impact of sweets. People who eat processed foods containing refined white sugar (as opposed to stevia or agave sweeteners) will lose some B vitamins, zinc, chromium, magnesium, and other minerals. Yep, that's right. White processed sugar is a drug mugger of minerals. And guess what? When you're chronically low in certain minerals, you develop blood sugar problems. Hello, diabetes. Supplementing with trace minerals is smart if you have an insatiable sweet tooth. Conversely, sugar cravings can actually be caused by mineral and B vitamin deficiencies.

Let's get back to vitamins. What exactly are they?

By themselves, vitamins don't give you energy. They merely participate in the chemical reactions in the body that produce energy. They also boost your immune system; help you grow; and allow you to think, move, and stay alive. Thanks to vitamins you can see the world in color instead of in black and white. You can read thanks to the power of vitamins. It takes certain vitamins and minerals to keep your skeleton and your teeth strong. Vitamins help determine your mood, your attention span, even how well you ward off major illnesses like cancer.

Certain vitamins can determine what color your hair is and may play a part in premature graying. Some vitamins keep you from bleeding to death when you get a small cut. Vitamins and minerals are also cofactors, which means that they assist enzymes in their job of digesting your food. Think of a cofactor as your good buddy.

The list goes on and on. If you think you can put just any old vitamin into your body and get good results, then I'm glad you're reading my book. Not all vitamins are created equal, as you will see. Think of a car: It needs gas to run well. Without enough fuel, it conks out. If you take cheap or second-rate vitamins, your body will conk out, too.

Think of banking, too. If you don't put away some money now, you won't have it to rely on later when you need it. It's the same with vitamins. If you don't store up a good nutritional stash that allows your cells to run optimally, how will you stay healthy in the long run? However, many vitamins—especially the water-soluble ones—are not stored in the body long-term. So you really do need to keep replenishing certain nutrients. In the case of calcium, for example, you need to bank enough of this mineral to help you maintain strong bones and teeth for a lifetime.

I'm not saying that vitamins and minerals are a cure-all, or that they prevent disease. But they are certainly a good place to start. They offer some insurance against the poor state of our food supply and the many drug muggers out there. Nutritional supplements should be considered one big piece of the health puzzle.

Apparently, I'm not alone in my thinking, because an estimated 50 to 60 percent of Americans take dietary supplements. If you've already recognized the importance of nutraceuticals, let me teach you how to pick high-quality supplements (and herbs, too).

Selecting a multivitamin presents a particular challenge. What makes the process so difficult and confusing is that many multivitamins are basically the same at their core. They all seem to contain a wide range of the B vitamins, some A, D, C, and E, and a few minerals. Brand after brand, you see the same basic stuff. But you can't read what's not printed on the label. You may not know that some nutrients—zinc and copper, for example— need to stay in balance with each other in a specific ratio. They are both extremely beneficial to the body, but they need to be taken properly. Taking a poorly formulated multivitamin could tilt your body chemistry in the wrong direction.

Of course, quality issues come up with all supplements, not just multi-vitamins. Just one example: You couldn't possibly know that some fish oils are taken from fish caught in contaminated waters, waters that contain PCBs, heavy metals, radioactive waste, and other toxins. This will not be on the label.

I feel a responsibility to share some of the secrets of this industry with you to help you get more supplement savvy. If you're going to spend the money and bother to take a supplement, you need to take a good one.

Making an Educated Choice

You need a well-rounded multivitamin to fuel your body and provide it with the nutrition it needs to carry out hundreds of chemical reactions every minute. You need a trustworthy supplement, and you may need to take it several times a day for the same reason that you eat several times a day. This is news to many people who take their multivitamins once daily. The reason is that your body takes what it needs of certain nutrients—the water-soluble vitamins—then you excrete the rest. With fat-soluble vitamins (like E, D, A, and K), it's a different story. You can store these for a while. So having a high-quality nutritional supplement on board is incredibly important to your general health and well-being.

The ideas that follow are going to raise some eyebrows because it's likely that they will raise some issues with your current multivitamin formula. I'm willing to bet there's a good chance that you're taking products that will not meet the standards outlined here. While most of these points are deal breakers for me, you may be willing to accept a lower-quality product because the price is lower, too. Just make sure that you don't fall for any of the worst tricks in the industry, which I'll get to after we look at some of the fairly common and less serious issues.

These Tricks Are Fairly Common

Here's an overview of vitamin industry negatives that you should know about and how to deal with them.

Don't take just 1 pill. Does your vitamin formula deliver all of its nutrition in a single dose? Multivitamins sometimes offer comprehensive once-daily tablets or softgels. Supplements and multivitamins that promise dozens of nutrients in one single dose can't possibly have the potency needed for good health or they would be humongous horse pills. You are being duped if you think you're getting the right amounts of all the essential nutrients needed for optimal health in a single pill. High-quality multivitamins may require 3 to 6 capsules a day to give you top protection 24/7.

Expect to pay. If you can get 1,000 pills for $9.99, how good can they be? Are you getting a great deal or a great deal of junk? I get especially irked when I see companies preying on the most vulnerable and sickly segment of our population, the elderly. They produce vitamins of poor quality and sell them very inexpensively. The elderly are the very group of people who need the best supplements, not the cheapest ones!

Remember, the cost to produce vitamin supplements includes the bottle, label, shipping, marketing, and distribution. I'm not a mathematical genius, but how much money was left to invest in the quality of those vitamins if they only cost $10?

Watch for additives. Many vitamins contain magnesium stearate, an inactive plant- or animal-based substance that is used widely in the manufacture of supplements. It has been used for decades, but it is usually not disclosed on the label if the level does not reach 1 percent of the total content. Let me just say up front that practically all supplements contain this, and I take supplements with this almost every day.

Magnesium stearate (a combination of magnesium and stearic acid) is often added to the formula to make it flow better during the manufacturing process. Some companies insist that stearates ensure proper encapsulation, although I disagree. I think you can have proper encapsulation without this additive. Some companies offer stearate-free supplements. But stearates increase profits for manufacturers because the company can generate more products in less time.

Even the best in the scientific field debate this issue as if it were politics. Some scientists insist that the magnesium stearate breaks down in the stomach, along with the rest of your supplement, when it meets strong acid and gets churned up for a while during digestion. Other scientists feel that magnesium stearate actually prevents proper breakdown and absorption of nutrients in your body. I'm undecided.

A study published in *Immunology* in 1990 suggested that stearic acid could suppress your immune system, making you more prone to infection. This study remains controversial to this day. Many scientists agree that it is a toxic substance, and others feel it is an innocuous additive. I doubt this issue will be settled in our lifetimes.

Some consumers are just plain sensitive to inactive ingredients like stearic acid, magnesium stearate, and ascorbyl palmitate. Supplement makers often call their products hypoallergenic or pure even though they contain manufacturing additives. It's confusing.

This particular additive is not a deal breaker for me. Some supplements containing magnesium stearate have otherwise fantastic formulas, and I've included them in this book. However, I recommend choosing supplements that are free of stearates if you have multiple chemical sensitivities or many allergies. Thorne Research has always boasted about its stearate-free product line (www.thorne.com).

Pay attention to allergens. Is your supplement free of common allergens? Whenever possible, you want your product to be free of wheat, gluten, dairy, corn, yeast, and soy. It should also be free of artificial colors, sweeteners, and preservatives. I've tried very hard to recommend products in each chapter that, to the best of my knowledge, are free of common additives and allergens.

Don't fall for the 100 percent claim. Your product may say that it provides 100 percent of the RDI (Reference Daily Intake) of key nutrients. The RDIs are based on the older term you may be more familiar with, the RDAs (Recommended Dietary Allowances). RDI values are the amounts that medical science says will keep you from dying of a disease. *Woo-hoo!* I say, "So what?" Even if the supplement offers 100 percent of the RDI, you are still getting a very small amount of the nutrient you need.

These Tricks Are Worse. Be Warned!

Some of the vitamin industry's practices present more cause for concern. Here's how to protect yourself.

Know that more is not necessarily better. Is your product selling you a bill of goods, putting in everything but the kitchen sink? Despite promotional claims on the box, some nutrients may be present in negligible amounts. You have to be aware that some ingredients may be included just for show.

Pay attention to the delivery system. Is your formula a tablet, capsule, or powder? Many tablets are difficult to dissolve and often contain binders and preservatives. Capsules, preferably vegetarian capsules, and powders are much easier for you to assimilate.

Select a biologically active formula. Is your product in the right form, a form that is biologically active? Many vitamins contain the wrong form of a nutrient. Manufacturers may use a less active form because it's cheaper to produce. For example, some vitamins exist in two forms, like mirror images of each other. Think of your left and right hands.

How do you know which is the correct form to buy? It's a question of educating yourself, and this book will help you do that. Let's look at vitamin E as an example of what I'm talking about. Your body wants the natural right-sided form (the right hand, if you will). This is designated with the letter "d." So you want your supplement to offer you vitamin E as "d-alpha-tocopherol," not the lab-created kind, "dl-alpha-tocopherol," which is cheaper to produce. It is more biologically active in its "d" form. The highest-quality vitamin E supplements contain d-alpha-tocopherol along with the seven other variations of vitamin E collectively called "mixed tocopherols and tocotrienols." Remember that vitamin E is the name given to a family of eight molecules. So the very best brands have all eight in their formulas. Read the label and see what you have. Vitamins that come in the wrong form are definitely deal breakers for me.

Pay attention to quality control. Was your product tested and guaranteed for safety, purity, and potency? If so, it should say so on the label, or the company that manufactures it should be able to give you those assurances. The testing doesn't necessarily have to be done by an independent testing company. I have seen some of those independent labs do a poor job, and some have questionable ethics.

Who manufactures the product? Is it contracted to the lowest bidder, or does the company selling the product actually make it? If it does, then ask if it follows the FDA's good manufacturing practices and if it tests its raw materials. If so, another good question is: "Do you test your finished product for purity, label potency, and identity?" I like to know that my product comes with good quality assurance. I expect you do, too.

These Are the Worst Tricks. Run!

Finally, there are several vitamin industry practices that should send you running.

Be careful of false claims. Selling unique nutrients or herbal products that aren't safe or well researched is deceptive advertising. Unfortunately, it's also fairly common. Let's consider horny goat weed as an example. Many men use this herb to ramp up their sex drive because they think it will help them get erections. I can't find a single well-designed clinical trial that supports its use in men with erectile dysfunction, but the name sounds good, doesn't it? And whether it works or not (because I'm not going to argue with you guys who rely on it), there was a study published in a 2004 issue of *Psychosomatics* that found a suspicious connection between the herb and two problems—racing, irregular heartbeat (tachyarrythmia) and an uncomfortable feeling of agitation or irritability (hypomania).

How do you know whether a company is making exaggerated or false claims about one of its products? Again, you need to educate yourself and not rely solely on advertising hype to make your purchasing decisions.

Check for dissolvability. Does your formula meet pharmaceutical standards for complete disintegration? If it does, that means it meets USP (United States Pharmacopeia) guidelines. On occasion, a manufacturer will put a notation on the bottle about USP. Nature Made products have the USP symbol of quality on the front of their product labels. By the way, the USP–National Formulary is kind of like a very thick cookbook of sorts that provides manufacturers and scientists with specific directions on manufacturing and testing all sorts of components, as well as information about how to test disintegration of a tablet. What I like about the USP certification process is that it is a third-party verification program that is recognized as a sign of quality in more than 30 countries worldwide. I always think it's better when someone other than the manufacturer is able to certify quality, purity, and potency. You can learn more at www.usp.org.

Be on the lookout for problem ingredients. Is your product's formula free of ingredients that may gather in your tissues and cause an overdose problem? For example, some ingredients, such as preformed vitamin A (retinol), can accumulate in your tissues. This can happen if you take large quantities (greater than 25,000 IU) every day. It's different with beta-carotene. This nutrient goes on to form vitamin A in your body, and your body controls the conversion, so it won't accumulate like preformed vitamin A. Beta-carotene is a safer way to supplement vitamin A.

The mineral iron is another example. It accumulates over time and can be harmful in large doses—even in a single dose if the dose is large enough.

Some Formulas Are More Usable Than Others

I've saved the very worst for last. I'm about to teach you how to become the smartest health advocate for yourself and develop what I call "supplement savvy." If you really, truly want to improve your health and get the best vitamins for yourself, read on.

It's always best if your product is completely free of corn, wheat, gluten, soy protein, yeast, milk/dairy, sugar, salt, artificial colors, artificial flavors, and preservatives. A definite no-no on my list is artificial sweeteners! I see artificial sweeteners in many green powdered drinks, liquid supplements, and chewable tablets. You have to read the label to ferret out these ingredients. Just be aware that some products are nutritious and completely natural and others aren't.

Vitamins Don't Work Until Your Body Activates Them

The ingredient list on that vitamin label may be impressive, but the nutrients you take do nothing until your body activates them. Vitamin B_{12}, for example, is better when formulated as methyl B_{12} or methylcobalamin, which your body can use immediately and to the fullest extent. So the question to ponder is "Is my supplement providing my nutrients in a healthy, body-ready, usable form?"

Many nutrients require this activation process. Sometimes it's done by acid in your stomach and sometimes it's another nutrient that's used as a cofactor. Either way, your body has to convert nutrients to an activated, usable form before they can be taken up by your cells. This process is complicated and requires stomach acid for absorption, something you may be suppressing with acid-blocking heartburn drugs.

You also need a strong, healthy gut that has a friendly camp of intestinal flora in order to make certain vitamins, such as folic acid, iron, CoQ10, riboflavin, and vitamin K. To make a long story short, your body goes through several processes including breakdown, absorption, activation, and microbial gut manufacturing just to make or fully use vitamins.

It's plain and simple. If you have health challenges, eat fast food, have gastrointestinal problems, or take acid blockers, then you are probably not able to activate or absorb all of your vitamins efficiently. This means that you are not getting as much benefit from them as you should. It also means that you may need higher doses than the general population. It would be ideal for you to upgrade the quality of your supplements so that your vitamins come in activated forms. Basically, this means that they are handed to you on a silver platter.

If you're taking individual nutrients for therapeutic reasons, you'll need to educate yourself on the best forms to take. The chapters on individual nutrients in this book were designed to help you do just that. Consider vitamin B_6 as an example. Does your vitamin B_6 come in its active, usable form, pyridoxal 5'-phosphate (P5P), or is it just pyridoxine hydrochloride? Pyridoxine is fine, and I've taken it myself, but P5P is a step up because it does not require riboflavin (a sister B vitamin) to activate it. Does your vitamin B_{12} supplement contain methylcobalamin (usable), or does it contain cyanocobalamin? Most brands contain cyanocobalamin, which is more difficult to use, so your body has to work harder to get to the active, healthy, usable form of the vitamin.

In Chapter 9, I went into great detail on folic acid. I did so because this nutrient protects unborn babies (our future generations), protects the heart, and guards against DNA damage, so it has some anticancer effects. You want to make sure you get enough folic acid, but not too much. Believe it or not, too much has the opposite effect and may contribute to cancer. That's the way it is when you get too much of a good thing; it backfires on you. So please use my information as guidance, but only take doses your doctor approves.

The point here is that folic acid isn't active until your body activates it. High-quality brands offer this nutrient in the active coenzyme form called folinic acid or the most active form, 5-methyltetrahydrofolate (5-MTHF). Those forms are easier to incorporate into your cells because they are body ready and instantly usable. Just to be clear, folic acid is *not* a questionable ingredient. It's totally fine. But 5-MTHF is better, but harder to find. The same is true of pyridoxine.

Who Wants to Eat Chalk, Then Get Cramps and Diarrhea?

Most vitamin companies maximize profits by using raw materials that are competitively priced. Is it the cheapest stuff they can get their hands on? On occasion. And it's not just the nutrients themselves that we need to be concerned about. The binders that manufacturers use can also be problematic. Most of the minerals in multivitamins and even stand-alone products, for example, are bound to inexpensive carriers to form a complex. That means that the mineral is chemically glued to another substance so that it can be made solid and put in a tablet or capsule. When a complex is delivered to your body, it gets broken down into its separate components. My issue with this is that most companies use the cheapest possible carriers. Some of these binders can have a negative impact on your health.

Calcium is found in many bone-building formulas, for example, but the type of calcium used is very inexpensive and bound to carbonate. You'll see it on the label as calcium carbonate. Sometimes you'll see it as bone meal, oyster shell, or dolomite. These forms of calcium salts are terribly tough for your body to absorb, and so very little calcium makes it into your bones, where you need it the most to prevent osteoporosis. They also require a great deal of stomach acid to break down. Many people don't produce enough acid in the first place, and others suppress their stomach acid with acid-blocking medications.

Calcium carbonate is the cheapest form of calcium to manufacture, and it's similar to the calcium carbonate that is used to make chalk for a chalkboard. When you buy calcium, you have to think of shopping. When you go shopping, you want the most bang for your buck. That's why you'll often choose a shirt or a belt that you can wear with many different outfits. It's the same with calcium and other minerals. You want the form of calcium that can be used in more than one place. Some high-quality companies offer a form of calcium that's chemically bound to another nutrient your body needs, usually an organic acid such as citrate, malate, aspartate, or gluconate. If you take calcium aspartate, the calcium goes to your bones and the organic acid (aspartate) is used to produce energy.

Choosing an intelligently formulated brand guarantees that you are getting a more biologically active and usable form of calcium. The easiest form of calcium to find is calcium citrate, but even this form can spark headaches and fatigue in certain sensitive people. Regardless, calcium citrate is much better for you than calcium carbonate since it gets to the bloodstream better.

You face the same kind of challenge when buying magnesium. Is it bound to oxide? Magnesium oxide is sold widely in most vitamin formulas, but it can cause diarrhea. Worse, it requires precious antioxidants from your cells to break down. What a useless way to spend your antioxidants, for breaking down a poor-quality product. You could buy magnesium amino acid chelate or spirulina, a superfood that is rich in this precious mineral. That's a smarter purchase. These formulas provide you with magnesium, which in turn lowers blood pressure, elevates mood, boosts energy, and relieves muscle aches and pains. It's a bargain if you think about what you're getting for your money. It's best to buy mineral supplements that confer multiple benefits.

You may also see magnesium chelate or sometimes magnesium glycinate on the ingredient label. Those are okay, too.

It should be noted that some people are sensitive to magnesium no matter what form it comes in and may experience diarrhea with any brand of magnesium. They should get it from a superfood or from leafy greens.

What Else Is in Your Formula?

We're not done yet. As I've already intimated, your supplements can contain a whole lot more than the simple nutrient or herbal formula you think you're purchasing. Here's a look at what else might be in there.

Coloring. It's shocking, but FDA-approved colorants include ground-up or powdered red beetles. No company would dare put that on the label. They camouflage it as carmine or cochineal extract, C.I. 75470, crimson lake, Natural Red 4, E120, or "natural color." These dyes impart the pretty pinkish or red color to almost all lipsticks. Yes, even natural ones. Aren't insects natural? You also find carmine in red-colored drinks, ice cream, frozen ice pops, candy, and yogurt. If I want pink yogurt, I'll add strawberries, thank you (!), because in my house I chase bugs down with a broom, not a spoon!

The artificial colors, designated as "FD&C" or "Lake," are hair raising, too. To their credit, the FDA has banned some of these. FD&C Yellow No. 5 (also called tartrazine) and FD&C Blue No. 1 and No. 2 are problematic and may trigger asthma attacks, hives, or deadly allergic

Make Sure Supplements Work for **You**

When you purchase a supplement, are you sure it contains ingredients appropriate for you and that the dose is correct? Most consumers don't know the answers to these questions. They trust that if an ingredient is on the label, it's present in the formula in substantial amounts. In the case of herbs, people just assume that they're extracted from the correct part of the plant. The active component of a plant differs from herb to herb. With saw palmetto, for example, the active part is extracted from the berries, not the root; but with ginger, it's the root that's most active.

Consider the hormone known as DHEA. Our bodies make this hormone. Companies also sell it in supplemental form. These are sometimes called "fountain of youth pills." But did you know that some products claim they work just like DHEA when they only contain wild yam? Wild yam does provide the starting materials for the body's synthesis of DHEA (and pregnenolone), but it doesn't act like DHEA. This conversion must take place in a lab!

The sleep hormone melatonin is not an herb, but where it's derived from certainly matters. Some "natural" forms of melatonin hormone are extracted from the brains of cows. Many people are allergic to this form, so in this case it's actually better to take a synthetic version. Another extremely popular dietary supplement, MSM (methylsulfonylmethane), is used for arthritis. This supplement should be derived from DMSO (dimethyl sulfoxide) in order to work properly.

Supplement makers know that consumers are generally not savvy, and they often list an ingredient even if it appears in a negligible amount or if it's extracted from the wrong portion of a plant. For example, unworthy supplements may state "ginkgo extract," whereas a high-quality supplement is proud to disclose the dosage as "40 mg ginkgo extract (leaf) standardized to 24 percent heterosides."

Bottom line: Educate yourself about the supplements you take. Then educate yourself some more. Let your health-care provider know about any supplements you take and find out whether there may be better choices to meet your needs.

reactions. As far back as 1978 we knew this. A study published in *Clinical Allergy* showed what could happen upon oral administration of tartrazine. Scientists gave it to 122 patients and took note of the disturbing reactions. Here are just a few: weakness, palpitations, sensations of heat, blurred vision, runny nose, feelings of suffocation, and itchiness. There was also a noticeable activation of inflammatory pathways known to cause uncomfortable allergic reactions in the body. I can't figure out why dyes like tartrazine are ever used in our foods when natural colors exist. A few of them include chlorophyll, beta-carotene, grape skin, natural astaxanthin, hibiscus, turmeric, annatto, and elderberry extract. There are also many others.

Flavoring. Artificial flavors that sort of taste like banana or bubble gum help parents get otherwise yucky medicine into their toddlers. Why do we need those when Mother Nature provides natural flavors like mint, lemon, chocolate, and vanilla?

Sweeteners. Natural sweeteners that I recommend include stevia, coconut nectar, unrefined agave nectar, and molasses. But most supplements don't use these sweeteners. Instead, they contain things like cane sugar, mannitol, xylitol, or sorbitol and lab-created sweeteners like aspartame (NutraSweet, Equal) and sucralose (Splenda). Some scientists feel they damage brain cells, impair thinking, and cause migraines. Truvia is the latest patented sweetener to hit the market. It is derived and extracted from one of the leaves of the stevia plant. See *Diabetes without Drugs* for more on natural sweeteners.

Binders. A binder makes everything stick together. Examples include dextrose (a sugar) and polyethylene glycol. Incidentally, throw out anything that has the binder diethylene glycol (DEG) in it. The FDA recalled cough syrups and toothpastes because of this poison, which is used in antifreeze.

Humectants. These substances are used to prevent loss of water or drying of the skin. They make your lotions and creams feel smooth on your skin. One, called polyethylene glycol (PEG), is used in toothpastes to keep the paste from gunking up and to help it stay smooth and uniform. It's found in popular laxatives and bowel evacuation drugs like Colyte and Golytely.

The humectant called propylene glycol is found in paint and industrial antifreeze as well as medicine, shampoo, body lotion, and deodorant. Some studies suggest it may lead to nervous system damage, kidney damage, liver problems, and skin rash. The material safety data sheet that goes with this chemical warns about avoiding skin contact. Maybe because of the liver damage? So when you shampoo your hair, you're supposed to make sure not to get it on your skin? Yeah, right. I think bypassing these products is a better option.

Lubricants. The most common of these are stearates such as magnesium stearate. It's most often found in tablets, but a lot of capsules contain it, too. Magnesium stearate is not the same thing as the nutrient magnesium. Stearates help speed up the flow of the nutrient powder that's made into tablets or put into capsules. This speeds up the production line, but may reduce your absorption of the active goodies in your supplement or medicine.

Disintegrators. These ingredients help break down tablets. Cellulose (plant derived) is common, and so is sodium lauryl sulfate (SLS), which is currently under fire for its possible association with kidney and bladder damage and cancer. This chemical is found in floor cleaners and engine degreasers as well as personal care products and toiletries. Shampoo and soap often contain SLS. According to the American College of Toxicology's "Final Report on the Safety Assessment of Sodium Lauryl Sulfate," which was published in 1983, SLS "had a degenerative effect on the cell membranes because of its protein denaturing properties. High levels of skin penetration may occur at even low use concentration."

Did you know that SLS is actually used in clinical trials around the world to induce skin irritation so studies can be performed? This is interesting also: Products intended for use on the skin should not contain more than 1 or 2 percent concentration of SLS, yet many shampoos, soaps, body washes, creams, and lotions have 10 to 20 percent!

Preservatives. These help to maintain freshness. It's worth watching out for anything containing parabens (propyl-, methyl-, butyl-, or ethyl-). A scientific screaming match about the use of parabens persists because some researchers still think they are safe despite emerging research that shows they disrupt human hormones and can even cause cancer. Other preservatives, including BHA, BHT, sorbic acid, and potassium sorbate, are also commonly found in supplements. Often they are in the raw materials used in a vitamin formula and are not listed on the label.

Fluoride. We find it in many products and even in the water system. Fluoride is prescribed to kids to protect their teeth and prevent cavities. Which reminds me, aren't virtually all toothpastes made with fluoride? Well, not all, but certainly most toothpastes contain it. As of April 7, 1997, the FDA requires that all fluoride toothpastes sold in the United States carry a poison warning on the label. It cautions users: "WARNING: Keep out of reach of children under 6 years of age. If you accidentally swallow more than used for brushing, seek professional help or contact a poison control center immediately."

What a disturbing surprise to learn that this chemical is also found in many roach-killing products, pesticides, and wood-preserving chemicals.

Buy Only from Trusted Sources

By now, you are probably either confused or upset. Call it tough love. That really wasn't my intention, but I do want to prompt you to think more about what you are putting into your body. For years I have been disturbed as I watched a multibillion-dollar industry take advantage of people. Consumers are willing to buy supplements because of great marketing campaigns, but what's inside the tablets they buy often comes up short. I bet you spend more time pondering what you'll order for dinner at a restaurant than you do deciding what brand of vitamins to take. If you are counting on the dietary supplement industry to support your health and produce top-notch products, you are going to be sorely disappointed. Some genuinely care; some don't.

Vitamin and supplement makers have businesses to run. Even though there are many companies offering high-quality products made with integrity and purity, there are just as many others who are unscrupulous and want to sell you garbage. You have to be smart enough to learn the basics and insist on the best supplement in your price range. Most companies are banking on naive consumers who will buy anything with a pretty label, nice Web site, or fascinating infomercial. Now you know what to look for.

Purchase your supplements only from trusted sources, and bear in mind that some high-quality supplements are sold only through physicians' offices. This is because large retailers are not willing to pay a higher price to get quality products into their stores because you, the consumer, are always looking for a bargain. This forces first-rate supplement makers to sell their products to licensed practitioners who want to carry the better products. It's not always this way, but it's a good rule of thumb. As you may have learned, many good-looking labels don't pack a punch.

What Should You Do?

Start reading labels with your newfound knowledge. Look for pure and unadulterated formulas that are free of artificial colors, sweeteners, fillers, preservatives, and other unnecessary ingredients. I want you to take only exceptional supplements. There are many companies that are authentic, pure, and reputable. I've spent many years in this business, and I've done some of the legwork for you. I've been brutal in assessing the formulas I've recommended in each chapter, but I'm sure I've missed some really decent companies. Use your judgment and intuition, and recommendations from your naturopathic doctor. And do read the Resources section, which starts on page 448, because I've highlighted various companies that really put their best foot forward and create innovative, high-quality supplements.

Daily Values

Some people are obsessed with meeting the USDA's Recommended Dietary Allowance (RDA) for each vitamin and mineral because they feel that getting 100 percent of the RDAs will equate to good health. Remember that I said in the previous chapter that the term RDA is outdated. It was used for many years, but you won't hear it much anymore. Scientists have begun referring to it as either the RDI (Reference Dietary Intake) or the DV (Daily Value). Here's a little bit more information about each of these terms.

RDI: Reference Dietary Intake

This is the minimum amount of a vitamin or mineral that the USDA recommends that a person consume each day. They feel it will cover virtually all American citizens' needs and prevent illnesses that result from deficiencies. For example, the RDI for vitamin C is about 100 mg per day. If you get that much, you won't develop scurvy, the deficiency disease. Just an FYI: You might also see RDI called DRI, for Dietary Reference Intake.

DV: Daily Value

This is just the RDI based on a 2,000-calorie-per-day diet. These recommendations were originally set up by government officials at the USDA. Some of them are nutritionists.

Looking Back in History

The RDA is a set of recommendations originally developed during World War II and is based on what our military needed. The suggested standards also applied to civilians and to people overseas. Scary as it sounds, food had to be rationed during the war, and nutritional guidelines took this into account when the USDA set up the original guidelines in the early 1940s.

By the 1950s, the USDA had created a new set of guidelines that included the number of servings of each food group needed in order for you to receive the recommended dosage of each nutrient.

The recommendations have evolved a little over the years. In the late 1990s, the RDA became part of a broader set of guidelines called the Reference Dietary Intake or the Daily Value. When you see 100 percent for the DV on any label, it certainly looks impressive, but many studies have shown the DV amounts to be woefully inadequate for certain needs.

Human beings have embedded genetic information about how much of any given vitamin they need. We are all genetically blueprinted, and some of us need more of one nutrient than other people. Individual needs are based on the genetic code, which contains SNPs ("snips"), or pieces of the code. My snip could mean that I need a hundred times more folate each day than your snip, which says you need less folate than the average person. It gets too complicated for this book, but the moral of the story is that each of us has unique nutrient needs.

Now look at the DVs on your typical multivitamin label (see page 330). It will likely say the product contains 100 percent of almost every nutrient. So it looks like a great supplement. But it's not necessarily so. Look closer. You might see that the product provides only 30 IU of vitamin E. Since this meets 100 percent of the DV, you think you're getting the right amount. But 100 percent of the DV for vitamin E doesn't offer adequate protection for your brain or heart. Many studies show that you need at least 200 IU per day, even 800 IU for certain conditions.

Furthermore, if that 100 percent is a synthetic form of vitamin E, it works only half as well as natural vitamin E. (You can tell it's synthetic if there's a "dl" prefix rather than just a "d" in front of "alpha-tocopherol." If the label says "d-alpha-tocopherol," it means the product contains natural vitamin E.)

Not to pick on the typical multivitamin, but it also likely contains 100 percent of the DV for vitamin B_{12} in the form of cyanocobalamin. It's better if that particular nutrient comes as methylcobalamin, not cyanocobalamin. (Read about methylcobalamin on page 193 to learn more about vitamin B_{12}.) That formula probably contains about 6 mcg of B_{12}. That's a miniscule amount, and it won't do your body much good. You need at least 100 mcg of B_{12}, in the right, methyl form. Still, that 100 percent looks really impressive, doesn't it? Why should you care? Because a study published in *Neurology* in September 2008 concluded that getting inadequate amounts of B_{12} can eventually shrink your brain. If you've been a subscriber to my syndicated column at www.dearpharmacist.com, you knew this 10 years ago. This study followed 107 men and women without cognitive decline. Annual MRI scans were used to evaluate brain volume and blood tests were used to measure B_{12} levels. At the end of 5 years, the study found that "subjects with the lowest levels of B_{12} lost twice as much

Supplement Facts

Serving Size 1 Tablet

	Amount Per Serving	% Daily Value
Vitamin A (as retinyl acetate and 50% as beta-carotene)	5000 IU	100%
Vitamin C (as ascorbic acid)	400 IU	100%
Vitamin D (as cholecalciferol)	600 IU	100%
Vitamin E (as dl-alpha tocopheryl acetate)	30 IU	100%
Thiamin (as thiamin mononitrate)	1.5 mg	100%
Riboflavin	1.7 mg	100%
Niacin (as niacinamide)	20 mg	100%
Vitamin B6 (as pyridoxine hydrochloride)	2.0 mg	100%
Folate (as folic acid)	400 mcg	100%
Vitamin B12 (as cynocobalamin)	6 mcg	100%
Biotin	30 mcg	10%
Pantothenic Acid (as calcium pantothenate)	10 mg	100%

Other ingredients: Gelatin, lactose, magnesium stearate, micocrystalline cellulose, FD&C Yellow No. 6, propylene glycol, propylparaben, and sodium benzoate.

brain volume regardless of age, gender, or previous educational status."

Now back to that typical multivitamin. It likely contains unnecessary additives. One of them is propylene glycol. This chemical is found in anti-freeze! I could go on and on. (Aren't you glad I'm on your side?) So let me share another problem I have with this typical formula. It's the colorant, FD&C Yellow No. 6. This yellow dye may not be as harmful as Yellow No. 5, which causes dermatitis, asthma, and hives in some people, but it has its own issues.

Yellow No. 6 is on the product label we're considering here. Scientists are always running tests on food colorants (including this one) to determine whether they cause cancer. So far, Yellow No. 6 is FDA approved and appears not to cause cancer in lab rats. But here's my point: If they have to test these artificial colorants (the key word here is *artificial*) and there's even a question about their safety, do you really want to consume them when you have the choice not to? High-quality supplement makers don't pretty up their pills with potentially harmful colorants or dyes. Case closed.

Are Megadoses the Answer?

Taking megadoses (doses way above the Daily Value) of vitamins and min-erals is not the answer either, and I certainly don't advocate it to any of my clients. I also don't advocate the one-pill-a-day concept that the makers of many multivitamins promote. My position is that the standards set by the RDIs for life-sustaining nutrients are extremely low and therefore are not enough to improve your health. The DV can serve as a starting point, but it's not the optimal amount you should have.

People get so hung up on these numbers and percentages, but they're only suggestions. Numbers aren't everything they're cracked up to be. In fact, numbers change at the convenience of big companies and organiza-tions who wish to sell you something. After all, medicine is a business and they need customers. What's normal today wasn't normal 10 years ago. Thresholds representing normal values change routinely, as is the case with cholesterol. Hasn't the threshold for high cholesterol come down every few years, conveniently allowing sales of statin cholesterol drugs to explode?

I think people are more likely to become sick from cholesterol-lowering medication than they are from having slightly high cholesterol levels. We will one day look back on the days of statin mania with great remorse. Statins are drug muggers of coenzyme Q10, vitamin D, and minerals, and you've learned how your body is affected by statin-induced depletion of these nutrients.

Why are so many Americans now taking statins? As I've said, I can't help but notice that the threshold for high cholesterol went way down as the statins came to market. Imagine that. Now there's a push to get 8-year-old kids on statins. When you reduce cholesterol, you also reduce the production of sex hormones. Here's what's next: Eighteen-year-old would-be studs who need Viagra to go with that statin.

But back to my point: I think people need much higher dosages of nutrients than the RDIs if they ever want to improve their health or reverse disease. Herein lies another issue. We have been indoctrinated to think that pills are the cure for every disorder. No matter what, we expect a prescription from the doctor. If he or she told us to go home, meditate, steam greens every day, and take up Pilates, we would be furious and find another doctor to give us a pill that lowers blood pressure.

As a pharmacist, I've noticed this exasperating trend. Some people want one magic pill to fix their poor lifestyle choices. There is no such pill at any pharmacy. We only have pills to mask the trouble, not fix it. If you continue to drink heavily, for example, doctors and pharmacists won't be able to do much for you once your pancreas and liver start failing. This is a pill-popping society, yet we have numerous campaigns that tell our children to "just say no" to drugs. Yeah, right, but first swallow your methylphenidate, which is an amphetamine similar to the street drug speed that is prescribed for hyperactivity disorders. But say no after that, okay, kiddies? *Puhleez.*

Our soils are virtually depleted of minerals and nutrients. Industrialization has contaminated our rain and our rivers. In case you haven't heard, many oceans and rivers are tainted with pharmaceuticals in addition to radioactive waste, mercury, and other toxins. Well, you can't live your life in fear, or in a glass bubble, but you can compensate and clean up your body. Eating right, exercising, and avoiding processed foods is a good start. That's why it's so important to supplement with high-quality nutrients. If you're going to make the effort and investment, choose a good vitamin that is pure and active.

Why I Pay No Attention to the Numbers

Since the RDI does very little to advance your health, I have deliberately not put the chart of current RDIs in this book. I feel it would be a poor use of space. That said, you've seen my recommended dosages for general health in each chapter along with dosages that offset the drug mugger effect. Where possible, I listed doses for specific conditions, too. These are guidelines. If your doctor has a different suggestion for you, follow his or her instructions. Now I will tell you why I pay no attention to the RDI numbers.

The DV is a rough guide. It is based on meeting the needs of your average healthy person. Helloooo? Many people are not really healthy. They are dealing with numerous problems in their cells, arteries, glands, and organs. Often those problems have not even manifested yet. Before an individual is diagnosed with cancer, for example, it may have been growing for years. Before an infection like tuberculosis is discovered, an individual can have it for about 2 years and not know. Before you experience a heart attack, your arteries have been clogged and your body inflamed for years. Doesn't your mind start slipping years before you are diagnosed with Alzheimer's disease? Your bones and fingernails become brittle long before you fall and break your hip. I made a list of 10 of my friends, and not one enjoys perfect health. So all of us are really average healthy people until that lab test comes back abnormal and then, all of a sudden, we are sick. The DV doesn't take these issues into account.

DVs ignore special needs. DV thresholds don't take into account the needs of the elderly, children, pregnant women, lactating mothers, or people with disease. There are tremendous differences in what each of these populations requires. How can the government think that an

80-year-old man in a nursing home needs just marginally more of a particular vitamin than an 18-year-old college student?

The DV is based on a 2,000-calorie-per-day diet. I visited the Web site for McDonald's, one of the world's most popular fast-food restaurant chains. It has a cool feature on its site that allows you to view ingredient information (a plus for those with allergies to wheat, soy, or dairy) and the nutritional content of its salads, sandwiches, breakfast meals, and the rest. When I viewed it recently, I found one Big Mac has 540 calories all by itself. If you order the Premium Crispy Chicken Club Sandwich instead, you're up to 630 calories. That's not including fries or a soda. And that's just one meal!

The science behind DVs is incomplete. The board that establishes DV recommendations admits that scientific knowledge of nutritional requirements is far from complete, that the requirements for many nutrients have not been established, and that many essential nutrients are not on the list. They suggest that we eat a varied diet and not depend on vitamins, pills, or processed foods. I agree with all of that. But even when we take all of that into account, I still have questions about those numbers.

Government studies have shown that the population nationwide is chronically deficient in magnesium. So I am at a loss to explain why the RDI for magnesium is only 420 for a male and 320 for a female over 31 years of age. (DVs, remember, are based on RDIs.)

Magnesium deficiency can cause high blood pressure, diabetes, depression, and heart attack. Does this sound like many residents of the United States? You bet it does. Just so you know, once flour is stripped and bleached to make all-purpose white flour, it no longer has nutritious levels of magnesium, and you need magnesium to control blood sugar. To make matters worse, many blood pressure pills, cardiac drugs, and diuretics are drug muggers of this mineral, which maintains normal heart rhythm, too.

Early signs of magnesium deficiency include fatigue, numbness or tingling, cramps, and irritability. Magnesium is needed to help regulate insulin, and a shortage will contribute to the development of diabetes. (See

Chapter 12 for more on magnesium.) And yet, despite the epidemic of diabetes and heart disease and the fact that some of these cases might be due to magresium deficiency, the government still suggests the measly Daily Value stated above. Furthermore, the board has not taken into account the needs of a population that is eating food grown in soils virtually devoid of minerals, especially important ones like magnesium.

The DV is not the same thing as personal nutritional requirements. People often confuse the two. There's no connection. Your genes dictate how much of a vitamin you need. Nutritional requirements vary from person to person. For example, some people have a tough time utilizing folate (a B vitamin) and therefore have deficiencies that result from their genetic makeup. A deficiency of this B vitamin leaves you prone to depression, heart disease, and a higher risk of cancer. It may also lead to birth defects in the babies of pregnant women. Supplementing with additional folic acid may prevent neural tube defects.

The RDI is based on people who live under normal circumstances. Unfortunately, our reality is one in which there is a lot of illness—cancer, heart disease, diabetes, autism. Our reality also includes being exposed to a boatload of environmental toxins starting the day we're born. We get vaccinated with multiple injections before we even leave the hospital as newborns, which taxes a brand-new, vulnerable immune system. It shocks me that many caring pediatricians recommend vaccines at birth, but advise against giving cereal to babies until they are 6 months old. It's not that I advocate cereal early on, because an infant's digestive process can't handle it. But I think that giving so many vaccines to infants should be approached with a shot of skepticism.

Our reality includes exposure to lots of chemicals. We ingest cancer-causing phthalates and bisphenol from plastics, chlorine from the water, bromide from bread, alloxan from white flour, parabens from our makeup and shampoo, and pesticides from our produce. The list goes on and on. It's unpleasant just thinking about it, but we cannot escape these toxins as long as we live in an industrialized country. This is why we have to take the best care possible of our bodies.

So you tell me: Is the minimum amount of a nutrient enough to counter all of this? Is the DV really enough to keep us healthy in this type of industrialized society? I think not. The good news is that with this book I have armed you with the best protection of all—knowledge, and knowledge is power. When you absorb the message of this book, you will not fall prey to many of the hazards and drug muggers out there. It will help you care for your body more attentively. Your body is sacred. Take good care of it! It will feel better and you will look better for years to come. I've listed excellent products in each chapter in Part II, and you can read more about many of the companies that make them in the Resources section later in this book.

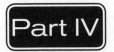

Where Do I Begin?

27

Where Do I Start to Stop a Drug Mugger?

Dealing with the drug mugging effects of medications—especially if you're faced with more than one disease and multiple medications—can seem daunting. This chapter answers questions you may have and also helps you pinpoint health challenges that may need the most attention. While you're sorting out these important first steps, I strongly recommend that you try the nutrient-boosting Total Body Tune-Up. This week-long program, which begins on page 357, will get you off to a positive start and will make a difference in your health almost from Day 1.

Please take the simple nutrient quiz that starts on the next page, and check off all the symptoms that apply to you. As you go through the quiz, be very honest. No one is going to check you or score you. If you are uncertain as to whether a particular symptom applies to you, check it if you experience it more than three times a week or if it has prevented you from doing a daily activity. Don't check it if it's rare. Even though there are dozens of symptoms associated with a particular nutrient deficiency, I've only selected a few to help you see a trend in your body. You may still have a vitamin/mineral deficiency even if you don't check off all the symptoms in a section. Do the best you can. You'll discover which of your body symptoms are in need of the most care. Although several nutrient deficiencies could cause a particular symptom, this questionnaire will at least help point you to appropriate chapters for more in-depth explanations about what is happening in your body. My sincere hope is that you experience an aha moment, along with a better sense of which nutrients you should target. The few minutes you spend taking this quiz will be worth your while. Besides, there are no wrong answers!

Take My Quiz on Necessary Nutrients

Think of this questionnaire as your body's GPS to put you on the road to faster recovery. Just check off any of the symptoms that apply to you, then read the assessment following the choices.

1. Calcium

_____ **I have a hard time losing even a few pounds.**

_____ **I have high blood pressure.**

_____ **I have osteopenia or osteoporosis.**

_____ **I often get muscle spasms or cramps.**

_____ **I experience mood swings or irritability.**

If you answered yes to 3 or more of these statements, you should read Chapter 7 on calcium. You may be suffering the drug mugging effect on this important mineral. Prescription and over-the-counter drugs rob calcium from the body, and the time frame can be as quick as 1 week or as long as 6 months of taking the drug. The time frame differs so much because certain drugs—like antacids—have an immediate action on the body. They work quickly to relieve heartburn by lowering your pH. So if you take antacids chronically for a week, within 1 week's time, your levels of calcium are being suppressed. (Many people abuse antacids or take acid blockers every single day, which has a similar outcome.) Other medications may take a bit longer to dampen nutrient levels because they work along metabolic pathways—so I've given 6 months as an outside range.

2. Riboflavin

_____ **I have daytime fatigue but "wake up" after 6:00 p.m.**

_____ **I have lots of stress in my life or find it hard to cope.**

_____ **I have watery, fatigued, or bloodshot eyes.**

_____ **I get headaches or migraines.**

_____ **I have iron deficiency anemia.**

If you answered yes to 3 or more of these statements, you should read Chapter 19 on riboflavin. You may be experiencing the drug mugging effect on this important B vitamin. Over time (as little as 1 week or up to 6 months), drugs wipe your body clean of riboflavin, and you need it for optimal health.

3. Probiotics

_____ I have constant diarrhea or constipation (or it alternates between the two conditions).

_____ I experience flatulence, cramps, belching, or other digestive problems.

_____ I get sick frequently or take antibiotics several times a year.

_____ I have an autoimmune disease.

_____ I am frequently tired.

If you answered yes to 3 or more of these statements, you Should read Chapter 17 on probiotics. You may be experiencing a drug mugging effect that has wiped out your healthy intestinal flora. Virtually all drugs scrub your colon clean of these vitally important microorganisms, which you need in order to make B vitamins. Since optimal health starts in the gut, this chapter could be among the most important for you—no matter what health condition you have.

4. Iron

_____ I fatigue easily or get short of breath with little exertion.

_____ Sometimes my heart beats unusually fast for no reason.

_____ I have hypothyroidism, Graves' disease, or Hashimoto's disease.

_____ I have pale skin or lips.

_____ I have heavy periods.

_____ I have brittle nails.

If you answered yes to 3 or more of these statements, you should read Chapter 11 on iron. You may be suffering the drug mugging effect on this crucial mineral. Iron helps your body breathe by making red blood cells. Drugs have the ability to squash levels of iron, but it's really easy to replenish them. Also, please read page 161 for information about serum ferritin blood tests.

5. Melatonin

_____ I have trouble going to sleep or staying asleep.

_____ I am depressed.

_____ I have a history of (or presently have) some type of cancer.

_____ I eat hot dogs, salami, or bologna.

_____ I feel fatigued much of the day.

If you answered yes to 3 or more of these statements, you should read
Chapter 13 on melatonin. It's possible that you are experiencing the drug
mugging effect on this valuable sleep hormone, which is made in your brain.
Melatonin helps your body respond to darkness by falling asleep. It also
makes immune-boosting chemicals that protect you. As we age, melatonin
production wanes. You'll be shocked at some of the medications that
suppress this hormone.

6. Coenzyme Q10

_____ **I have high cholesterol.**

_____ **I have heart disease (any type, including abnormal heart
rhythm, heart failure, or angina).**

_____ **Muscle cramps or spasms are just a part of my life now.**

_____ **I am tired all the time.**

_____ **I am forgetful, and my memory is not as sharp as it used to be.**

If you answered yes to 3 or more of these statements, you should read
Chapter 8 on coenzyme Q10. It's likely that you are clean out of this powerful antioxidant or experiencing the drug mugging effect on CoQ10. This is
really important because your heart and brain both need this nutrient in
order to function properly. In fact, the medication you use for high cholesterol might very well be the drug that is mugging you! There are more than
200 other medications in multiple drug classes that rob your body of this
essential nutrient.

7. Thiamine

_____ **I feel pins and needles, numbness, or burning pain in my hands
or feet.**

_____ **I attract mosquitoes and gnats, while the people I'm with don't
even get bit.**

_____ **I like to drink red wine with dinner at night.**

_____ **I am an alcoholic.**

_____ **I have a malabsorption disease (such as celiac, Crohn's, or
colitis).**

_____ **I have memory problems.**

_____ **I am always on a diet.**

If you answered yes to 3 or more of these statements, you should read Chapter 21 on thiamine. You are likely dealing with the drug mugging effect on this phenomenal B vitamin. It helps your body make memory chemicals in the brain, digest food properly, and protect your nerves. Drugs have the ability to banish this precious B vitamin. Even though true deficiencies are rare, a low-level deficiency can make you miserable from head to toe.

8. Magnesium

_____ **I get tearful and feel anxious or depressed.**

_____ **I get panic attacks.**

_____ **I have high blood pressure.**

_____ **I have an irregular heartbeat.**

_____ **I have a child with attention-deficit disorder or hyperactivity.**

If you answered yes to 3 or more of these statements, you should read Chapter 12 on magnesium. You (or your child) could be suffering from the drug mugging effect on this amazing mineral, known to support mood, circulation, and heart and brain function. This could be the missing link in what ails you. More than 250 drugs can steal it. Magnesium deficiency is ridiculously common, and unless doctors measure it properly (in the red blood cell), you can fall through the cracks and get on a medication merry-go-round.

Your Questions, My Answers

I want results as much as you do. I need to make a connection with you, if only through this book. I want you to feel as close to me as possible, as if I were holding your hand through this transition period. Since there are millions of you reading this and I can't possibly respond to all of you, the best I can do is head off your questions by answering them now. Please take a few more minutes to read the next section, because it should answer your most immediate questions, even those you haven't thought of at the moment. Let the healing begin!

Q: Do certain medical conditions (or disease states) make you more susceptible to the drug mugging effect?

A: Yes, certain conditions cause your body to react differently than a completely healthy person. Be realistic. If you have fragile health or a serious medical condition such as kidney failure, heart disease, pancreatitis, seizure disorder, and so forth, be more careful about diving into high dosages or doing a complete juice fast. Obviously, your fragile health may be the result of taking multiple medications, so keep that in mind and make sure you remain supervised by a physician. For example, digestive disorders can affect the gastrointestinal tract and make it harder for you to extract and absorb all the micronutrients you need from your food. These conditions include celiac disease, Crohn's disease, ulcerative colitis, irritable bowel syndrome, gluten and wheat allergies, pancreatitis, and yeast overgrowth. If you have any of these conditions, you may be more likely to run low on zinc, selenium, vitamin B_{12}, magnesium, and beta-carotene.

These shortages can cause all sorts of mishaps that could be diagnosed as a new disease instead of being diagnosed as a digestive disorder. Let me give you a few examples, because this can be a huge barrier to your getting a proper diagnosis. When you run low on the following minerals, these are the diseases you might be diagnosed with.

Nutrient Deficiency	Potential Diagnosis
Zinc	Prostate disease
Selenium	Hypothyroidism
Vitamin B$_{12}$	Multiple sclerosis
Magnesium	High blood pressure
Beta-carotene	Macular degeneration
Thiamine	Alzheimer's disease
Riboflavin	Migraines
Pyridoxine	Peripheral neuropathy
Coenzyme Q10	Congestive heart failure

Imagine, all these potential diseases waiting in the wings simply because you are clean out of certain essential nutrients, and the real culprit may be an undiagnosed digestive disorder that has just become part of your life.

So, the answer is yes. Certain medical conditions or diseases can mean that you suffer more drug mugging effects than a family member or a friend who takes the same medication.

Q: Are the diseases caused by nutrient depletion real?

A: Yes, the disorders are real enough. It's important to realize, however, that sometimes the road to healing involves replacing missing nutrients rather than taking medications that mask symptoms. I'm not a doctor, and I'm not trying to be one. But *you*, on the other hand, need to educate yourself and partner with your doctor to find the best treatment to meet your individual needs. Knowledge is power, and in the case of your health, the information in this book can spare you much suffering and perhaps get you on the right road to spectacular health.

Q: Should I take all the supplements I need at once or take one at a time?

A: My rule of thumb is to bring in one supplement at a time. Individual supplements can make a huge difference in your health. Even one supplement can, in some cases, alter your need for some of the medications you may be taking. It's important for you to pay attention to how supplements affect your body. It's a lot easier to do this when you bring just one supplement on board at a time.

The one exception here is with B vitamins, which work in tandem with each other. If you want to start taking several different B vitamins, your best bet is to take a B complex supplement that supplies the Bs at once.

When starting new supplements to combat drug mugging effects, add them to your diet at least 1 week apart. Keep a notepad handy and jot down anything different in your daily health (such as diarrhea, headache, nausea). If you have new symptoms, you may need to experiment to see if the change is related to the vitamins you've added. Always take vitamins with food.

Also, you may notice that I've suggested adding new supplements on many of the days in the Total Body Tune-Up. While it seems counter to my advice here about adding new supplements slowly, the Tune-Up supplements are targeting cleansing and nourishing, so you can add them more quickly. Just be aware that as you add more supplements into your daily regimen, your body may begin clearing toxins faster. This means that you may feel one of two ways: Either you'll feel temporarily weakened for a few days as your body dumps stored chemicals, or you'll feel energized as your body improves at a cellular level. There's no way to tell because everyone is unique. Most of my readers have had good experiences.

I can tell you that any discomfort you feel should be relatively slight and short-lived; the integration of high-quality supplements is intended to help you, not harm you. In fact, it can help you remain compliant with your medications because you will have no annoying or disabling side effects.

As the weeks progress, your medication dose may need to be lowered or perhaps eliminated. Ask your doctor to closely monitor you if you take medications that draw a fine line between therapeutic and dangerous. These medications have what pharmacists call a narrow therapeutic index and are used for blood thinning, seizure disorders, bipolar disorder, hypertension, or cardiac arrhythmias. You must be monitored more closely because you will become more sensitive to the effects of your medications as your body heals and your cells get the food they've been hungry for. For instance, if you eat foods from my Side-Effect Solution diet and install a tight nutrient security system based on the medication you take, your blood pressure may fall lower than normal, and you may feel dizzy. It's a good thing in the sense that you can get your physician's approval to reduce your dosage or discontinue your medication. As your healing progresses, today's dark days will be nothing more than a faint memory.

Q: If I need to take several supplements, which ones are most important?

A: Try to begin with the supplements that affect larger parts of your system and form the foundation for better health. For example, if you realize that you are deficient in thiamine, probiotics, and vitamin C, then take the probiotics first because this forms a healthier environment in your digestive tract, making it easier for you to absorb everything else that you take afterward. Allowing the probiotics to take effect for a few weeks lays a good foundation because these microorganisms help extract nutrients from your food and dietary supplements.

After that, I would begin taking thiamine because healthy intestinal microflora support the B vitamins and even help you propagate them.

And finally, vitamin C, a water-soluble antioxidant, will sweep away free radicals in your body that cause DNA disruption and that increase your risk for dozens of disorders including Alzheimer's, Parkinson's disease, high blood pressure, diabetes, heart attack, stroke, and cancer. These are all tied to free radical damage and DNA damage, and vitamin C helps you.

Here's another example: If you find that you are deficient in either beta-carotene, vitamin D, glutathione, melatonin, or probiotics, begin by adding probiotics for overall gut health. Then start taking glutathione to keep your liver healthy and to help with detoxification (healthy livers help to activate vitamin D supplements). After probiotics, bring in the melatonin. This hormone helps you sleep, and restorative sleep is crucial to one's health. (You'd be surprised at how many diseases are tied to insomnia and the resulting chronic sleep deprivation.) Then, after you've gauged how you're feeling, start taking vitamin D and beta-carotene together. I think these two fat-soluble nutrients are fine together because neither usually causes any noticeable side effects or problems; they are both fat soluble and best taken with food.

In summary, you need to view your body as a whole, but pay attention to the individual systems. Correcting shortages that impact your digestive tract and liver would come first. Remember, these organ systems allow you to absorb all other nutrients and to activate the basic nutrients you get from food and sunshine and turn them into powerful biologically active forms that your cells are hungry for.

One example of this is vitamin D, which you get from UV rays of the sun. Your liver (and kidneys) need to activate that to calcitriol. Vitamin D does nothing on its own. Coenzyme Q10 is another good example. The body-ready form that is biologically active is called ubiquinol. You can buy that as a supplement, of course, but your liver—if it's healthy—can make it for you. And speaking of CoQ10, your heart health is important, too, and that's where most of the CoQ10 in your body resides. So if you are missing CoQ10 (read Chapter 8), then that supplement should be near the top of the list but after supplements for the intestines and liver.

Okay, I recognize that for many people, especially those who are dealing with multiple conditions and many medications, figuring out the order in which to begin new supplements may simply be too daunting. If this is the case for you, don't worry. You can't go wrong here. You may be lucky enough to have a doctor or other health-care provider who can advise you. Or you can rely on your intuition. Read the descriptions of the nutrients and what they do, and simply select the one that feels right to you.

You cannot hurt yourself doing things your way. Follow your gut feeling and your doctor's advice, even if it's different from what I've suggested here.

Q: Is it better to take multiple doses of a single supplement in a day or to simply take a higher dose once a day?

A: Usually it's better to take multiple doses of a single supplement spread throughout the day. Your body is constantly creating new cells. Millions are born each day, and millions more die. Your body is always in flux. Think of it this way: Every hour you give birth to new cells. They will be born at a higher level of functioning if you have the proper nutrients on board.

Take the example of vitamin C, a water-soluble antioxidant. Because it plays a role in protecting your DNA, it helps slash your risk for infection and cancer. If you plan on taking 1,000 mg daily, it's better to take 250 mg four times daily rather than 1,000 mg all at once. When I say four times a day, I don't expect you to wake up at night, I just mean every 3 to 4 hours while awake. When I say three times a day, you could take the supplement every 5 or 6 hours. For a twice-daily recommendation, you could take the supplement in the morning and at dinnertime.

Read the information in this book on each particular nutrient to find out if it's best to take it with food or on an empty stomach. By and large, most nutrients should be taken with food. They are, after all, "food in a pill" in the loosest sense of the term.

I believe that it's a good idea to split the dosages to allow your body to have optimum nourishment on board throughout the day. Most nutrients don't linger like relatives you don't like; they do their job then make a fast exit. They're in and out quickly. Sometimes an antioxidant only sweeps away free radicals (toxins) for 1 or 2 minutes, then the party's over. So by taking your vitamins in smaller doses throughout the day, you give your newborn cells a better chance at thriving. Remember, you are constantly exposed to all sorts of damaging things from the environment, diet, stress, and so on, so it's good to have essential nutrients on standby all day.

Here's just one more example of how this works. Let's look at what happens with calcium. Some experts feel that the body cannot take up more than 600 mg at a time and that if you take higher amounts, the full amount may not even make it into the cells. So follow your physician's orders or your gut feeling about supplementation. Whenever I'm short on calcium, I break up the dose myself and take it with food. (See Chapter 7 for more on calcium.)

Q: What kinds of side effects may I encounter?

A: Each nutrient has its own potential side effects, so please refer to the respective chapters on those. Most frequent side effects include nausea, cramps, bloating, stomach upset, and indigestion. This is because some micronutrients, especially minerals, are just plain hard to digest. The following suggestions may help you mitigate side effects from supplements.

Don't take supplements on an empty stomach. Take them either with a meal or with a small snack.

Time the occurrence of side effects. You might try taking supplements at night so you sleep through some of the side effects. But be careful not to take stimulating nutrients—such as vitamin B$_6$—at night or you'll be tossing and turning rather than sleeping.

Try switching brands. I've provided lengthy lists of supplements that I recommend, including many that I've tried myself, to help you select those that are easiest on the tummy and that are free of additives and artificial colors.

Take digestive enzymes. People who experience chronic indigestion with their vitamins and minerals and have a lot of sensitivities to foods or to vitamin brands are almost always deficient in digestive enzymes. You can buy these over the counter for less than $20 at any health food store. Sometimes they are labeled "digestive enzymes" and sometimes you will find a similar formula called "pancreatic enzymes." You may have to experiment with the brands, but this is usually the cure for people who have a tough time with supplements or who have a lot of allergies. You can take digestive enzymes with any nutrient that I've mentioned in this book.

Q: Isn't diet also important?

A: In a word, yes! It's good to eat more foods rich in particular nutrients if you have been mugged by a drug or lifestyle choice. In fact, I think it's the *best* way to install a tight nutrient security system. That's why in the Total Body Tune-Up in Chapter 28, I've given you a special menu for the week, as well as a daily smoothie recipe (and a daily juice recipe if you prefer to drink juice).

I could write a whole book about the way our food choices impact our health (hey, that's a great idea for my next book). It's that important. So I really want to emphasize this. The way you eat absolutely impacts how well you absorb nutrients and also how fast you restore them when you take drug mugging medications. If you are a soda pop junkie, for example, you're getting a huge burden of sugar each day, and the soda is wiping you clean of important minerals. Plus, soda doesn't have any health benefits associated with it. It's going to be harder for you to replenish what your soda (a drug mugger) steals when you're robbing yourself every day.

Coffee is another culprit. I know that you're going to continue drinking it even though it's thought to be a drug mugger of iron and other minerals. I totally understand! Coffee does have some health benefits (if you don't mess it up with 2,000 calories from candy flavorings and sugar). I drink coffee myself, and I've been told that I'm deficient in iron. But I take care to supplement daily with spirulina and iron glycinate to offset the drug mugging effect of my dietary choices.

So even though what you eat is important, the occasional unhealthy choice is not a deal breaker, because you can offset the effects if you know what you're doing.

Q: Are there any supplements and superfoods that can help me cover all my bases at once?

A: Sure, spirulina is one. It's a blue-green algae that has been around for eons. It is a rich source of beta-carotene and all the minerals listed in this book. Talk about a lot of bang for your buck. I take this superfood every single day. Why? Because there are more than 500 scientific studies tying spirulina to better health. It is a powerhouse at reducing inflammation. One 2009 study found that spirulina was able to block the production of pain-causing chemicals. This means it could actually be helpful for all sorts of aches, pains, and joint problems.

Spirulina is an amazing source of minerals, so it can help reduce muscle cramps and spasms. The mineral content can also support mood and pancreatic function (think diabetes). And it's energizing. It is great for stamina and endurance because it has a lot of B vitamins, which help nourish the adrenal glands. The chlorophyll in spirulina is fantastic for cleaning out the digestive tract. It also works like probiotics, helping to plant healthy microorganisms in your gut.

Most people don't like the flavor of powdered blue-green algae, which is how many companies sell it. I've found it in a tasteless tablet form (Spirulina Pacifica by Nutrex Hawaii), and it's a relatively small tablet to swallow. You just have to be creative and find supplements that come in forms you can tolerate.

There are other superfoods in my kitchen cabinet. Chia seeds are great because they contain healthy essential fatty acids that work in tandem with vitamin D and vitamin A, two commonly drug mugged nutrients. I also like coconut oil, a potent antifungal oil rich in healthy micronutrients. Pomegranate juice and coconut water are good because they contain powerful antioxidants and micronutrients that charge our electrical system (think heart). And don't forget chocolate! It's high in phytonutrients that protect our heart and brain. It affects the brain center by making endorphins (those wonderful feel-good chemicals).

Q: Should I consult my physician before doing any of this?

A: Yes, by all means. Far be it from me to give you advice without asking you to consult your doctor. Of course, you should tell your doctor what you want to do and make sure you get his or her blessing. One reason to do this is because it helps educate physicians. The more they understand, the more they can help others. I like the pay-it-forward principle because there is a trickle effect. For example, if you tell your doctor that you think you have leg cramps as a result of your statin medication and that you want to take coenzyme Q10, then your physician may begin recommending this nutrient to all patients who get a prescription for a statin drug, thereby sparing others from unnecessary pain.

Also, it's entirely possible that your doctor will *not* want you to undertake a new vitamin regimen for a particular reason. If you're undergoing chemotherapy, for example, your oncologist may not want you to take vitamins, minerals, or superfoods while being treated. I cannot decide for you what is right; only your physician can do that.

In any case, do have a frank discussion with your doctor. If you meet with resistance, I will not suggest that you find another doctor, but I am suggesting you have an honest conversation and let your doctor know that you're enthusiastic about taking natural supplements. Lots of doctors don't even realize that their patients are taking vitamins, minerals, and other supplements. You may even get a pleasant surprise and find that your doctor can give you some helpful advice about what to take. These days increasing numbers of doctors are educating themselves about the benefits of supplements.

Q: *Are there nutritional tests that I could take that will tell me exactly *what I am deficient in?

A: Yes, there are several excellent tests available to the public. You can ask your doctor about those. Please realize, however, that most physicians are in the habit of determining which medication, not which vitamin, is right for you.

Nutritional deficiencies can actually be tested with special micronutrient blood tests. There are three tests that I've taken myself: Comprehensive Nutritional Panel by SpectraCell Labs, NutrEval by Genova Diagnostics, and the Cardio/ION from Metametrix. Healthcare practitioners with appropriate licenses can become providers with these companies and order tests immediately.

Q: *Can I hurt myself with supplements?*

A: Unfortunately, the answer is yes. It's possible that you could be harmed by tilting your nutrients completely out of whack by taking too much of a single supplement. If you take too much of a single B vitamin, for example, and don't get enough of the other Bs, you could get yourself into trouble.

Consulting with your doctor may help keep you safe. If you like my natural health message, you can receive my syndicated column "Dear Pharmacist," which is available to the public for free by signing up at my Web site (www.dearpharmacist.com). I know for a fact that many people take supplements indiscriminately without telling their doctor because many readers who write to me with questions tell me this. Always discuss your health concerns and your supplements with your doctor.

Q: If I suffer from drug mugging effects of prescription and over-the-counter medications and follow your advice on replacing nutrients, how long should it take until I start to see a difference in my well-being?

A: Once you've made the decision to protect your body and replenish what the drug muggers may have stolen, it could take a matter of days to weeks for you to feel a difference. Most people notice some effect during the first month; I've also had people write me within a week of starting a nutrient to say they've noticed a change. It all depends on how long you've been taking your medicine and how severe your symptoms are. It also depends, in part, on the quality of the nutrients you purchase and the nutrient density of the foods you buy. Once you have the mind-set and the intention of getting well, you've started the domino effect—change your mind, change your body, change your life. I'm still so amazed that every day I get dozens of e-mails and social network comments on how well people are doing. You can have the life you dream of, you can participate in the activities you desire, and you can take back your life—you just have to have a little information to do that. I hope that you feel empowered to stay with it. Don't ever give up. If you don't get a response immediately, stay with it. Then you might want to switch to another supplement brand; it's often a case of trial and error.

The laws of nature govern that if you are deficient in a certain nutrient and you replenish that nutrient, wellness should occur on some level. Naturally, there may be several conditions layered on top of one another, and teasing this out can be difficult. But you have to know and believe that healing can take place and you can be well again. Your body wants to heal. Here's a supersimple example: Watch your finger after you cut yourself. The body makes an immediate effort to close the wound and protect it. Within a few days, new skin is growing there. It's a miracle that our body wants to—and can—heal so miraculously. We just have to allow it.

By putting back what medication stole, the body will get what it's hungry for, and wellness and nutritional balance will follow. In time, you will feel better and you'll be amazed at how easy it is to take back your life.

28

The Total Body Tune-Up

Are you ready for a total body tune-up? Whether you are suffering from the drug mugging effects of medications, from a particular illness or disease, or from a lifestyle choice, you've taken the first step to get well. Good for you! The rest is going to be relatively easy. You'll notice improvements in your health right from the start with this nutrient-booster program, and those improvements will motivate you to stick with it. This Total Body Tune-Up, which lasts just 1 week, will start you on a new way of living, a journey that will allow you to continue using necessary medications without suffering their drug mugging effects. In some cases, it may even allow you to put those medications behind you completely.

The Benefits to You

The Total Body Tune-Up will help you focus on the kinds of foods that you should be eating. It's a program meant first to sweep your cells clean of all the chemical gunk that has been stuck in there, then to replenish healthy, vital nutrients to those same cells so that you feel well again. Additionally, you *may* very well lose weight following this 7-day program. In fact, I expect you *will* lose weight, although that is not the intention or focus of the tune-up. It is not a fad diet designed to help you lose weight; it is a health-changing program that can improve the quality of your daily life.

If you follow the Total Body Tune-Up for 7 days, here's what the plan will do for you:

Reduce inflammation and pain-causing chemicals in your body. This happens because you will consume a lot of antioxidants on Days 2 and 3. Plus, I've included a smoothie that is made with fresh

357

pineapple, which contains bromelain, an enzyme that reduces pain and inflammation.

Cause cancer cells to actually commit suicide. This process is known as apoptosis, and it happens because of the rich supply of supplements such as spirulina and bioflavonoids.

Create more energy. This is accomplished by taking B vitamins, vitamin C, and spirulina.

Improve your mood. Vitamin C and the glutathione precursors (protein powders) will help you make happy brain chemicals. As an added benefit, the glutathione also helps to sweep toxic residue from your liver.

Reduce your cholesterol. This happens for two reasons. First, there's no refined sugar in the recipes; too much sugar causes high cholesterol. Also, you'll start taking detoxification supplements and making recipes with lots of fiber that focuses on binding cholesterol and taking it out of the gut. I'll also introduce you to a supplement from traditional Indian medicine known as triphala.

The truth is you could do a cleansing and detoxification on your own; my advice and nutrient-boosting recipes are just suggestions. If you follow this plan, you will eat only certain types of food to help clean out your body. The key is to remember that you are giving your body a TUNE-UP:

T—Total cleansing

U—Unsticking pollutants

N—Nourishing cells

E—Energizing

and

UP—Unleashing your potential!

What to Expect

Here's a quick summary of what to expect during your week-long tune-up, followed by a detailed description of what to do for each day.

Day 1: Total Cleansing

The idea behind a cleansing diet is that the body needs a rest and needs time to heal. So Day 1 is devoted to gently clearing your gut, even the tiny folds. If you have constipation, you'll get relief. The point of a cleansing diet isn't starvation. Go ahead and eat when you are hungry, and stick to raw, unprocessed foods as much as you can, as well as those recipes listed on pages 360–362.

Days 2 and 3: Unsticking Pollutants

We are assaulted daily by toxic materials, whether from pollution, medication (drug muggers), junk food, old pots and pans, or plastic products. This part of the week allows the body to expel those toxins from the body. They happen to occupy space in your cells, and your cells don't like it because the toxins can damage DNA and lead to cancer in some cases. We want them OUT.

Days 4, 5, and 6: Nourishing Cells

This part of the booster week has to do with quickly replenishing what the drug mugger stole and nourishing the cells. The recipes and supplements that I suggest have lots of antioxidants and minerals to rapidly restore your cells to a higher functional level. The idea here is to give the body what it has been starving for. You will definitely feel a positive impact and a sense of feeling lighter, happier, and stronger.

Day 7: Energizing

Making the decision to get healthy is revitalizing and energizing, and by Day 7 you will definitely be on the right path. You have the power within you to get well. Your body seeks wellness. You just have to remind yourself that you—not the drugs, not the pain, and not the past—are in charge now. Move forward, taking baby steps if you have to, and you will eventually get where you wish to be.

The 7-Day Tune-Up Menu

The Total Body Tune-Up focuses on the kinds of foods that you should eat to restore balance in your system. First, it will sweep your cells clean of all chemical debris. Second, it will replenish healthy, vital nutrients to those cells. You will know this is happening as you feel well again—like your old self, only better. This health-changing program will literally improve the quality of your daily life and give you unbelievable energy.

These menus are offered only as guidelines, so if you don't like or are allergic to a particular ingredient, feel free to substitute with an ingredient that offers similar nutrients. Each day of the week includes a smoothie recipe and juicing recipe specifically designed to achieve the tune-up goals of the day.

Day 1 Total Cleansing

Today's eating plan is all about cellular housekeeping. Be kind to your body and cleanse your system on a relaxed, stay-at-home day so you can be near the bathroom. My Carrot Parrot Juice is great for all kinds of digestive problems including constipation, Crohn's disease, and ulcerative colitis.

Strawberry Sweetness Smoothie

FEATURED NUTRIENT: VITAMIN C (100%)

Makes 1 serving

1 cup fresh strawberries

1 cup crushed ice

½ cup vanilla almond milk or hemp milk

1 tablespoon liquid aloe vera

2 teaspoons ground flaxseed

1 tablespoon raw cane sugar, turbinado, agave syrup, or honey

1 teaspoon fresh lemon juice

In a blender, combine the strawberries; ice; milk; aloe vera; flaxseed; sugar, turbinado, syrup, or honey; and lemon juice. Blend for 1 to 2 minutes, or until smooth.

Per serving: *Calories 166; Protein 3 g; Carbohydrates 32 g; Fiber 4 g; Fat 4 g; Saturated Fat 0 g; Sodium 83 mg; Vitamin C 93 mg*

Carrot Parrot Juice

FEATURED NUTRIENT: VITAMIN A (80%)

Makes 1 serving

3 or 4 carrots

2 kale leaves

¹/₂ cup fresh pineapple

2 Granny Smith apples

¹/₂ cup parsley

In a juicer, according to the manufacturer's directions, combine the carrots, kale, pineapple, apples, and parsley. Process until juiced.

Per serving: *Calories 279; Protein 5 g; Carbohydrates 72 g; Fiber 14 Fat 1g; Saturated Fat 0 g; cholesterol 0 mg; Sodium 161 mg; Vitamin A 3,832 IU*

Day 1 Menu

Breakfast

1 serving steel-cut oatmeal with 1 teaspoon ground flaxseed, ¹/₄ cup blueberries, ¹/₄ cup raspberries, 1 tablespoon chopped walnuts, a sprinkling of ground cinnamon, and a drizzle of maple syrup

¹/₂ cup plain yogurt

1 wedge honeydew topped with sliced strawberries

Herbal tea (tulsi or rooibus)

Snack

1 serving Carrot Parrot Juice (above)

Lunch

1 serving Tomatoes Stuffed with Basil Salmon (page 433)

1 whole grain gluten-free crispbread

1 pear

Sparkling or pure filtered water with a wedge of lime or lemon

Dinner

1 serving Walnut Chicken with Snow Peas (page 435)

¹/₂ cup cooked brown rice

1 serving Carrots with Citrus and Jalapeño (page 394)

Sparkling or pure filtered water with a wedge of lime or lemon

Snack

1 serving Strawberry Sweetness Smoothie (opposite page)

Supplement

Today, start taking a daily probiotics supplement. Probiotics are great for your general health and especially for digestion. They drive out *Candida* yeast and other pathogens from the gut. Take them on an empty stomach. Follow the manufacturer's suggested dosage or your physician's orders.

Stay on these for at least the entire week if not indefinitely. Make sure you choose a good brand (see Chapter 17).

Day 2 Unsticking Pollutants

Building on the supercleansing of Day 1, you'll begin to detoxify your system with nutrient-dense foods containing B vitamins, vitamin C, and those rich in chlorophyll to support heavy metal detoxification.

Piña Colada Smoothie

FEATURED NUTRIENT: VITAMIN C (100%)

Makes 1 serving

1 cup coconut water

1 cup frozen coconut-based sorbet, gelato, or ice cream

½ cup vanilla almond milk or hemp milk

¾ cup fresh pineapple chunks

1 banana

¼ cup dried unsweetened coconut flakes

In a blender, combine the water; sorbet, gelato, or ice cream; milk; pineapple; banana; and coconut. Blend for 1 to 2 minutes, or until smooth.

Per serving: *Calories 692; Protein 6 g; Carbohydrates 122 g; Fiber 11 g; Fat 23 g; Saturated Fat 18 g; Sodium 371 mg; Vitamin C 75 mg*

Detox on the Rocks

FEATURED NUTRIENT: VITAMIN A

Makes 1 serving

1 cucumber (with peel)

2 celery stalks

2 kale leaves

2 romaine leaves

½ cup green cabbage

¼ inch ginger

4 stems cilantro (or parsley)

1 or 2 pears (or apples) to sweeten

In a juicer, according to the manufacturer's directions, combine the cucumber, celery, kale, romaine, cabbage, ginger, cilantro, and pears. Process until juiced. Serve over ice.

Per serving: *Calories 225; Protein 6 g; Carbohydrates 55 g; Fiber 14 g; Fat 1 g; Saturated Fat 0 g; Sodium 143 mg; Vitamin A 7,999 IU*

Day 2 Menu

Breakfast

1 serving Italian Scrambled Eggs (page 419)

1 slice whole grain gluten-free toast

1 tangerine

1 cup milk or milk substitute

Coffee or herbal tea (tulsi, rooibos, or peppermint)

Snack

1 serving Detox on the Rocks (opposite page)

Lunch

1 serving Chicken, Bell Pepper, and Apple Salad (page 394)

$^{1}/_{2}$ cup red grapes

Sparkling or pure filtered water with a wedge of lime or lemon

Dinner

1 serving South-of-France Baked Cod (page 426)

1 serving Green Beans with Cashews and Chiles (page 399)

1 serving Honeyed Summer Fruit Bowl (page 442)

Sparkling or pure filtered water with a wedge of lime or lemon

Snack

1 serving Piña Colada Smoothie (opposite page)

Supplement

Start taking triphala, a complete body cleanser and detoxifier for the colon. Triphala also purifies the blood, removes toxins from the liver, and helps reduce cholesterol. No matter what the damage done by drug muggers, triphala helps to wipe the slate clean over time.

I've tried many of the brands and seem to get the best effect with the Organic India. Finish the first bottle at the recommended dosage on the label. After that, take 1 capsule daily for maintenance.

Day 3 Detoxing with Antioxidants

Today, you'll continue with the essential process of restoring lost nutrients while supporting detoxification. Day 3 is devoted to replenishing antioxidants with a special focus on vitamin C.

Banana Blue Smoothie

FEATURED NUTRIENT: VITAMIN C (100%)

Makes 1 serving

½ cup coconut water

1 cup frozen coconut-based sorbet, gelato, or ice cream

1 cup vanilla almond milk or hemp milk

½ cup organic frozen blueberries

1 cored fresh pineapple

2 scoops hemp or whey protein powder

1 tablespoon ground flaxseed

2 teaspoons lemon juice

In a blender, combine the coconut water; sorbet, gelato, or ice cream; milk; blueberries; pineapple; hemp or whey protein powder; flaxseed; and lemon juice. Blend for 1 to 2 minutes, or until smooth.

Per serving: *Calories 953; Protein 15 g; Carbohydrates 206 g; Fiber 23 g; Fat 15 g; Saturated Fat 5 g; Sodium 335 mg; Vitamin C 441 mg*

Juice C Juice

FEATURED NUTRIENT: VITAMIN C (100%)

Makes 1 serving

1 apple

1 cup grapes

½ small sweet red bell pepper

¼ lemon, peeled but pith remaining

1 kiwifruit

½ small navel orange, peeled but pith remaining

In a juicer, according to the manufacturer's directions, combine the apple, grapes, bell pepper, lemon, kiwifruit, and orange. Process until juiced.

Per serving: *Calories 276; Protein 3 g; Carbohydrates 72 g; Fiber 11 g; Fat 1 g; Saturated Fat 0 g; Sodium 8 mg; Vitamin C 181 mg*

Day 3 Menu

Breakfast

1 serving cooked gluten-free rice cereal with ½ cup plain yogurt, 2 tablespoons chopped dates, 1 tablespoon chopped pecans, and a sprinkling of cinnamon

1 wedge cantaloupe garnished with a squeeze of lemon juice and 1 teaspoon honey

Coffee or herbal tea (tulsi, rooibus, or rose hips)

Snack

1 serving Juice C Juice (opposite page)

Lunch

1 serving Cold Tomato and Cucumber Soup (page 387)

1 serving Black Bean, Rice, and Pepper Salad (page 391)

1 kiwifruit

Sparkling or pure filtered water with a wedge of lime or lemon

Dinner

1 serving Chicken-and-Bean Enchilada Bake (page 413)

1 serving Collard Greens with Tomato and Balsamic (page 396)

1 serving Baked Coconut Custards (page 439)

Sparkling or pure filtered water with a wedge of lime or lemon

Snack

1 serving Banana Blue Smoothie (opposite page)

Supplement

Continue taking triphala and probiotics. This supplement originated in India and is a combination of extracts from the harada, amla, and bihard fruits. Harada (*Terminalia chebula*) is known for its laxative effect. Amla (*Emblica officinalis*) is high in vitamin C—about 20 times higher than citrus fruit. Bihara (*Terminalia bellerica*) is particularly high in omega-3 fatty acids. Follow the manufacturer's suggested dosage or your physician's orders.

Day 4 Feed Your Cells

Today we'll focus on meals that provide powerful antioxidants as well as potassium. This mineral is known to improve blood pressure, heart disease, and leg cramps. The juice below, Potassium Splash, is great for people with anxiety, neuropathy, carpal tunnel, mouth sores, and diarrhea.

Berry Berry Good Smoothie

FEATURED NUTRIENT: VITAMIN B$_{12}$ (100%)

Makes 1 serving

1$^1\!/_2$ cups mixed berries (blackberries, raspberries, and blueberries)

1 cup plain yogurt

$^1\!/_2$ cup coconut water

2 scoops whey protein powder, any flavor

1 cup crushed ice

1 tablespoon maple syrup or honey

1 teaspoon hulled hemp seeds

1 teaspoon aloe vera juice

In a blender, combine the berries, yogurt, water, whey protein, ice, syrup or honey, seeds, and juice. Process for 1 to 2 minutes, or until smooth.

Per serving: *Calories 461; Protein 35 g; Carbohydrates 64 g; Fiber 8 g; Fat 8 g; Saturated Fat 2 g; Sodium 308 mg; Vitamin B$_{12}$ 4.25 mcg*

Potassium Splash

FEATURED NUTRIENT: POTASSIUM (33%)

Makes 1 serving

$^1\!/_2$ bunch parsley

4 carrots

2 celery ribs

$^1\!/_2$ papaya

$^1\!/_4$ cantaloupe, peeled

In a juicer, according to the manufacturer's directions, combine the parsley, carrots, celery, papaya, and cantaloupe. Process until juiced.

Per serving: *Calories 245; Protein 4 g; Carbohydrates 60 g; Fiber 13 g; Fat 1 g; Saturated Fat 0 g; Sodium 334 mg; Potassium 1,198 mg*

Day 4 Menu

Breakfast

1 whole grain gluten-free English muffin, toasted, spread with 2 tablespoons cashew butter

$\frac{1}{2}$ cup fresh cherries

1 cup milk or milk substitute

Coffee or herbal tea (tulsi or pau d'arco)

Snack

1 serving Berry Berry Good Smoothie (opposite page)

Lunch

1 serving Greek Chicken and Cauliflower Salad with Tomato Vinaigrette (page 398)

1 Pear, Date, and Walnut Muffin (page 444)

Sparkling or pure filtered water with a wedge of lime or lemon

Snack

1 serving Potassium Splash (opposite page)

Dinner

1 serving Chicken Braised with Port and Prunes (page 414)

1 serving Strawberry and Red Onion Salad (page 407)

$\frac{1}{2}$ cup cooked brown rice

$\frac{1}{2}$ cup steamed spinach

Supplement

Today, start taking two more supplements: ubiquinol, 50 to 100 mg daily, and vitamin E, 400 IUs mixed tocopherols (natural). This will support blood pressure, heart health, and muscle health (leg cramps), and will simultaneously offer you powerful antioxidant protection.

Day 5 The Magic of Minerals

Minerals such as iron, potassium, and zinc are rich in healing nutrients. We can take comfort in the fact that the foods containing these energizing minerals support good mood, pancreatic health, and boundless energy.

Go Green Smoothie

FEATURED NUTRIENT: VITAMIN D (37%)

Makes 1 serving

1 cup vanilla yogurt

1 banana, cut into chunks

½ cup coconut water

½ cup almond or hemp milk

½ cup ice cubes

1 scoop vanilla whey protein powder

½ teaspoon spirulina

1 teaspoon vanilla extract

In a blender, combine the yogurt, banana, water, milk, ice, protein powder, spirulina, and vanilla. Process for 1 to 2 minutes, or until smooth.

Per serving: *Calories 501; Protein 34 g; Carbohydrates 81 g; Fiber 5 g; Fat 6 g; Saturated Fat 3 g; Sodium 429 mg; Vitamin D 154 IU*

Iron Bonanza

FEATURED NUTRIENT: IRON (20%)

Makes 1 serving

½ cup fresh spinach leaves

1 golden beet, peeled, plus some beet greens

2 kale leaves

4 carrots

½ cup broccoli florets with a little stem

1 navel orange, peeled but pith remaining

In a juicer, according to the manufacturer's directions, combine the spinach, beet and beet greens, kale, carrots, broccoli, and orange. Process until juiced.

Per serving: *Calories 236; Protein 8 g; Carbohydrates 55 g; Fiber 15 g; Fat 1 g; Saturated Fat 0 g; Sodium 273 mg; Iron 3.74 mg*

Day 5 Menu

Breakfast

1 serving Tomato and Spinach Crustless Quiche (page 432)

1 slice whole grain gluten free bread, toasted

$^1/_2$ cup blueberries

Coffee (This is okay with me only if you need to avoid the caffeine headache, but coffee is a drug mugger of iron.)

Tea (Alvita brand makes two iron-rich teas, alfalfa leaf and horsetail grass. You can also drink rooibos or tulsi tea today. Note: Avoid peppermint, spearmint, green, black, and yerba maté, as they will chelate iron from the body. They are considered gentle drug muggers, like coffee.)

1 cup milk or milk substitute

Snack

1 serving Iron Bonanza (opposite page)

Lunch

1 serving Mediterranean Vegetable Salad Platter (page 400)

2 crispbreads

Sparkling or pure filtered water with a wedge of lime or lemon

Snack

1 serving Go Green Smoothie (opposite page)

Dinner

1 serving Spicy Bean Pancakes with Tomato-Pepper Sauce (page 428)

1 serving Summer Squash alla Parmigiana (page 431)

1 cup mixed salad greens tossed with 1 baby carrot, grated; $^1/_2$ tablespoon grape seed oil; and 1 teaspoon wine vinegar

Sparkling or pure filtered water with a wedge of lime or lemon

1 serving Watermelon-Cranberry Granita (page 447)

Supplement

This begins your burst of energy. Start taking spirulina, a blue-green algae superfood that is extremely rich in protein, minerals, vitamins, and anti-oxidants. In studies, spirulina has been shown to suppress allergies, enhance immunity, and lower triglycerides and harmful LDL cholesterol in the blood. Dietitians and nutritionists recommend 6 to 8 servings of fruits and vegetables each day; spirulina offers people an option to get one of those servings in a convenient pill. Take 2 tablets (500 mg per dose) two or three times a day without regard to meals.

Spirulina is very well tolerated in normal dosages. Its primary side effect is wellness. But some people will experience inability to sleep at night if they take it too close to bedtime (it is energizing). Spirulina is also called blue-green algae and contains natural pigments (blue and green); in high dosages, this can affect the color of your stool, but it's a harmless discoloration. Also, you may experience night sweats, a very slight fever, or a sensation that the skin is warm. This is possible because spirulina contains proteins and other nutrients that help you burn off fat, and this thermogenesis naturally creates heat in the body as the calories burn.

Day 6 Cell Genesis

By this point in your tune-up week, your cells will be restored to a higher functional level. The focus today is to provide all the micronutrients to help you with problems such as a sluggish liver, skin issues, cataracts, vision problems, fungal infections, and low bile flow. The primary nutrient that supports this day is beta-carotene, which forms vitamin A in the body.

Celebration Smoothie

FEATURED NUTRIENT: VITAMIN B_{12} (100%)

Makes 1 serving

1 cup hemp milk

¼ cup pomegranate juice

½ cup organic pear juice

1 teaspoon liquid aloe vera

1 cup coconut-based yogurt (any flavor)

1 scoop egg white, hemp, or whey protein powder

Ice cubes

In a blender, combine the milk, pomegranate juice, pear juice, aloe, yogurt, powder, and ice cubes. Process for 1 to 2 minutes, or until smooth.

Per serving: *Calories 502; Protein 12 g; Carbohydrates 83 g; Fiber 9 g; Fat 13 g; Saturated Fat 9 g; Sodium 134 mg; Vitamin B_{12} 3.9 mcg*

Apple Carrot Cocktail

FEATURED NUTRIENT: FOLATE (35%)

Makes 1 serving

1 apple

3 large carrots

1 golden beet, peeled and with some greens

3 kale leaves

In a juicer, according to the manufacturer's directions, combine the apple, carrots, beet, and kale. Process until juiced.

Per serving: *Calories 235; Protein 5 g; Carbohydrates 57 g; Fiber 13 g; Fat 12 g; Saturated Fat 0 g; Sodium 229 mg; Folate 146 mcg*

Day 6 Menu

Breakfast

1 breakfast sandwich made with 1 toasted whole grain gluten-free English muffin, 1 egg cooked over easy, 1 slice tomato, 1 slice Cheddar cheese or 1 ounce goat cheese

½ pink grapefruit drizzled with 1 teaspoon honey

1 cup milk or milk substitute

Coffee or herbal tea (pau d'arco, tulsi, or goji)

Snack

1 serving Apple Carrot Cocktail (above)

Lunch

1 serving White Bean Salad with Tiny Pasta (page 408)

4 cherry tomatoes

1 crispbread

Sparkling or pure filtered water with a wedge of lime or lemon

Snack

1 serving Celebration Smoothie (page 370)

Dinner

1 serving Cold Tomato and Cucumber Soup (page 387)

1 serving Warm Grilled Beef with Quinoa Salad (page 436)

1 serving Cherry Pudding Cake (page 442)

Cooking Dried Beans and Lentils

For convenience, cook dried beans and lentils ahead of time. Dried beans require soaking before cooking. Lentils do not require soaking.

The Basic Cooked Beans recipe works for any type of dried bean such as cannellini, great Northern, black, pinto, or kidney. The Basic Cooked Lentil recipe works best with the most common brown lentil.

Store the cooled, cooked beans or lentils in a covered container in the refrigerator for up to 5 days or in freezer containers for up to 3 months. If freezing beans or lentils, it makes sense to divide them into recipe-ready portions, such as 1 cup.

Basic Cooked Beans

Makes 5 cups

1 pound dry beans, picked over

1 rib celery, cut into chunks

1 carrot, cut into chunks

1 small onion, halved

1 bay leaf

Place beans in a large bowl with enough cold water to rise 2" over the tops of the beans. Set aside to soak overnight.

Drain the beans and transfer to a large pot. Cover with enough cold water to rise 2" over the tops of the beans. Cover and cook over high heat for about 10 minutes, or until almost to a boil. Reduce the heat to medium-low. Add the celery, carrot, onion, and bay leaf. Partially cover

Supplement

Continue taking your spirulina. It is an excellent source of natural carotenoids. It has a positive impact on obesity and diabetes. Plus, spirulina contains chlorophyll, so it will continue the detoxification that you started on Days 2 and 3. Take 2 tablets, two or three times a day.

the pot. Cook, skimming off and discarding any foam, for about 2½ hours, or until the beans are tender. Check occasionally to make sure the water covers the beans. Add additional hot water to cover, if needed.

Remove from the heat and set aside to cool. Remove and discard the celery, carrot, onion, and bay leaf. Transfer the beans and cooking liquid to a storage container.

Basic Cooked Lentils

Makes 5 cups

1 pound dry brown lentils, picked over and rinsed

9 cups vegetable broth, chicken broth, or water

1 rib celery, cut into chunks

1 carrot, cut into chunks

1 small onion, halved

1 bay leaf

In a large pot over high heat, combine the lentils, broth or water, celery, carrot, onion, and bay leaf. Bring the mixture to a boil. Cover the pot and reduce the heat to medium-low. Cook for 20 to 25 minutes, or until tender. Drain any excess liquid. Remove and discard the celery, carrot, onion, and bay leaf.

Remove from the heat and set aside to cool. Transfer the lentils to a storage container.

Day 7 Energizing

Fat-soluble vitamins D and essential fatty acids finish your week with a kickstart to your immune system. Be sure to choose wild-caught salmon for your dinner. It's rich in omega-3s. My Fruitylicious Enzyme Juice will help you beat allergies, improve immunity, relieve joint pain, and improve digestion. You'll crave this every day.

Chocolate Banana Smoothie

FEATURED NUTRIENT: VITAMIN D (25%)

Makes 1 serving

1 cup vanilla almond milk
1 banana
1 tablespoon maple syrup

1 teaspoon unsweetened cacao powder
$^1/_2$ teaspoon ground cinnamon
Ice

In a blender, combine the milk, banana, syrup, cocoa, and cinnamon. Process for 1 to 2 minutes, or until smooth.

Per serving: *Calories 213; Protein 3 g; Carbohydrates 46 g; Fiber 6 g; Fat 4.5 g; Saturated Fat 1 g; Sodium 183 mg; Vitamin D 100 IU*

Fruitylicious Enzyme Juice

FEATURED NUTRIENT: VITAMIN C

Makes 1 serving

2 carrots
1 papaya, pitted
$^1/_2$ cup fresh pineapple

$^1/_4$ cup blueberries
$^1/_2$ cup fresh spinach leaves
1 pear

In a juicer, according to the manufacturer's directions, combine the carrots, papaya, pineapple, blueberries, spinach, and pear. Process until juiced.

Per serving: *Calories 356; Protein 3 g; Carbohydrates 92 g; Fiber 16 g; Fat 0.5 g; Saturated Fat 0 g; Sodium 117 mg; Vitamin C 240 mg*

Day 7 Menu

Breakfast

1 serving Sam's Fruit and Nut Medley (page 446)
$^1/_2$ cup black raspberries

1 cup milk or milk substitute

Coffee or herbal tea (blueberry, tulsi, or raspberry leaf)

Snack

1 serving Fruitylicious Enzyme Juice (opposite page)

Lunch

1 serving Crab, Avocado, and Pomelo Salad (page 416)

1 crispbread

Sparkling or pure filtered water with a wedge of lime or lemon

Dinner

1 serving Honey-Mustard Salmon (page 418)

1 serving New Potato and Asparagus Salad (page 402)

1 serving Cherry-Berry Almond Fruit Cake (page 441)

Sparkling or pure filtered water with a wedge of lime or lemon

Snack

1 serving Chocolate Banana Smoothie (opposite page)

Supplement

Start taking a good source of essential fatty acids. I recommend taking 1 softgel of either Nordic Naturals Ultimate Omega or Essential Living Oils by Dr. Ohhira once or twice a day with food. Follow the manufacturer's dosage. Also start taking vitamin D_3, 1,000 to 2,000 IU daily.

In Closing

Once you finish the Total Body Tune-Up, you should be feeling better than you have in many years in terms of energy, pain levels, and outlook. Try to slowly transition back into a more normal but still healthy diet. After the tune-up, you may find that you don't like things as sweet anymore or that soda suddenly feels intolerable. Maybe you'll be proud of the fact that you lost a few inches here or there, and you'll want to continue by incorporating a detox day once a week or one weekend of every month. This can only help you.

In an earlier chapter, I suggested that you take time adding supplements to your diet. In this tune-up chapter, I'm pushing you a little: Many of you are already taking supplements and are veterans. You have likely been seeking better health, so your body is used to nutrients. In that case, I think it's okay to integrate these supplements more frequently than earlier recommended.

You have to use good judgment and base your booster-week plan on how your body typically responds to major changes. If you are a sensitive individual, perhaps you should stretch my weeklong suggestions into a month. That's fine by me; I just want you to get well. If you are a hard-core health nut like myself, then you can integrate much of what you've read here during the first week and feel wonderful for doing so. If you are chronically ill, you may just want to change only a few things, using my booster-week plan as a suggestion. If you are one of those people who has been struggling for a long time, and you just want to dive in, I would still advise you to reevaluate the plan every day based on how you're reacting. You can even pick one or two components of the plan to get started. Try just the smoothie (or the juice recipe) each day, or eat the way you normally do and just integrate the supplements. My chapter is a guideline; you do not need to do everything at once because this may create some serious detoxing (and means time spent on the potty that would be better spent doing chores and watching Jimmy Fallon on TV).

Be gentle with yourself. If you break down and have a sweet treat every now and then, it's okay. Life is about treats and about treating yourself with love. Just don't make that treat a cinnamon bun with a soda every day for breakfast. That will get you into trouble in a hurry.

I hope that after the weeklong Total Body Tune-Up you'll feel inspired to take better care of yourself. Consider having blood tests done to determine which nutrients you really need. This way, you can customize your vitamin and mineral regimen based on black-and-white data. You can also track how well you are doing if you retest every few months or twice a year. This will prevent you from oversupplementing and throwing off your ratios for B vitamins or minerals. Life is about balance, and I hope this plan helps you achieve your goals.

29

Recipes for Restoring Health with Every Bite

We all try our best to eat for optimal health. But if we don't pay attention to also restoring nutrients depleted by the drug mugging effects of our medications, our good intentions may not be enough. In this chapter, I'll escort you into the kitchen to share the fun of creating amazing meals that will have you feeling better than you have in years.

You'll find 100 recipes to nourish yourself for breakfast, lunch, dinner, and even for snacks. In the Total Body Tune-Up chapter, I've created even more recipes for smoothies and juices with powerful antimugging ingredients. The quickie recipes in the Tune-Up chapter are so nutrient packed that you'll want to make them part of your daily fare.

Along with these delicious recipes, I'd like to share my food philosophy so you better understand the basis and benefits of eating for maximum nutrition.

Go natural. Choose foods that are as close to their harvested state as possible rather than foods that are heavily refined, processed, or laden with additives. Whole, unprocessed foods are more nutrient dense, and that's exactly what you need as you go about freeing yourself from the drug mugging effects of medications and nonbiodegradable chemicals in your body.

Avoid genetically modified foods. Genetically modified organisms (GMOs) are created by scientists when they transplant genetic material from one organism to another, creating a new plant or animal with new traits. Simply put, it means scientists change the core makeup of a plant or animal to create one that is no longer the way nature intended it to be. I believe we should eat foods in their natural state rather than participate in this scientific experiment.

While it's nearly impossible to avoid GMO foods altogether unless you're extremely vigilant (GMO soybeans and corn have been available in the marketplace for many years), you can make educated choices to eat organic and avoid processed foods, where GMOs often lurk among the ingredients.

Choose organic. Whether you're eating a diet with meat or a vegetarian diet, choose foods that have been raised or grown organically. You'll avoid most of the pitfalls of artificial growth hormones, steroids, antibiotics, pesticides, herbicides, and synthetic chemical fertilizers. It's impossible to eliminate them entirely, however. With fruits and vegetables, organic is the best choice because it's not always possible to completely scrub pesticides from conventionally cultivated produce, and many of them disrupt the human endocrine system, thereby raising the risk for cancer.

Shop at the farmers' market in season. Fruits and vegetables that go directly from the field to your mouth are optimal. With just one degree of separation, your locally grown produce is packed with nutrients that far outweigh the diminishing nutrient levels in foods that have traveled long distances or languished at the supermarket for weeks. And locally grown foods are much less likely to have been coated with a layer of oil or wax for a longer shelf life.

Get an oil change. Buy oils that are nutrient dense and more healthful. These include cold-pressed coconut oil, cold-pressed olive oil, grape seed oil, almond oil, apricot oil, avocado oil, sunflower oil, hemp seed oil, sesame oil, and flaxseed oil. You need healthy fats for a well-rounded diet, so don't skimp on the price. Buy top-quality and organic oils as often as possible. Store these oils in a dark container in a cool spot to protect the nutrients, which are susceptible to light and heat.

You may also cook with butter. Select pure butter or clarified butter (ghee) instead of a butter alternative. Margarine and other processed fat substitutes are drug muggers for fat-soluble vitamins. Those need to go.

Avoid gluten. Almost all people who have health problems related to eating gluten don't even know it. They think their poor health or their

My Preferred Nutrient-Boosting Ingredients

Beans, dry, home-cooked, loose-pack frozen, or commercially packed in jars

Beef, preferably grass-fed and organic

Berries, fresh or loose-pack frozen

Broth, homemade, commercially packed in aseptic containers, or MSG-free cubes

Butters, nut, almond or cashew; avoid peanut butter because of its allergic component and mold content

Chicken, preferably organic free-range

Fish, wild-caught

Flour, almond or brown rice

Fruits, fresh, loose-pack frozen, or commercially packed in jars with juice

Honey, raw

Mayonnaise, grape seed

Milk/milk substitutes, organic dairy, almond, coconut, rice

Oils, cold-pressed coconut oil, cold-pressed olive oil, grape seed oil, almond oil, apricot oil, avocado oil, sunflower oil, hemp seed oil, sesame oil, and flaxseed oil

Pork, preferably organic

Salt, sea

Sugar, raw or turbinado

Syrup, agave, raw

Syrup, maple, pure

Tamari, wheat-free; or Bragg's Aminos

Tomatoes, cooked fresh, or commercially packed in aseptic containers or jars

Vegetables, fresh, loose-pack frozen, or commercially packed in jars with minimal additives

Yogurt, plain (coconut or dairy)

disease is related to something else, not gluten sensitivity. Gluten, a composite protein found predominantly in wheat, has been tied to migraines, schizophrenia, bipolar disease, irritable bowel syndrome, psoriasis, Sjogren's syndrome, brain fog, fibromyalgia, arthritis, chronic fatigue, coordination problems, neuropathy, and dozens of other hard-to-pin-down disorders. Avoiding gluten is easy. Cook with brown rice flour or almond flour instead of all-purpose wheat flour. For thickening, replace wheat flour with tapioca starch or potato starch. Instead of traditional soy sauce, which contains some wheat, use Bragg's Liquid Aminos or wheat-free tamari soy sauce to spice your dishes.

Use fresh, not canned. Whenever possible, purchase fresh fruits and vegetables. Next best alternatives are loose-pack plain frozen produce, produce in glass jars, or aseptic-packed produce. Avoid produce packed in cans. You don't want to ingest any potentially harmful bisphenol A. BPA is a controversial industrial chemical found in epoxy resins used to line the insides of metal-based food and beverage cans and in baby bottles. Even though the FDA decided not to ban BPA in January 2011, it still sparks anxiety among health-seeking individuals who prefer not to ingest added chemicals. The chemical has been suspiciously linked to breast and prostate cancer, as well as obesity, infertility, early puberty in girls, and attention-deficit/hyperactivity disorder. Proponents say that BPA is cleared from the body quickly and that you may get more "estrogenic" hormone disruption from eating tofu (as one example). But let's just forget BPA for a moment because I'd like to appeal to your common sense: Using fresh produce from your garden, farmers' market, or grocery store is always better than fruits and veggies stored in a can for a year or two. Period.

Minimize grains. These are high-carb foods, such as pasta, cereal, muffins, bread, and rice. High-carb foods have been linked to obesity, primarily because starchy foods cause your body to release a lot of insulin, which promotes fat production in the body. Grains often spark digestive problems and fungal overgrowth in the gut, making it difficult to absorb nutrients from the vitamins or minerals you take. Make sure the carbohydrates you do eat are made from whole grains.

Don't eat corn. Almost all the corn you buy today is genetically modified. Also avoid products and ingredients made from corn, including high fructose corn syrup, corn oil, and corn syrup.

Eat soy only occasionally. I do not eat soy, and I know many others who avoid it. If you want to make soy part of your diet, I'd like to suggest that you limit consumption of soy foods, such as tofu, soy flour, soy oil, lecithin, and soy protein isolate. Please make sure any soy foods you eat are organic because nonorganic soy foods are likely to be a GMO product. In addition, soy is a goitrogen—a substance that can lower your thyroid hormone levels. Low thyroid hormone can cause chronic fatigue and overweight.

Don't eat fake food. Eat real food. Don't buy fake hot dogs, turkey tofu, cheese food products, veggie burgers, and so forth. Most of these foods are loaded (and I mean *loaded*) with fillers, artificial colors, and artificial flavors to make them look and taste like the real thing. Food manufacturers morph their goop into flavors and shapes that make it seem relatively edible in order to attract people who don't know any better but seek a healthy alternative. There's nothing healthy about fake food. I'd prefer you eat a 100 percent beef burger because you are getting one ingredient—meat. This is better than eating a fake burger with 20 or more ingredients. Eating these bizarre wanna-be foods alters normal digestion because your body has to figure out how to eliminate all the additives, chemicals, nitrates, sulfites, colorants, MSG, and whatever else the food manufacturer can think of to make it taste good enough for you to consume. Just buy the real stuff.

Switch to sea salt. Forget about white, iodized salt, which has been stripped of its minerals. Some salt brands contain cornstarch to make it pour easily, and cornstarch is a likely GMO ingredient.

Eat more plant-based foods. The idea is to tilt your diet into a more living palette rather than a dead one. This means the amount of meat and protein that you eat will likely be somewhat smaller than it probably is now. I shoot for a diet that contains 70 percent vegetables, 20 percent starches, and 10 percent meat. So what I'd like to see on your plate is a big fresh salad, a small dollop of brown basmati rice, and a little bit of meat sprinkled on top.

Forget about soda. Soda pop steals minerals. Instead, drink pure, filtered water, fresh-squeezed juice, coffee, or tea. My goal is to get you completely away from high fructose corn syrup, which has been shown to promote obesity.

Look into juicing. Buying a juicer is a fabulous investment for better health. You are able to make fresh, organic juices that help unstick pollutants and restore your system with healthy nutrients. Juicers are a must for anyone with high cholesterol, high blood pressure, or high blood sugar.

I have a Hurom juicer, which allows me to easily make fresh almond milk, too. It's an amazing new product that I found at the company's Web site, www.slowjuicer.com. I love this juicer because it uses a blade that presses and grinds the greens, veggies, and fruits. Traditional juicers work with a centrifuge system, rapidly spinning the vegetables. This doesn't work well with parsley, cilantro, kale, sprouts, or other greens. I also have a Vita-Mix, which I use to make fresh soup, protein shakes, and smoothies; but juicing with a Vita-Mix won't be palatable to newbies because it leaves the juice very "chewy." Go with a juicer that strains all the fiber.

When you juice, be sure to include a variety of fresh fruits, herbal greens (cilantro, parsley, and dandelion), and salad greens (kale, spinach). These green juices produce immediate results. Newbies don't have to down an entire glassful; it may be too much. So you can start with $\frac{1}{3}$ cup and see how you feel. Put the rest in the fridge for later.

Bear in mind that the healthy enzymes in juices deteriorate after 6 to 8 hours, so you can't store fresh juices in the fridge for very long. The juice recipes I've provided in the 7-Day Tune-Up Menu (page 360) will help your body burn more fat for fuel.

Banish mercury. Eliminate all foods considered high in mercury. This is mainly seafood. Mercury, which is a metal, is also a drug mugger for most of your healthy minerals. It interferes with thyroid function, causing hypothyroidism. It can also cause chronic fatigue by sneaking into your Krebs cycle and displacing minerals that otherwise help you make ATP (energy). You need to make sure that you are not taking it into your body anymore, or at least in the lowest possible amount.

The fish considered highest in mercury are tuna (ahi, yellowfin, blue, and canned albacore), swordfish, shark, orange roughy, salmon (farmed and Atlantic), mackerel (king, gulf, and Spanish), bluefish, blue crab, Chilean sea bass, grouper, and tilefish.

Love your diet. Love yourself. Good food should—and does—taste wonderful. It restores your soul as much as it restores nutrients. I always want you to make the best possible choices for yourself when it comes to your diet. So, find a recipe that appeals to your tastebuds and start loving your diet and yourself. When you're shopping for ingredients for my recipes, refer to "My Preferred Nutrient-Boosting Ingredients," page 379, to make the best choices.

The Side-Effect Solution Diet

I want you to get on the fast track to vibrant health. For years, you've been eating foods that send the wrong signals to your immune system and blood vessels, foods that tire your liver and pancreas, causing you to wrinkle, feel tired, and get sick. It's time to change all that and start eating meals that reduce inflammation, improve blood flow, make your skin glow, and fight free radicals.

I've compiled some delicious recipes based specifically on nutrient categories so that you can start eating what the drug muggers stole. These recipes are your side-effect solution. The recipes that follow include appetizers, main meals, desserts, and beverages. It's okay to use recipes from all the nutrient sections but to focus on folate, for example, if that's the nutrient you need the most. You'll find that many of my recipes are either gluten free or dairy free and very low in sugar. Make appropriate substitutions for your taste preferences and food sensitivities. Buy organic when possible; it really does make a difference. Store your fresh produce in those amazing green bags from www.greenbags.com.

Beverages

Almond Energy Drink

FEATURED NUTRIENT: NIACIN

Makes 2 servings

1 cup almond milk

$\frac{1}{2}$ cup plain yogurt

1 banana, sliced

$\frac{1}{4}$ cup fresh blueberries

$\frac{1}{2}$ cup fresh papaya, diced

2 tablespoons almond butter

1 tablespoon ground flaxseed

2 tablespoons whey protein powder

$\frac{1}{4}$ teaspoon spirulina powder
(optional)

In a blender, combine the milk, yogurt, banana, blueberries, papaya, almond butter, flaxseed, protein powder, and spirulina powder (if using). Blend for about 30 seconds, or until smooth.

Per serving: *Calories 305; Protein 18 g; Carbohydrates 31 g; Fiber 5 g; Fat 14 g; Saturated Fat 2.5 g; Sodium 209 mg; Niacin 2 mg*

Avocado-Kiwifruit Smoothie

FEATURED NUTRIENT: BIOTIN

Makes 2 servings (2$\frac{1}{2}$ cups total)

1 ripe avocado, cut into chunks

1 ripe kiwifruit

$\frac{1}{2}$ cup plain yogurt

$\frac{1}{2}$ cup milk or milk substitute

1 tablespoon honey or agave syrup

$\frac{1}{2}$ teaspoon grated fresh ginger

4–5 ice cubes

In a blender, combine the avocado, kiwi, yogurt, milk or milk substitute, honey or syrup, ginger, and ice. Blend for 1 to 2 minutes, or until smooth.

Per serving: *Calories 292; Protein 6 g; Carbohydrates 28 g; Fiber 8 g; Fat 19 g; Saturated Fat 4.5 g; Sodium 62 mg; Biotin 5.76 mcg*

Banana Smoothie

FEATURED NUTRIENT: IRON

Makes 2 servings

1 cup milk or milk substitute

½ cup plain yogurt

½ cup coconut water

1 ripe banana

2 tablespoons whey protein powder

2 tablespoons maple syrup or honey

1 teaspoon vanilla extract

½ teaspoon spirulina powder

In a blender, combine the milk or milk substitute, yogurt, water, banana, protein powder, syrup or honey, vanilla, and spirulina powder. Blend for about 30 seconds, or until smooth.

Per serving: *Calories 293; Protein 18 g; Carbohydrates 41 g; Fiber 2 g; Fat 7 g; Saturated Fat 4 g; Sodium 172 mg; Iron 0.81 mg*

Mango-Pineapple Smoothie

FEATURED NUTRIENT: FOLATE

Makes 1 serving

1 mango, cut into chunks

1 cup plain yogurt

½ cup pineapple chunks

½ cup crushed ice

1 teaspoon coconut extract

1 teaspoon ground flaxseed

In a blender, combine the mango, yogurt, pineapple, ice, coconut extract, and flaxseed. Process for about 1 minute, or until smooth.

Per serving: *Calories 335; Protein 11 g; Carbohydrates 58 g; Fiber 6 g; Fat 9 g; Saturated Fat 5 g; Sodium 121 mg; Folate 61 mcg*

Tea Latte

FEATURED NUTRIENT: GLUTATHIONE

Makes 1 serving

1 cup water

¼ cup milk or milk substitute

2 bags white, green, or chai tea

1 medium banana, cut into chunks

2 tablespoons whey protein powder

2 teaspoons almond or cashew butter

In a microwaveable measuring cup, combine the water and milk or milk substitute. Cook in the microwave oven on high power for about 90 seconds, or until very hot. Submerge the tea bags into the mixture. Let steep for 4 minutes. Squeeze the excess water from the bags. Remove and discard.

In a blender, combine the banana, protein powder, nut butter, and tea mixture. Blend for about 30 seconds, or until smooth.

Per serving: *Calories 323; Protein 27 g; Carbohydrates 37 g; Fiber 4 g; Fat 10 g; Saturated Fat 2 g; Sodium 120 mg*

Veggie Punch

FEATURED NUTRIENTS: BETA-CAROTENE, VITAMIN A

Makes 2 servings

3 large carrots

3 ribs celery

1 Granny Smith apple

½ cup pineapple chunks

½ bunch fresh parsley

1 wedge lime

In a juicer, combine the carrots, celery, apple, pineapple, parsley, and lime according to the manufacturer's directions. Process until juiced.

Per serving: *Calories 113; Protein 2 g; Carbohydrates 28 g; Fiber 6 g; Fat 0.5 g; Saturated Fat 0 g; Sodium 128 mg; Beta-carotene 9,483 mcg; Vitamin A 1,894 IU*

Appetizers

Black Bean Soup

FEATURED NUTRIENT: FOLATE

Makes 10 servings

4 cups chicken broth

$3^{1}/_{2}$ cups chunky tomato sauce

2 cups cooked black beans, rinsed and drained (page 372)

1 large onion, chopped

$1^{1}/_{2}$ tablespoons ground cumin

1 clove garlic, minced

$^{1}/_{4}$ teaspoon salt

$^{1}/_{4}$ teaspoon ground black pepper

In a large pot over medium heat, combine the broth, tomato sauce, beans, onion, cumin, garlic, salt, and pepper. Bring to a boil. Reduce the heat to low. Cover and cook, stirring occasionally, for 35 minutes, or until the flavors are blended.

Transfer the soup to a blender or the bowl of a food processor, in batches if necessary. Process until smooth.

Per serving: *Calories 83; Protein 5 g; Carbohydrates 16 g; Fiber 5 g; Fat 1 g; Saturated Fat 0 g; Sodium 736 mg; Folate 54 mcg*

Cold Tomato and Cucumber Soup

FEATURED NUTRIENT: VITAMIN C

Makes 4 servings

2 pounds ripe tomatoes, peeled and cut into chunks

1 large clove garlic

1 large cucumber, peeled, halved, seeded, and finely chopped

1 cup tomato juice

$^{1}/_{2}$ cup finely chopped fresh basil

1 tablespoon olive oil

1 tablespoon red wine vinegar

$^{1}/_{2}$ teaspoon salt

$^{1}/_{4}$ teaspoon ground black pepper

In a food processor, combine half of the tomatoes and the garlic. Process until smooth. Transfer to a bowl. Add the remaining tomatoes. Process until smooth and transfer to a mixing bowl.

(continued)

Add the cucumber, juice, basil, oil, vinegar, salt, and pepper to the bowl. Cover and chill for at least 3 hours, or until very cold and the flavors blend.

Per serving: *Calories 98; Protein 3 g; Carbohydrates 14 g; Fiber 4 g; Fat 4 g; Saturated Fat 0.6 g; Sodium 375 mg; Vitamin C 37.25 mg*

Hummus with Tahini

FEATURED NUTRIENT: IRON

Makes 12 servings (4 tablespoons per serving)

2 cloves garlic

2½ cups cooked chickpeas with cooking liquid (see Basic Cooked Beans, page 372)

½ cup tahini

⅓ cup fresh lemon juice

2 tablespoons olive oil

½ teaspoon sea salt

Pinch of paprika

Dash of hot-pepper sauce

1 tablespoon finely chopped parsley

With a food processor running, drop the garlic through the feed tube to mince. Turn off the processor. With a slotted spoon, transfer the chickpeas to the food processor. Reserve the cooking liquid.

Process, scraping the sides of the bowl occasionally, for about 2 minutes, or until coarsely ground. Add the tahini, juice, oil, salt, paprika, and hot-pepper sauce. Process for about 1 minute, or until smooth. Add a few tablespoons of the reserved cooking liquid (the remainder may be reserved as a base for soup) and process if the mixture seems too dry. Transfer to a serving dish and sprinkle with the parsley.

Per serving: *Calories 136; Protein 5 g; Carbohydrates 13 g; Fiber 4 g; Fat 8 g; Saturated Fat 1 g; Sodium 77 mg; Iron 1.3 mg*

Icy Watermelon Soup

FEATURED NUTRIENT: VITAMIN A

Makes 4 servings

2 cups chopped watermelon

2 cups orange juice

1 tablespoon frozen orange juice concentrate

Fresh mint sprigs for garnish (optional)

In a food processor or blender, combine the watermelon, juice, and concentrate. Process for about 1 minute, or until smooth. Place the processor bowl or blender jar in the refrigerator for at least 1 hour.

Return the bowl or blender to the stand. Pulse briefly to remix the ingredients.

Pour into chilled bowls and garnish with mint sprigs (if using).

Per serving: *Calories 85; Protein 1 g; Carbohydrates 21 g; Fiber 0.5 g; Fat 0 g; Saturated Fat 0 g; Sodium 8 mg; Vitamin A 449.26 IU*

Pinto Bean and Spinach Soup

FEATURED NUTRIENT: FOLATE

Makes 4 servings

1 tablespoon olive oil

2 onions, chopped

3 cloves garlic, minced

1½ to 2 cups chicken broth, divided

1½ cups cooked pinto beans (page 372)

1 cup milk or milk substitute

¼ teaspoon dried thyme

¼ teaspoon sea salt

¼ teaspoon ground black pepper

2 cups loosely packed baby spinach, chopped

Juice of 1 lemon (3–4 tablespoons)

4 tablespoons plain yogurt

Heat the oil in a large saucepan over medium-high heat. Add the onions and garlic. Cook, stirring occasionally, for about 10 minutes, or until golden.

Add 1½ cups of the broth, the beans, milk or milk substitute, thyme, salt, and pepper. Cook over medium heat, stirring occasionally, for about 10 minutes, or until the flavors blend.

Transfer the soup, in batches if necessary, to a blender or food processor. Process until smooth. Return to the pot. Stir in the spinach. Cook over medium heat for about 2 minutes, or until the spinach is wilted. Add up to ½ cup of the remaining broth, if needed, to thin the soup. Remove from the heat. Stir in the juice. Serve topped with the yogurt.

Per serving: *Calories 209; Protein 10 g; Carbohydrates 30 g; Fiber 8 g; Fat 6.5 g; Saturated Fat 2 g; Sodium 368 mg; Folate 127 mcg*

Side Dishes

Asian Spinach

FEATURED NUTRIENT: CALCIUM

Makes 4 servings

1 teaspoon grape seed oil

1 sweet onion, thinly sliced

2 cloves garlic, sliced

1 small jicama, cut into matchsticks

1 bag (10 ounces) baby spinach

2 teaspoons wheat-free tamari

$^1\!/_2$ teaspoon grated fresh ginger

1 teaspoon toasted sesame oil

Warm the grape seed oil in a skillet over medium-low heat. Add the onion and garlic. Cook, stirring occasionally, for about 10 minutes, or until the onion is soft.

Increase the heat to medium-high. Add the jicama. Cook, tossing occasionally, for about 4 minutes, or until the jicama is hot. Add the spinach, tamari, and ginger. Toss.

Cover and cook, tossing occasionally, for 2 to 3 minutes, or until the spinach is wilted. Remove from the heat and drizzle with the sesame oil.

Per serving: *Calories 115; Protein 3 g; Carbohydrates 22 g; Fiber 9 g; Fat 2.5 g; Saturated Fat 0 g; Sodium 280 mg; Calcium 80 mg*

Asparagus with Feta Cheese

FEATURED NUTRIENT: FOLATE

Makes 4 servings

$^1\!/_4$ cup water

1 tablespoon olive oil

1 clove garlic, minced

Pinch of sea salt

1 pound asparagus, ends trimmed

2 tablespoons crumbled feta cheese

In a large skillet over high heat, combine the water, oil, garlic, and salt. Cover and bring to a boil. Place the asparagus in the pan. Cover and cook, shaking the pan occasionally, for about 3 minutes, or until the asparagus turns bright green. Uncover the pan and cook, tossing occasionally, for 1 to 2 minutes, or until the water evaporates and the asparagus is tender-crisp. Place the asparagus on a serving dish. Sprinkle with the cheese.

Per serving: *Calories 66; Protein 3 g; Carbohydrates 5 g; Fiber 2 g; Fat 4.5 g; Saturated Fat 1.2 g; Sodium 104 mg; Folate 60 mcg*

Avocado-Tomato Salad with Goat Cheese and Capers

FEATURED NUTRIENT: GLUTATHIONE

Makes 4 servings

2 avocados, sliced

2 tomatoes, sliced

1 cucumber, sliced

1 tablespoon olive oil

1 tablespoon red wine vinegar

$\frac{1}{4}$ cup (1 ounce) goat cheese, crumbled

2 teaspoons capers, rinsed and drained

On a platter, arrange the avocados, tomatoes, and cucumber by alternating the slices. Drizzle with the oil and vinegar. Scatter the cheese and capers on top.

Per serving: *Calories 236; Protein 5 g; Carbohydrates 13 g; Fiber 8 g; Fat 20 g; Saturated Fat 4 g; Sodium 58 mg*

Black Bean, Rice, and Pepper Salad

FEATURED NUTRIENT: SELENIUM

Makes 6 servings

1 red bell pepper, cut into strips

2 light green frying peppers (such as Italian or Cubanalle), cut into strips

1 small fresh hot chile pepper, seeded and finely chopped (optional) (wear plastic gloves when handling)

2 cups cooked black beans, rinsed and drained (page 372)

$\frac{1}{2}$ cup olive oil

2 tablespoons red wine vinegar

2 tablespoons fresh lemon juice

3 scallions, thinly sliced

$\frac{1}{4}$ cup chopped fresh basil leaves

2 cloves garlic, minced

1 bay leaf

4 tablespoons finely chopped parsley, divided

1 cup long-grain brown rice

Place the bell and frying peppers and the chile pepper (if using) in a strainer and then set into a bowl. Pour boiling water over the peppers (enough to cover) and let steep for 30 seconds. Remove the strainer and turn the peppers out onto several layers of paper towels to dry. Transfer the peppers to a large bowl.

Add the beans, oil, vinegar, juice, scallions, basil, garlic, bay leaf, and 2 tablespoons of the parsley. Toss to mix thoroughly. Set aside to marinate for 1 hour.

(continued)

Meanwhile, in a medium saucepan, cook the rice according to package directions.

Add the hot rice to the salad and toss. Remove and discard the bay leaf. Serve hot or at room temperature, sprinkled with the remaining 2 tablespoons parsley.

Per serving: *Calories 371; Protein 9 g; Carbohydrates 42 g; Fiber 7 g; Fat 19 g; Saturated Fat 3 g; Sodium 9 mg; Selenium 8.12 mcg*

Broccoli Cashew Salad

FEATURED NUTRIENT: MAGNESIUM

Makes 4 servings

3 tablespoons mayonnaise

1 tablespoon red or white wine vinegar

$\frac{1}{8}$ teaspoon salt

2 cups broccoli florets, cut into small pieces

$\frac{1}{2}$ cup roasted unsalted cashews

$\frac{1}{4}$ cup slivered red onion

$\frac{1}{4}$ teaspoon red-pepper flakes

In a large serving bowl, combine the mayonnaise, vinegar, and salt. Whisk until smooth. Add the broccoli, nuts, onion, and red-pepper flakes. Toss to coat.

Per serving: *Calories 150; Protein 4 g; Carbohydrates 10 g; Fiber 2 g; Fat 12 g; Saturated Fat 2 g; Sodium 140 mg; Magnesium 54.34 mg*

Brown and Green Rice with Snow Peas

FEATURED NUTRIENT: RIBOFLAVIN

Makes 6 servings

$2\frac{1}{2}$ cups water

1 cup long-grain brown rice

4 large shallots or small onions, finely chopped

2 tablespoons unsalted butter

$\frac{1}{2}$ teaspoon grated fresh ginger

1 package (10 ounces) frozen baby peas, thawed

$\frac{1}{2}$ cup finely chopped parsley

1 tablespoon wheat-free tamari

Pinch of ground red pepper

12 fresh snow peas

In a saucepan, combine the water, rice, shallots or onions, butter, and ginger. Place over medium heat and bring to a boil. Stir once and then cover. Reduce the heat to medium-low and cook for 25 minutes, or until most of the liquid is absorbed. Remove from the heat and add the baby peas, parsley, tamari, and pepper. Fluff with a fork. Cover the pot and cook over medium-low heat for 5 minutes. Remove from the heat and let stand, covered, for 10 minutes.

Mound the rice on a platter and place the snow peas around the edges.

Per serving: *Calories 228; Protein 7 g; Carbohydrates 40 g; Fiber 4 g; Fat 4.8 g; Saturated Fat 2.6 g; Sodium 165 mg; Riboflavin 0.09 mg*

Caribbean Black Bean Salad

FEATURED NUTRIENT: VITAMIN C

Makes 8 servings

2 cups cooked black beans, rinsed and drained (page 372)

2 roasted red bell peppers, chopped

3 plum tomatoes, chopped

$\frac{1}{2}$ small red onion, quartered and thinly sliced

$\frac{1}{2}$ cucumber, halved, seeded, and chopped

3 tablespoons fresh lime juice

2 tablespoons finely chopped fresh cilantro

$1\frac{1}{2}$ teaspoons grape seed oil

$1\frac{1}{2}$ teaspoons flaxseed oil

2 cloves garlic, minced

$\frac{1}{4}$ teaspoon sea salt

In a large bowl, combine the beans, peppers, tomatoes, onion, cucumber, juice, cilantro, oils, garlic, and salt. Toss to coat well. Let stand for at least 15 minutes to allow the flavors to blend.

Per serving: *Calories 92; Protein 5 g; Carbohydrates 14 g; Fiber 5 g; Fat 2 g; Saturated Fat 0 g; Sodium 52 mg; Vitamin C 44.44 mg*

Carrots with Citrus and Jalapeño

FEATURED NUTRIENT: VITAMIN A

Makes 4 servings

1 pound carrots, cut into matchsticks

Juice of 2 limes (4–6 tablespoons)

1 teaspoon honey

1 red bell pepper, chopped

1 jalapeño chile pepper, seeded and finely chopped (wear plastic gloves when handling)

1 tablespoon chopped fresh cilantro

Set the carrots in a strainer. Pour boiling water over them for about 5 seconds. Drain well.

In a medium bowl, combine the juice and honey. Whisk to blend. Add the peppers, cilantro, and carrots. Toss to mix. Serve at room temperature or chilled.

Per serving: Calories 69; Protein 2 g; Carbohydrates 16 g; Fiber 4 g; Fat 0.4 g; Saturated Fat 0 g; Sodium 104 mg; Vitamin A 1,992 IU

Chicken, Bell Pepper, and Apple Salad

FEATURED NUTRIENT: VITAMIN B_6

Makes 6 servings

4 boneless, skinless chicken breast halves

$\frac{1}{3}$ cup olive oil

$\frac{1}{4}$ cup orange juice

$\frac{1}{2}$ teaspoon ground black pepper

$\frac{1}{4}$ teaspoon salt

1 red bell pepper, thinly sliced

1 yellow bell pepper, thinly sliced

1 orange bell pepper, thinly sliced

1 onion, thinly sliced

1 Golden Delicious apple, chopped

Place a steamer basket or wire rack in a large pot with 2" of water. Bring to a boil over high heat. Place the chicken in the basket or rack. Cover and steam for about 10 minutes, or until a thermometer inserted in the thickest portion registers 160°F and the juices run clear. Remove the chicken to a plate to cool.

In a mixing bowl, combine the oil, juice, black pepper, and salt. On a cutting board, chop the chicken. Transfer to the bowl. Add the bell peppers, onion, and apple. Toss to coat the ingredients with the dressing.

Per serving: *Calories 237; Protein 18 g; Carbohydrates 10 g; Fiber 2 g; Fat 14 g; Saturated Fat 2 g; Sodium 160 mg; Vitamin B₆ 0.76 mg*

Chinese Slaw

FEATURED NUTRIENT: VITAMIN A

Makes 4 servings

⅓ cup rice wine vinegar or white wine vinegar

2 tablespoons wheat-free tamari

1 tablespoon grated fresh ginger

1 tablespoon toasted sesame oil

½ head Chinese cabbage, shredded (about 1 pound)

2 carrots, shredded

3 scallions, sliced

1 red bell pepper, cut into thin strips

2 tablespoons chopped fresh cilantro

2 teaspoons sesame seeds, toasted (see note)

In a large bowl, combine the vinegar, tamari, ginger, and oil. Whisk to blend. Add the cabbage, carrots, scallions, pepper, and cilantro. Toss to coat well. Sprinkle with the seeds. Let stand for at least 15 minutes for the flavors to blend.

Note: *To toast the seeds, place them in a dry skillet over medium heat. Toast, shaking the pan often, for 2 to 3 minutes, or until lightly browned.*

Per serving: *Calories 104; Protein 4 g; Carbohydrates 14 g; Fiber 3 g; Fat 4.6 g; Saturated Fat 0.55 g; Sodium 752 mg; Vitamin A 1,086.4 IU*

Collard Greens with Tomato and Balsamic

FEATURED NUTRIENT: VITAMIN B$_6$

Makes 4 servings

1 tablespoon olive oil

1 small onion, finely chopped

1 tomato, chopped

1 pound collard greens (tough stems removed), chopped

$\frac{1}{4}$ cup water

$\frac{1}{8}$ teaspoon salt

$\frac{1}{8}$ teaspoon ground black pepper

1 tablespoon balsamic vinegar

Red-pepper flakes (optional)

Warm the oil in a large skillet set over medium heat. Add the onion and cook, stirring occasionally, for about 5 minutes, or until soft. Add the tomato. Cook for about 3 minutes, or until it starts to soften. Add the greens, water, salt, and pepper. Stir. Cover and increase the heat to high. Cook for about 2 minutes, or until the greens wilt. Remove the lid and reduce the heat to medium-high. Cook, tossing, for 2 to 3 minutes, or until the greens are tender-crisp. Drizzle lightly with the vinegar and sprinkle with red-pepper flakes (if using).

Per serving: *Calories 81; Protein 3 g; Carbohydrates 10 g; Fiber 5 g; Fat 4 g; Saturated Fat 0.54 g; Sodium 79 mg; Vitamin B$_6$ 0.21 mg*

Creamy Tomato Dressing

FEATURED NUTRIENT: PROBIOTICS

Makes 16 servings (4 tablespoons per serving)

2 ripe tomatoes, peeled, seeded, and chopped

1 clove garlic, minced

1 teaspoon dried basil or dillweed

1 cup kefir

In a food processor or blender, combine the tomatoes, garlic, and basil or dillweed. Process until smooth. Add the kefir. Pulse briefly until smooth.

Per serving: *Calories 12; Protein 1 g; Carbohydrates 1 g; Fiber 0 g; Fat 0.5 g; Saturated Fat 0 g; Sodium 8 mg*

Fresh Fig Salad with Kiwifruit Lime Dressing

FEATURED NUTRIENT: CALCIUM

Makes 4 servings

2 cups halved fresh figs

1 cup blueberries

½ cup honeydew melon balls

½ cup sliced strawberries

2 tablespoons lime juice, divided

2 cups torn lettuce leaves

1 small kiwifruit, quartered

2 tablespoons mayonnaise

2 tablespoons sour cream or plain yogurt

1 tablespoon honey

1 tablespoon chopped pecans

In a medium bowl, combine the figs, blueberries, melon, strawberries, and 1 tablespoon of the juice. Toss gently to combine. Divide the lettuce among 4 plates. Spoon the salad onto the lettuce.

In a food processor or blender, combine the kiwi, mayonnaise, sour cream or yogurt, honey, and the remaining 1 tablespoon juice. Process for about 1 minute, or until smooth. Drizzle on the salads. Sprinkle with the pecans.

Per serving: *Calories 186; Protein 2 g; Carbohydrates 36 g; Fiber 5 g; Fat 5.5 g; Saturated Fat 1.5 g; Sodium 66 mg; Calcium 57.65 mg*

Greek Chicken and Cauliflower Salad with Tomato Vinaigrette

FEATURED NUTRIENT: FOLATE

Makes 6 servings

Vinaigrette

¼ cup tomato juice

¼ cup fresh lemon juice

¼ cup grape seed oil

2 tablespoons balsamic vinegar

1 clove garlic, crushed

¾ teaspoon Greek seasoning

¼ teaspoon sea salt

Salad

2 cups cauliflower florets, cut into small pieces

½ pound boneless, skinless chicken breast

½ cup shredded carrot

⅓ cup thinly sliced scallions

⅓ cup grape or cherry tomatoes, halved

¼ cup pitted kalamata olives

¼ cup crumbled feta cheese

3 tablespoons chopped pistachios

3 cups mixed baby greens

To make the vinaigrette: In a large bowl, combine the juices, oil, vinegar, garlic, seasoning, and salt. Whisk to blend. Set aside.

To make the salad: Place a steamer basket or wire rack in a large pot with 3" of water. Bring to a boil over high heat. Place the cauliflower in the basket or on the rack. Cover and cook for about 5 minutes, or until tender-crisp. Remove the cauliflower and set aside to cool.

Place the chicken in the basket or rack. Cover and steam for about 10 minutes, or until a thermometer inserted in the thickest portion registers 160°F and the juices run clear. Remove the chicken to a plate to cool. Chop the chicken.

Whisk the reserved vinaigrette. Add the chicken, cauliflower, carrot, scallions, tomatoes, olives, cheese, and pistachios. Line 6 plates with the greens. Spoon the salad on top of the greens.

Per serving: *Calories 205; Protein 11 g; Carbohydrates 9 g; Fiber 2 g; Fat 14 g; Saturated Fat 2.5 g; Sodium 433 mg; Folate 64 mcg*

Green Beans with Cashews and Chiles

FEATURED NUTRIENT: IRON

Makes 4 servings

1 pound green beans, trimmed

2 tablespoons grape seed oil

2 cloves garlic, lightly crushed

2 small dried hot chile peppers

2 tablespoons ($\frac{1}{2}$ ounce) cashews

1 teaspoon toasted sesame oil

Bring a large covered pot of water to a boil. Add the beans. Cover and return to a boil for 1 minute. Drain the beans and pat very dry. Set aside.

Heat a wok or large skillet over high heat for about 30 seconds, or until very hot. Add the oil and heat for 20 seconds. Add the garlic and peppers. Cook for 10 seconds, taking care not to let the garlic burn. Add the cashews and the reserved beans. Cook, tossing constantly, for 30 seconds. Remove from the heat. Remove and discard the peppers and garlic. Drizzle with the oil. Toss gently.

Per serving: *Calories 128; Protein 3 g; Carbohydrates 10 g; Fiber 3 g; Fat 9.8 g; Saturated Fat 1 g ; Sodium 8 mg; Iron 1.45 mg*

Kale-Fried Rice with Goat Cheese

FEATURED NUTRIENT: RIBOFLAVIN

Makes 4 servings

$\frac{1}{2}$ cup brown rice

2 tablespoons olive oil

$\frac{1}{2}$ cup chopped onion

2 cloves garlic, minced

1 pound kale (tough stems removed), chopped

$\frac{1}{4}$ cup water

$\frac{1}{8}$ teaspoon salt

$\frac{1}{8}$ teaspoon ground black pepper

2 tablespoons crumbled goat cheese

2 tablespoons dried cranberries

1 tablespoon hulled hemp seeds

In a medium saucepan, cook the rice according to package directions.

Meanwhile, warm the oil in a large skillet set over medium heat. Add the onion and cook, stirring occasionally, for about 5 minutes, or until soft. Add the garlic and cook for 1 minute. Add the kale and water. Stir, cover, and increase the heat to high. Cook for 2 minutes, or until the kale wilts. Remove the lid and reduce the heat to medium-high. Cook, tossing, for 2 to 3 minutes, or until the kale is tender-crisp. Sprinkle the kale with the salt and pepper.

(continued)

Remove the pan from the heat. Add the cheese, cranberries, and cooked rice. Toss gently to combine. Sprinkle with the seeds.

Per serving: *Calories 270; Protein 9 g; Carbohydrates 35 g; Fiber 4 g; Fat 11.8 g; Saturated Fat 3 g; Sodium 126 mg; Riboflavin 0.26 mg*

Kidney Bean Salad with Dill Dressing

FEATURED NUTRIENT: RIBOFLAVIN

Make 6 servings

Dressing

½ cup plain yogurt

2 tablespoons olive oil

1 scallion, minced

1 tablespoon finely chopped fresh dill

1 tablespoon fresh lemon juice

⅛ teaspoon ground black pepper

Salad

2 cups cooked red kidney beans, rinsed and drained (page 372)

2 tomatoes, diced

2 cups baby spinach

½ cup coarsely grated carrot

½ cup finely chopped scallions

¼ teaspoon ground black pepper

To make the dressing: In a blender, combine the yogurt, oil, scallion, dill, juice, and pepper. Process for 1 minute, or until smooth. Refrigerate for 1 hour for the flavors to blend.

To make the salad: In a large bowl, combine the beans, tomatoes, spinach, carrot, scallions, and pepper. Add the dressing and toss gently.

Per serving: *Calories 146; Protein 7 g; Carbohydrates 19 g; Fiber 6 g; Fat 5.6 g; Saturated Fat 1 g; Sodium 34 mg; Riboflavin 0.09 mg*

Mediterranean Vegetable Salad Platter

FEATURED NUTRIENT: GLUTATHIONE

Makes 4 servings

1½ cups hummus

1 ripe avocado, sliced

1 cucumber, sliced

1 ripe tomato, sliced

¼ cup grated smoked Gouda cheese

2 tablespoons mixed olives

1 tablespoon fresh cilantro

⅛ teaspoon sea salt

1 tablespoon balsamic vinegar

Spoon the hummus onto the center of a serving platter. Surround with the avocado, cucumber, and tomato. Scatter the cheese, olives, and cilantro on top. Sprinkle with the salt and drizzle lightly with vinegar.

Per serving: *Calories 287; Protein 11 g; Carbohydrates 21 g; Fiber 10 g; Fat 19.5 g; Saturated Fat 4 g; Sodium 596 mg*

Mixed-Grain Almond Pilaf

FEATURED NUTRIENT: BIOTIN

Makes 4 to 6 servings

¹/₂ cup sliced almonds

2 tablespoons grape seed oil

6 ounces uncooked long-grain
  brown rice

¹/₄ cup chopped onion

¹/₄ cup shredded raw beet

¹/₂ teaspoon ground black pepper

3 cups low-sodium vegetable broth

¹/₂ teaspoon turmeric

¹/₂ cup quinoa

In a medium saucepan, combine the almonds and oil over medium heat. Cook, stirring with a fork, for 2 minutes, or until the almonds are golden. Use the fork to transfer the almonds to a plate, leaving the oil in the pan.

Add the rice, onion, beet, and pepper to the pan. Cook, stirring, for 2 minutes, or until the rice is glazed. Add the broth and turmeric. Bring almost to a boil. Reduce the heat to medium-low. Cover and cook for 30 minutes.

Add the quinoa and stir. Cover and cook for 10 minutes, or until all the grains are cooked and the broth is absorbed. Sprinkle with the almonds.

Per serving: *Calories 264; Protein 7 g; Carbohydrates 36 g; Fiber 4 g; Fat 11 g; Saturated Fat 1 g; Sodium 80 mg; Biotin 6.74 mcg*

New Potato and Asparagus Salad

FEATURED NUTRIENT: POTASSIUM

Makes 4 servings

Dressing

3 tablespoons olive oil

2 tablespoons vegetable broth or water

1 tablespoon finely chopped parsley

1 tablespoon red wine vinegar

2 teaspoons Dijon mustard

¾ teaspoon chopped fresh thyme

⅛ teaspoon sea salt

Pinch of ground black pepper

Salad

3 eggs in the shell

½ pound small red potatoes, quartered

2 pinches of salt, divided

1 pound asparagus, ends trimmed, cut into 2" lengths

1 bag (5 ounces) baby spinach

½ cup sliced radishes

½ cup halved grape tomatoes

3 scallions, thinly sliced

Ground black pepper

To make the dressing: In a small jar, combine the oil, broth or water, parsley, vinegar, mustard, thyme, salt, and pepper. Tightly close the jar lid. Shake vigorously to blend. Set aside.

To make the salad: Place the eggs in a small saucepan with cold water to cover by 1". Cook over high heat until the water boils. Reduce the heat to low and simmer for 10 minutes. Carefully drain most of the water and set the pan under a faucet. Run cold water over the eggs to stop the cooking. Let the eggs sit in the cold water for 10 minutes to cool.

Meanwhile, place the potatoes in a medium saucepan with cold water to cover and a pinch of salt. Cover the pan and cook over high heat until the water boils. Uncover and reduce the heat to medium. Cook for 8 to 10 minutes, or until tender. Drain and cool briefly under cold running water. Set aside.

Add 1" of water to the same pan. Set over high heat until the water boils. Add the asparagus and the remaining pinch of salt. Cook for 3 to 4 minutes, or until bright green and tender-crisp. Drain and cool briefly under cold running water.

On a platter, make a bed of the spinach. Shell the eggs and cut into wedges. Place the eggs, potatoes, asparagus, radishes, and tomatoes in mounds on the spinach. Sprinkle with the scallions. Shake the reserved dressing and drizzle over the salad. Season to taste with pepper.

Per serving: *Calories 235; Protein 10 g; Carbohydrates 21 g; Fiber 6 g; Fat 14 g; Saturated Fat 2.7 g; Sodium 378 mg; Potassium 616 mg*

Oven-Roasted Tomatoes with Pesto

FEATURED NUTRIENT: THIAMINE

Makes 4 servings

12 plum tomatoes, halved lengthwise

1 tablespoon olive oil

1 clove garlic, minced

$\frac{1}{8}$ teaspoon red-pepper flakes

$\frac{1}{4}$ teaspoon sea salt

$\frac{1}{4}$ cup basil pesto

Preheat the oven to 325°F. Coat a baking pan with cooking spray. Scatter the tomatoes on the pan. Drizzle with the oil, garlic, red-pepper flakes, and salt. Toss to coat the tomatoes. Spread them out on the pan.

Bake for about 35 minutes, or until the tomatoes are very soft but still hold their shape.

Transfer the tomatoes to a serving platter. Top each with $\frac{1}{2}$ teaspoon of the pesto. Serve warm or at room temperature.

Per serving: *Calories 142; Protein 5 g; Carbohydrates 9 g; Fiber 3 g; Fat 11 g; Saturated Fat 2.5 g; Sodium 227 mg; Thiamine 0.08 mg*

Sautéed Cabbage, Apple, and Leeks

FEATURED NUTRIENT: GLUTATHIONE

Makes 4 servings

1 tablespoon olive oil

1 leek, white and light green parts only, chopped

$\frac{1}{4}$ teaspoon salt

6 cups finely sliced cabbage (about $1\frac{1}{2}$ pounds)

1 unpeeled Gala apple, diced

$\frac{1}{2}$ teaspoon dried thyme

Ground black pepper to taste

Warm the oil in a large skillet over medium heat. Add the leek and salt. Cook, stirring occasionally, for about 5 minutes, or until soft. Add the cabbage, apple, thyme, and pepper. Cook, stirring frequently, for 8 to 10 minutes, or until the apple is just tender.

Per serving: *Calories 93; Protein 2 g; Carbohydrates 15 g; Fiber 4 g; Fat 4 g; Saturated Fat 0.5 g; Sodium 122 mg*

Savory Sweet Potato Pancakes with Cranberries

FEATURED NUTRIENTS: VITAMIN A, BETA-CAROTENE

Makes 4 servings (2 pancakes per serving)

1¼ cups brown rice flour

⅓ cup dried cranberries

2 tablespoons ground flaxseed

1 teaspoon baking powder

1 cup shredded raw sweet potatoes

¾ cup milk or milk substitute such as
    unsweetened almond milk

2 eggs, beaten

2 tablespoons minced scallions

1 teaspoon grated fresh ginger

4 tablespoons plain yogurt or sour
    cream

In a large bowl, combine the flour, cranberries, flaxseed, and baking powder. Stir to mix.

In another bowl, combine the potatoes, milk or milk substitute, eggs, scallions, and ginger. Stir to mix. Add the dry ingredients and stir just until no dry ingredients are visible.

Preheat a nonstick skillet or griddle over medium-high heat. Coat with cooking spray. Heat for 1 minute. For each pancake, spoon 2 generous tablespoonsful of the batter onto the pan. Cook for about 2 minutes, or until browned on the bottom. Flip and cook for about 2 minutes, or until heated through. Remove and serve with the yogurt or sour cream. Continue cooking with the remaining batter.

Per serving: *Calories 330; Protein 10 g; Carbohydrates 58 g; Fiber 5 g; Fat 6.5 g; Saturated Fat 2.2 g; Sodium 222 mg; Vitamin A 4,954 IU; Beta-carotene 2,854 mcg*

Southwestern Vegetable Cheese Gratin

FEATURED NUTRIENT: FOLATE

Makes 8 servings

2 yellow summer squash, sliced

2 zucchini, sliced

2 cups cooked red beans or kidney beans, rinsed and drained (page 372)

1 bag (16 ounces) frozen baby lima beans, thawed

1 bag (16 ounces) frozen corn kernels

1 large jicama, quartered and sliced

$\frac{1}{4}$ cup water

$\frac{1}{2}$ teaspoon ground cumin

$\frac{1}{4}$ teaspoon sea salt

$\frac{1}{4}$ teaspoon ground black pepper

1 cup (4 ounces) shredded Monterey Jack cheese

$\frac{1}{2}$ cup chopped fresh cilantro

Preheat the oven to 350°F. Coat a 13" × 9" baking dish with cooking spray.

In a large, deep skillet, combine the squash, zucchini, beans, corn, jicama, water, and cumin. Cover and bring to a boil over medium-high heat. Reduce the heat to medium. Cover and cook, stirring occasionally, for about 15 minutes, or until the squash and zucchini are tender. Drain.

Transfer the mixture to the prepared dish. Add the salt and pepper and toss to mix. Scatter the cheese evenly on top. Bake for 10 to 15 minutes, or until the cheese melts and lightly browns. Sprinkle with the cilantro before serving.

Per serving: *Calories 308; Protein 15 g; Carbohydrates 52 g; Fiber 16 g; Fat 5.4 g; Saturated Fat 3 g; Sodium 303 mg; Folate 186 mcg*

Spiced Rice with Cashews

FEATURED NUTRIENT: BIOTIN

Makes 6 servings

$\frac{1}{2}$ tablespoon grape seed oil

1 onion, chopped

1 cup brown basmati or long-grain brown rice

$\frac{1}{2}$ teaspoon ground cardamom

$\frac{1}{4}$ teaspoon ground cinnamon

$\frac{1}{4}$ teaspoon sea salt

2 cups chicken broth

$\frac{1}{3}$ cup unsalted cashews, toasted (see note)

Warm the oil in a large saucepan over medium heat. Add the onion and cook, stirring frequently, for 4 minutes, or until soft. Add the rice, cardamom, cinnamon,

(continued)

and salt. Stir to coat the rice with the seasonings. Cook, stirring, for 2 minutes, or until the rice is glazed. Add the broth and bring to a boil over high heat. Reduce the heat to low. Cover and cook for 50 minutes, or until the liquid is absorbed and the rice is tender.

Stir in the cashews. Remove from the heat and let stand 5 minutes.

Note: *To toast nuts, place them in a dry skillet over medium heat. Toast, shaking the pan often, for 3 to 5 minutes, or until lightly browned.*

Per serving: *Calories 158; Protein 4 g; Carbohydrates 25 g; Fiber 2 g; Fat 5.6 g; Saturated Fat 1 g; Sodium 257 mg; Biotin 1.6 mcg*

Stir-Fried Orange Asparagus with Pine Nuts

FEATURED NUTRIENT: THIAMINE

Makes 4 servings

2 pounds asparagus, trimmed and cut into 2½" pieces

2 cloves garlic, minced

¼ teaspoon salt

Dash of ground red pepper (optional)

¼ cup orange juice

½ cup (2 ounces) pine nuts, toasted (see note)

Bring 1" of water to a boil in a large pot over high heat. Add the asparagus and cook for 2 minutes, or until bright green. Drain and pat dry.

Coat a large nonstick skillet with cooking spray. Add the asparagus, garlic, salt, and pepper (if using). Cook, tossing occasionally, over medium-high heat, for 2 minutes, or until the garlic is lightly browned.

Add the juice and cook, stirring, for 3 minutes, or until the juice reduces slightly and the asparagus is tender. Scatter the pine nuts on top.

Note: *To toast nuts, place them in a dry skillet over medium heat. Toast, shaking the pan often, for 3 to 5 minutes, or until lightly browned.*

Per serving: *Calories 168; Protein 8 g; Carbohydrates 13 g; Fiber 5 g; Fat 12 g; Saturated Fat 1 g; Sodium 104 mg; Thiamine 0.40 mg*

Strawberry and Red Onion Salad

FEATURED NUTRIENT: VITAMIN C

Makes 4 servings

3 tablespoons strawberry all-fruit spread

2 teaspoons balsamic vinegar

1 teaspoon grape seed oil

1 teaspoon flaxseed oil

1/8 teaspoon sea salt

1/8 teaspoon red-pepper flakes

1 pound fresh strawberries, sliced

1/4 cantaloupe, cut into 1/4" chunks

1/2 small red bell pepper, finely chopped

1/2 small red onion, finely chopped

1 head escarole, torn (about 3 cups)

1/2 ripe avocado, cut into 1/4" chunks

Ground black pepper

In a medium glass bowl, combine the spread, vinegar, oils, salt, and red-pepper flakes. Whisk to blend. Add the strawberries, cantaloupe, bell pepper, and onion. Mix gently. Cover and let stand for 15 minutes to allow the flavors to blend.

Place the escarole in a serving bowl. Add the avocado and reserved strawberry mixture. Toss to coat well. Season to taste with black pepper.

Per serving: *Calories 171; Protein 3 g; Carbohydrates 28 g; Fiber 9 g; Fat 6.6 g; Saturated Fat 1 g; Sodium 91 mg; Vitamin C 102.03 mg*

Balsamic Lentil Salad

FEATURED NUTRIENT: IRON

Makes 4 servings

2 cups cooked brown lentils (page 373)

1/2 cup finely chopped red onion

1/2 cup chopped carrot

1/2 cup chopped celery

1/2 cup chopped red bell pepper

1/4 cup chopped fresh basil

3 tablespoons balsamic vinegar

2 tablespoons olive oil

1 tablespoon capers, rinsed and drained

1/2 teaspoon sea salt

1/4 teaspoon ground black pepper

In a large bowl, combine the lentils, onion, carrot, celery, bell pepper, basil, vinegar, oil, capers, salt, and pepper. Toss to mix. Serve chilled or at room temperature.

Per serving: *Calories 209; Protein 10 g; Carbohydrates 27 g; Fiber 9 g; Fat 7.3 g; Saturated Fat 1 g; Sodium 269 mg; Iron 3.75 mg*

Watermelon Salad

FEATURED NUTRIENT: THIAMINE

Makes 4 servings

1 bag (4 ounces) baby arugula, stems removed and roughly torn

2 cups cubed watermelon

1 package (3 ounces) feta cheese, crumbled

2 tablespoons olive oil

Ground black pepper

1 tablespoon dried currants

In a large bowl, combine the arugula, watermelon, cheese, and oil. Gently toss to combine. Season to taste with pepper. Transfer to serving plates and sprinkle with the currants.

Per serving: *Calories 152; Protein 4 g; Carbohydrates 9 g; Fiber 1 g; Fat 12 g; Saturated Fat 4 g; Sodium 246 mg; Thiamine 0.07 mg*

White Bean Salad with Tiny Pasta

FEATURED NUTRIENT: POTASSIUM

Makes 4 servings

$\frac{1}{2}$ cup gluten-free ditalini, acini di pepe, or orzo

1 tablespoon olive oil

2 teaspoons fresh lemon juice or white wine vinegar

$\frac{1}{2}$ teaspoon dried thyme

$\frac{1}{8}$ teaspoon sea salt

$\frac{1}{8}$ teaspoon ground black pepper

2 cups cooked great Northern beans, rinsed and drained (page 372)

$\frac{1}{3}$ cup finely chopped celery

$\frac{1}{3}$ cup finely chopped red bell pepper

$\frac{1}{3}$ cup minced scallions

In a small saucepan, cook the pasta according to package directions. Drain and rinse with cold water. Drain and set aside.

In a serving bowl, combine the oil, juice or vinegar, thyme, salt, and black pepper. Add the beans, celery, bell pepper, scallions, and reserved pasta. Toss gently to combine. Serve at room temperature or chilled.

Per serving: *Calories 194; Protein 8 g; Carbohydrates 32 g; Fiber 7 g; Fat 4 g; Saturated Fat 0.6 g; Sodium 60 mg; Potassium 421 mg*

Wild Rice Stuffing with Apricots and Pistachios

FEATURED NUTRIENT: COENZYME Q10

Makes 8 servings

1 cup vegetable broth

$\frac{1}{2}$ cup orange juice

$\frac{2}{3}$ cup wild rice

2 teaspoons olive oil

1 Gala apple, chopped

1 small onion, chopped

1 rib celery, chopped

$\frac{1}{2}$ teaspoon dried thyme

$\frac{1}{2}$ teaspoon dried sage

$\frac{1}{2}$ cup dried apricots, cut into strips

$\frac{1}{4}$ cup (1 ounce) pistachios

$\frac{1}{8}$ teaspoon sea salt

$\frac{1}{8}$ teaspoon ground black pepper

1 tablespoon chia seeds

Preheat the oven to 325°F. Coat a 1-quart baking dish with cooking spray. Set aside.

In a medium saucepan, combine the broth and juice. Bring to a boil.

Stir in the rice and return to a boil. Reduce the heat to medium-low. Cover and simmer for 45 to 50 minutes, or until the rice is tender and the liquid is absorbed.

Meanwhile, warm the oil in a large skillet over medium heat. Add the apple, onion, celery, thyme, and sage. Cook, stirring occasionally, for about 4 minutes, or until the onion is translucent. Add the apricots, pistachios, salt, and pepper. Cook, stirring, for 2 minutes for the flavors to blend. Add the seeds and cooked rice. Toss to mix thoroughly. Spoon the mixture into the prepared dish. Cover with foil.

Place in the oven and bake for about 30 minutes, or until heated through.

Per serving: *Calories 116; Protein 4 g; Carbohydrates 19 g; Fiber 3 g; Fat 4 g; Saturated Fat 0.5 g; Sodium 424 mg*

Main Dishes

All-American Pot Roast

FEATURED NUTRIENT: COENZYME Q10

Makes 6 servings

¼ cup brown rice flour

¾ teaspoon dried oregano

½ teaspoon dried thyme

½ teaspoon salt

¼ teaspoon ground black pepper

1½ pounds beef boneless eye-of-round roast, trimmed of all visible fat

2 cups beef broth

½ cup red wine or nonalcoholic wine (optional)

1 teaspoon Worcestershire sauce

2 teaspoons olive oil

1 bay leaf

¾ pound red potatoes, unpeeled, cut into eighths

¾ pound turnips, cut into eighths

1 cup frozen pearl onions, thawed

1 cup carrots, cut into 1" chunks

Preheat the oven to 400°F.

In a large bowl, combine the flour, oregano, thyme, salt, and pepper. Dredge the meat to coat, shaking off the excess, and transfer to a plate. Whisk the broth, wine (if using), and Worcestershire sauce into the remaining flour mixture until smooth.

Heat the oil in a large ovenproof pot over medium-high heat. Add the meat and cook for 2 minutes per side, or until browned. Remove the pot from the heat and stir in the broth mixture and bay leaf.

Cover and bake for 1½ hours. Add the potatoes, turnips, onions, and carrots. Cover and return to the oven. Bake for 45 to 55 minutes, or until the meat and vegetables are tender. Remove and discard the bay leaf.

Per serving: *Calories 367; Protein 26 g; Carbohydrates 22 g; Fiber 3 g; Fat 19 g; Saturated Fat 7.5 g; Sodium 517 mg*

Baked Basil-Garlic Oysters

FEATURED NUTRIENT: ZINC

Makes 4 servings

$\frac{1}{2}$ cup brown rice

3 cups shucked oysters

$\frac{1}{2}$ cup oyster liquor (juice)

3 tablespoons finely chopped fresh
   basil

1 tablespoon olive oil

1 clove garlic, minced

$\frac{1}{4}$ teaspoon grated lemon peel

$\frac{1}{4}$ teaspoon red-pepper flakes

Preheat the oven to 375°F. Coat a 1-quart baking dish with cooking spray.

Cook the rice according to package directions.

Meanwhile, in the baking dish, combine the oysters, liquor, basil, oil, garlic, peel, and pepper. Toss gently to mix. Cover the dish.

Bake for about 10 minutes, or until the oysters are opaque. Serve with the rice.

Per serving: *Calories 245; Protein 15 g; Carbohydrates 26 g; Fiber 1 g; Fat 8 g; Saturated Fat 2 g; Sodium 459 mg; Zinc 169 mg*

Bean and Veggie Burgers

FEATURED NUTRIENT: VITAMIN B_6

Makes 6 servings

Burgers

1 small onion, finely chopped

$\frac{3}{4}$ cup shredded zucchini

$\frac{1}{2}$ cup shredded carrot

$\frac{1}{2}$ cup chopped red bell pepper

3 cloves garlic, minced

2 cups chopped spinach

$1\frac{1}{2}$ teaspoons ground cumin

$\frac{1}{2}$ teaspoon sea salt

4 ounces firm tofu

2 cups cooked chickpeas, rinsed and
   drained (page 372)

1 egg, beaten

$\frac{1}{4}$ cup ground flaxseed

6 gluten-free whole grain buns, split

Sauce

$\frac{1}{3}$ cup plain yogurt

3 tablespoons chopped fresh cilantro

1 scallion, finely chopped

1 jalapeño chile pepper, seeded and
   finely chopped (wear plastic gloves
   when handling)

$\frac{1}{8}$ teaspoon sea salt

6 leaves green lettuce

1 tomato, sliced

(continued)

To make the burgers: Preheat the oven to 400°F. Coat a baking sheet with cooking spray. In a large nonstick skillet over medium heat, combine the onion, zucchini, carrot, bell pepper, and garlic. Cook, stirring frequently, for 5 to 8 minutes, or until the vegetables are tender-crisp. Increase the heat to medium-high. Stir in the spinach, cumin, and salt. Cook for 2 minutes, or until the spinach wilts. Cool for 10 minutes.

Pat the tofu dry with paper towels. Crumble the tofu into a large bowl and add the chickpeas. With a potato masher or food processor, mash until smooth. Add the egg and vegetable mixture, and stir to mix well. Shape into 6 burgers (3" diameter). Coat with the flaxseed. Place on the prepared baking sheet.

Bake for 10 minutes. Coat the burgers with cooking spray and turn over. Bake for 15 minutes, or until browned.

To make the sauce: Meanwhile, in a small bowl, combine the yogurt, cilantro, scallion, chile pepper, and salt. Stir until blended.

Serve each burger on a bun with lettuce, tomato, and sauce.

Per serving: *Calories 436; Protein 21 g; Carbohydrates 75 g; Fiber 12 g; Fat 5.6 g; Saturated Fat 1 g; Sodium 212 mg; Vitamin B$_6$ 0.27 mg*

Calf's Liver Italiano

FEATURED NUTRIENT: VITAMIN D

Makes 6 servings

½ cup brown rice flour or cornstarch

¼ teaspoon ground black pepper

2 pounds thinly sliced calf's liver

3 tablespoons grape seed oil

2 cloves garlic, halved

2 tablespoons butter

¼ cup fresh lemon juice

1 lemon, sliced

Parsley sprigs

On a plate, combine the flour or cornstarch and pepper. Toss to mix. Dip the meat in the mixture to coat both sides. Shake off the excess.

Warm the oil in a large skillet over medium-low heat. Add the garlic. Cook, stirring occasionally, for about 2 minutes, or until golden. Increase the heat to medium-high. Place the meat in the pan, taking care not to crowd the slices. Cook for about 2 minutes on each side, or just until golden brown. Transfer to a heated serving platter and cover to keep warm. Repeat cooking the remaining meat and transfer to the platter. Remove and discard the garlic.

Set the pan over medium-low heat. Add the butter and juice. Stir with a wooden spoon, scraping up any browned bits on the bottom. Pour the pan juices over the meat. Garnish with lemon slices and parsley sprigs.

Per serving: *Calories 353; Protein 32 g; Carbohydrates 18 g; Fiber 1 g; Fat 16.5 g; Saturated Fat 5 g; Sodium 107 mg; Vitamin D 77 IU*

Chicken-and-Bean Enchilada Bake

FEATURED NUTRIENT: IRON

Makes 8 servings

1 pound boneless, skinless chicken breast halves, cut into bite-size pieces

2 teaspoons olive oil

1 large onion, chopped

3 tablespoons chicken broth or water

2 cloves garlic, minced

1 large green bell pepper, chopped

2 cups tomato sauce

1 cup mild picante sauce

1½ teaspoons ground cumin

1 teaspoon chili powder

2 cups cooked kidney beans, rinsed and drained (page 372)

10 corn tortillas (6" diameter)

1½ cups finely shredded Cheddar cheese, divided

½ cup sour cream

1 large tomato, chopped

Preheat the oven to 350°F.

Coat a large skillet with cooking spray. Place over medium heat and add the chicken. Cook, stirring, for 10 minutes, or until no longer pink. Remove and set aside.

Add the oil to the skillet and warm over medium heat. Add the onion, broth or water, and garlic. Cook, stirring occasionally, for 5 minutes, or until the onion is tender.

Stir in the pepper, tomato sauce, picante sauce, cumin, and chili powder. Add the beans and reserved chicken. Bring to a boil. Reduce the heat and simmer for 5 minutes for the flavors to blend.

(continued)

Spread half of the mixture evenly in a 13" × 9" nonstick baking dish. Place the tortillas on top, overlapping them to cover the surface. Sprinkle with ¾ cup of the cheese. Top with the remaining mixture.

Cover with foil and bake for 30 to 35 minutes, or until heated through. Sprinkle with the remaining ¾ cup cheese. Bake, uncovered, for 5 minutes, or until the cheese partially melts.

To serve, use a sharp knife to cut the mixture into 8 pieces. Use a wide spatula to transfer the pieces to dinner plates. Top each serving with the sour cream and tomatoes.

Per serving: *Calories 440; Protein 27 g; Carbohydrates 48 g; Fiber 9 g; Fat 15 g; Saturated Fat 6.8 g; Sodium 854 mg; Iron 2.3 mg*

Chicken Braised with Port and Prunes

FEATURED NUTRIENT: POTASSIUM

Makes 4 servings

16 pitted prunes, chopped

¾ cup port wine

4 chicken breasts (4 ounces each)

½ teaspoon sea salt, divided

1 tablespoon butter, divided

¼ cup finely chopped leek

¼ cup finely chopped carrot

¼ cup finely chopped celery

1 teaspoon chopped fresh thyme

½ cup beef broth

1 tablespoon red currant jelly
   or apricot preserves

⅛ teaspoon ground black pepper

In a medium saucepan over medium-low heat, combine the prunes and port. Bring to a simmer. Cook for 7 to 10 minutes, or until the prunes are plump. Remove from the heat.

Sprinkle the chicken with ¼ teaspoon of the salt. In a large nonstick skillet over medium-high heat, melt ½ tablespoon of the butter and add the chops. Cook for 1 minute per side, or until lightly browned. Remove the pork from the pan.

Reduce the heat to medium and add the leek, carrot, celery, and thyme. Cook, stirring occasionally, for 4 to 5 minutes, or until the vegetables are lightly browned. Add the broth and the prune mixture. Bring to a simmer. Reduce the heat to medium-low. Place the chicken in the pan and cook for 5 to 7 minutes, or until a thermometer inserted in the center of a chop registers 160°F and the juices run clear. Remove the chicken to a plate and keep warm.

Increase the heat to high and bring to a boil. Boil for 3 to 4 minutes, or until the mixture starts to thicken slightly. Remove from the heat and stir in the jelly or preserves, pepper, and the remaining $^{1}/_{2}$ tablespoon butter and $^{1}/_{4}$ teaspoon salt. Spoon the sauce and prunes over the chicken.

Per serving: *Calories 339; Protein 26 g; Carbohydrates 35 g; Fiber 3 g; Fat 6 g; Saturated Fat 2.5 g; Sodium 443 mg; Potassium 809 mg*

Chicken Pesto

FEATURED NUTRIENT: CALCIUM

Makes 4 servings

4 plum tomatoes

$^{1}/_{2}$ cup mozzarella cheese, shredded

2 tablespoons ($^{1}/_{2}$ ounce) grated Parmesan cheese

8 thinly sliced chicken breast cutlets (2 ounces each)

$^{1}/_{4}$ teaspoon salt

$^{1}/_{4}$ teaspoon red-pepper flakes

2 tablespoons prepared pesto sauce

Preheat the broiler. Coat a rimmed baking sheet with cooking spray.

Cut the skin from 2 opposite sides of each tomato. Discard the skin. Cut each tomato into 4 slices. In a small bowl, combine the cheeses and toss to mix. Set the tomatoes and cheeses aside.

Arrange the cutlets on the prepared pan. Sprinkle with the salt and pepper. Spread each with equal amounts of pesto.

Broil the cutlets 3" from the heat for 5 minutes, or until no longer pink and the juices run clear.

Remove from the broiler. Top each cutlet with 2 tomato slices, overlapping if necessary, and sprinkle evenly with the cheeses. Broil for 1 to 2 minutes, just until the cheese melts.

Per serving: *Calories 230; Protein 31 g; Carbohydrates 3 g; Fiber 1 g; Fat 19 g; Saturated Fat 3 g; Sodium 391 mg; Calcium 95 mg*

Chinese Braised Mackerel

FEATURED NUTRIENT: VITAMIN D

Makes 4 servings

¼ cup rice wine vinegar

3 thin slices fresh ginger, cut into matchsticks

3 cloves garlic, minced

½ teaspoon wheat-free tamari

1 pound mackerel fillets

1 cup chicken broth

3 white icicle radishes, cut into matchsticks

1 large carrot, cut into matchsticks

5 scallions, cut into matchsticks

In a glass baking dish, combine the vinegar, ginger, garlic, and tamari. Add the fish, skin side up, in a single layer. Marinate for at least 10 minutes.

Bring the broth to a boil in a large nonstick skillet over high heat. Reduce the heat to medium-low. Add the fish, skin side up, and the marinade. Cover and cook for 5 minutes.

Add the radishes and carrot. Cover and cook for 2 to 3 minutes, or until the fish is opaque. With a slotted spoon, transfer the fish and vegetables to a serving platter.

Boil the liquid until reduced by half. Pour over the fish. Sprinkle with the scallions.

Per serving: *Calories 272; Protein 23 g; Carbohydrates 9 g; Fiber 1 g; Fat 16 g; Saturated Fat 4 g; Sodium 442 mg; Vitamin D 729 IU*

Crab, Avocado, and Pomelo Salad

FEATURED NUTRIENT: ZINC

Makes 4 servings

2 tablespoons orange juice

2 tablespoons white wine vinegar

1½ tablespoons olive oil

2 teaspoons finely chopped fresh tarragon or fresh chervil

½ teaspoon grated orange peel

½ teaspoon salt

¼ teaspoon dry mustard

¼ teaspoon ground black pepper

2 heads butterhead lettuce, separated into leaves

2 sweet onions, sliced

2 pomelos, peeled and cut into sections (see note)

1 avocado, sliced

1 cup lump crabmeat

1 tablespoon (½ ounce) chopped blanched hazelnuts, toasted (see note)

In a large bowl, combine the juice, vinegar, oil, tarragon or chervil, peel, salt, mustard, and pepper. Whisk until blended.

Add the lettuce, onions, and pomelos. Toss to coat with the dressing. Mound onto 4 plates. Fan out a quarter of the avocado on top of each salad and top with the crabmeat and hazelnuts.

Notes: *Grapefruit may be substituted for the pomelos. To toast nuts, place them in a dry skillet over medium heat. Toast, shaking the pan often, for 3 to 5 minutes, or until fragrant and golden.*

Per serving: *Calories 454; Protein 14 g; Carbohydrates 75 g; Fiber 12 g; Fat 15 g; Saturated Fat 2 g; Sodium 461 mg; Zinc 2.5 mg*

Curried Eggs and Avocados

FEATURED NUTRIENT: VITAMIN D

Makes 6 servings

12 eggs

1 cup brown rice

3 tablespoons butter

¼ cup finely chopped onion

3 tablespoons rice or almond flour

2 teaspoons curry powder

2 cups milk or milk substitute

2 avocados, thickly sliced

1 tablespoon finely chopped parsley or fresh cilantro

Place the eggs in a large saucepan with cold water to cover by 1". Cook over high heat until the water boils. Reduce the heat to low and cook for 10 minutes. Carefully drain most of the water and set the pan under a faucet. Run cold water over the eggs to stop the cooking. Let the eggs sit in the cold water for 10 minutes to cool.

Meanwhile, cook the rice according to package directions.

Shell the eggs. Quarter the eggs and set aside.

Melt the butter in a medium skillet over medium heat until bubbling. Add the onion. Cook, stirring occasionally, for about 5 minutes, or until soft.

Add the flour and curry powder. Stir to make a paste. Add the milk or milk substitute gradually while stirring constantly. Cook, stirring constantly, for about 8 minutes, or until the mixture thickens. Add the eggs and avocados. Stir gently just until heated through.

Serve over the rice. Sprinkle with the parsley or cilantro.

Per serving: *Calories 488; Protein 20 g; Carbohydrates 39 g; Fiber 6 g; Fat 29 g; Saturated Fat 10 g; Sodium 184 mg; Vitamin D 96 IU*

Fish Cakes

Makes 4 servings

1 pound haddock or salmon

³⁄₄ cup ground almonds

2 tablespoons ground flaxseed

2 tablespoons finely chopped onion

2 tablespoons finely chopped celery

2 tablespoons finely chopped red bell
pepper

2 tablespoons finely chopped parsley

2 eggs, lightly beaten

2 teaspoons fresh lemon juice

¹⁄₂ teaspoon hot-pepper sauce

¹⁄₄ teaspoon ground black pepper

2 tablespoons grape seed oil, divided

Place a steamer basket or wire rack in a large pot with 2" of water. Bring to a boil over high heat. Place the fish in the basket or rack. Cover and steam for about 10 minutes, or until the fish is opaque. Remove from the pan and set aside to cool.

Place the fish in a medium bowl and flake with a fork. Add the almonds, flaxseed, onion, celery, bell pepper, parsley, eggs, juice, hot-pepper sauce, and black pepper. With clean hands or 2 forks, toss until thoroughly mixed.

Shape the mixture into 8 cakes (3" diameter). In a large skillet over medium heat, warm half of the oil. Add the cakes and cook for 3 to 4 minutes per side, or until golden and heated through. Repeat with remaining fish cakes.

Per serving: *Calories 318; Protein 30 g; Carbohydrates 7 g; Fiber 4 g; Fat 19 g; Saturated Fat 2 g; Sodium 132 mg; Biotin 22.26 mcg*

Honey-Mustard Salmon

Makes 4 servings

1¹⁄₂ tablespoons honey

1¹⁄₂ tablespoons Dijon mustard

4 salmon fillets (4 ounces each)

Preheat the oven to 375°F. Line a rimmed baking pan with foil.

In a small bowl, combine the honey and mustard. Whisk until smooth.

Place the fillets, skin side down, on the pan. Spread the honey-mustard mixture evenly on the tops.

Roast for 10 to 12 minutes, or until the fish is opaque.

Per serving: *Calories 163; Protein 23 g; Carbohydrates 8 g; Fiber 0 g; Fat 4 g; Saturated Fat 1 g; Sodium 211 mg; Vitamin B$_{12}$ 3.4 mcg*

Italian Scrambled Eggs

FEATURED NUTRIENT: VITAMIN B$_{12}$

Makes 4 servings

2 tablespoons olive oil	$^1/_4$ cup water
1 small green bell pepper, diced	$^1/_2$ teaspoon oregano
1 small red bell pepper, diced	$^1/_4$ teaspoon salt
1 onion, diced	8 slices (4 ounces) Provolone cheese
4 tomatoes, diced	$^1/_2$ avocado, diced
8 eggs	

Heat the oil in a large skillet over medium-high heat. Add the peppers, onion, and tomatoes. Cook, stirring occasionally, for about 10 minutes, or until the vegetables are tender.

Meanwhile, in a bowl, combine the eggs, water, oregano, and salt. Beat with a fork until the eggs are well blended. Add to the pan. Cook, stirring occasionally, for about 4 minutes, or until the eggs are set but not dry. Top with the cheese. Cover and reduce the heat to low. Cook for 1 to 2 minutes, or until the cheese melts. Garnish with the avocado.

Per serving: *Calories 482; Protein 29 g; Carbohydrates 14 g; Fiber 4 g; Fat 36 g; Saturated Fat 14 g; Sodium 740 mg; Vitamin B$_{12}$ 2.11 mcg*

Japanese Salmon and Vegetable Soup

FEATURED NUTRIENT: ZINC

Makes 4 servings

4 skinless salmon fillets (3 ounces each)

1 tablespoon wheat-free tamari

2 tablespoons miso paste, preferably organic, divided

1 tablespoon grape seed oil

2 cloves garlic, minced

1½ teaspoons finely chopped fresh ginger

3 cups low-sodium vegetable broth

2 tablespoons shao hsing cooking wine or dry sherry (optional)

1 head bok choy, sliced ¼" thick

6 ounces sugar snap peas

6 ounces asparagus, cut into 1" lengths

2 carrots, cut into matchsticks

1 bunch scallions, diagonally sliced

Preheat the broiler. Line a broiler pan with foil. Place the fish on the pan. Set aside.

In a cup, combine the tamari and 1 tablespoon of the miso paste. Spread over the top of the salmon. Set aside.

Place the oil, garlic, and ginger in a large saucepan over medium heat. Cook, stirring, for 1 to 2 minutes, or until fragrant.

Add the broth and shao hsing or sherry (if using). Increase the heat to high. Cover and bring to a boil. Reduce the heat to medium. Add the bok choy, peas, asparagus, and carrots. Cover and cook for 5 to 6 minutes, or until tender-crisp. Add the scallions and remove from the heat. Stir in the remaining 1 tablespoon miso paste and cover to keep warm.

Meanwhile, set the reserved pan in the broiler 5" from the heat source. Cook for 8 to 10 minutes, or until browned on top and opaque in the center. Transfer the salmon to large soup bowls. Ladle the soup on top.

Per serving: *Calories 261; Protein 25 g; Carbohydrates 21 g; Fiber 8 g; Fat 9 g; Saturated Fat 1 g; Sodium 876 mg; Zinc 1.4 mg*

Moo Shu Pork

FEATURED NUTRIENT: THIAMINE

Makes 4 servings

2 cloves garlic, minced

½ teaspoon finely chopped fresh ginger

1 teaspoon cornstarch

1 teaspoon wheat-free tamari

¾ pound lean pork, thinly sliced across the grain

8 small gluten-free tortillas (6" diameter)

1 tablespoon grape seed oil

1 cup coarsely shredded Chinese cabbage

3 scallions, cut into 1" lengths

¼ cup chicken broth

2 tablespoons gluten-free oyster sauce

In a medium bowl, whisk the garlic, ginger, cornstarch, and tamari. Place the meat in the bowl. Toss and set aside for 15 minutes.

Meanwhile, preheat the oven to 250°F. Wrap the tortillas tightly in foil. Place in the oven for 15 minutes, or until hot.

Heat a wok or skillet over high heat for about 2 minutes. Add the oil and swirl to coat the pan. Add the reserved meat with the seasonings. Cook, tossing frequently, for about 3 minutes, or until no longer pink. Add the cabbage, scallions, and broth. Toss to combine.

Carefully unwrap the tortillas. Brush some oyster sauce on each tortilla. Fill each with some of the meat mixture. Wrap and eat by hand.

Per serving: *Calories 400; Protein 23 g; Carbohydrates 51 g; Fiber 5 g; Fat 10 g; Saturated Fat 1 g; Sodium 739 mg; Thiamine 0.9 mg*

Roasted Ratatouille

FEATURED NUTRIENT: POTASSIUM

Makes 4 servings

1 eggplant (about 1 pound), trimmed, peeled, and cut into $\frac{1}{2}$" pieces

1 zucchini (about 8 ounces), trimmed and cut into $\frac{1}{2}$" pieces

1 onion, chopped

1 red bell pepper, seeded and cut into $\frac{1}{2}$" pieces

$\frac{1}{2}$ bulb fennel, cored and thinly sliced

1 tablespoon olive oil

1 tablespoon chopped fresh thyme

$\frac{1}{2}$ teaspoon chopped fresh rosemary

2 tomatoes, diced

2 cloves garlic, minced

$1\frac{1}{2}$ teaspoons chopped fresh oregano

$\frac{1}{2}$ teaspoon sea salt

$\frac{1}{4}$ teaspoon ground black pepper

1 tablespoon ($\frac{1}{2}$ ounce) grated Parmesan cheese

Preheat the oven to 400°F. Coat a 9" × 9" baking dish with cooking spray.

In a large bowl, combine the eggplant, zucchini, onion, bell pepper, fennel, oil, thyme, and rosemary. Toss to coat the vegetables. Spread the mixture evenly in the prepared dish.

Roast, stirring occasionally, for 50 to 55 minutes, or until the vegetables are lightly browned and tender. Add the tomatoes, garlic, oregano, salt, and black pepper. Mix well to combine. Sprinkle with the cheese.

Roast for 20 to 22 minutes, or until the mixture bubbles and thickens.

Per serving: *Calories 115; Protein 4 g; Carbohydrates 18 g; Fiber 7 g; Fat 4.5 g; Saturated Fat 1 g; Sodium 243 mg; Potassium 775 mg*

Salmon with Creamy Avocado Sauce

FEATURED NUTRIENT: NIACIN

Makes 6 servings

6 wild-caught salmon fillets (6 ounces each)

¼ teaspoon salt

¼ teaspoon ground black pepper

½ large avocado, quartered

¼ cup sour cream

1 tablespoon mayonnaise

1 teaspoon fresh lemon juice

1 clove garlic, minced

¼ teaspoon hot-pepper sauce

¼ teaspoon Worcestershire sauce

Preheat the broiler. Line a rimmed baking pan with foil. Place the fish, skin side down, on the pan. Coat the fish with cooking spray. Sprinkle with some of the salt and pepper.

Place the fish in the broiler about 5" from the heat source. Cook for 8 to 10 minutes, or until the fish is opaque.

Meanwhile, in a food processor, combine the avocado, sour cream, mayonnaise, juice, garlic, hot-pepper sauce, Worcestershire sauce, and the remaining salt and pepper. Process, scraping down the bowl occasionally, until the mixture is smooth. Transfer the fish to plates. Spoon some of the sauce next to each fillet.

Per serving: *Calories 299; Protein 35 g; Carbohydrates 3 g; Fiber 1 g; Fat 16 g; Saturated Fat 3 g; Sodium 170 mg; Niacin 20 mg*

Sesame Beef and Cauliflower Stir-Fry

FEATURED NUTRIENT: COENZYME Q10

Makes 6 servings

1 cup brown rice

1$\frac{1}{2}$ cups chicken broth

2 tablespoons cornstarch

1 tablespoon wheat-free tamari

$\frac{1}{2}$ teaspoon toasted sesame oil

4 scallions, thinly sliced

1 teaspoon grape seed oil

1 pound beef top round, trimmed of all
   visible fat and cut into bite-size pieces

2 large cloves garlic, minced

2 teaspoons grated fresh ginger

1 large head cauliflower, cut into
   bite-size florets

1 red bell pepper, sliced

1 tablespoon sesame seeds, lightly
   toasted (see note)

In a saucepan, cook the rice according to package directions.

Meanwhile, in a small bowl, combine the broth, cornstarch, tamari, and sesame oil. Whisk to mix well. Stir in the scallions and set aside.

Warm the grape seed oil in a wok or large skillet over medium-high heat. Add the meat, garlic, and ginger. Cook, tossing constantly, for 3 to 4 minutes, or until the meat is no longer pink. Transfer to a bowl and set aside.

Add the reserved broth mixture to the wok or skillet. Cook, stirring constantly, for 2 to 3 minutes, or until the mixture thickens. Add the cauliflower and pepper. Reduce the heat to low. Cover and cook for 8 minutes, or until the cauliflower is tender-crisp. Add the reserved meat. Cook for 1 to 2 minutes, or until the meat is heated through. Serve over the rice. Sprinkle with the seeds.

Note: *To toast the seeds, place them in a dry skillet over medium heat. Toast, shaking the pan often, for 2 to 3 minutes, or until lightly browned.*

Per serving: *Calories 338; Protein 23 g; Carbohydrates 36 g; Fiber 1 g; Fat 11 g; Saturated Fat 3.5 g; Sodium 384 mg*

Shrimp and Broccoli Pasta Salad

FEATURED NUTRIENT: VITAMIN A

Makes 4 servings

8 ounces gluten-free small shell pasta

1½ cups broccoli florets, cut into small pieces

1 carrot, sliced

1 red bell pepper, sliced

1 tablespoon olive oil

2 cloves garlic, minced

1 scallion, minced

12 ounces large shrimp, peeled, deveined, and halved lengthwise

1 cup cherry or grape tomatoes

½ cup buttermilk

2 tablespoons red wine vinegar

1 tablespoon flaxseed oil

1 tablespoon Dijon mustard

1 teaspoon ground black pepper

½ teaspoon salt

Prepare the pasta according to package directions, adding the broccoli, carrot, and bell pepper during the last 5 minutes of cooking.

Meanwhile, warm the olive oil in a large skillet over medium heat. Add the garlic and scallion and cook for 1 minute. Add the shrimp and cook, stirring frequently, for 3 minutes, or until the shrimp are opaque. Add the tomatoes and cook for 1 minute. Remove from the heat.

Meanwhile, in a large bowl, combine the buttermilk, vinegar, flaxseed oil, mustard, black pepper, and salt. Add the shrimp mixture and pasta mixture. Toss to coat well.

Per serving: *Calories 415; Protein 24 g; Carbohydrates 54 g; Fiber 5 g; Fat 11 g; Saturated Fat 2 g; Sodium 482 mg; Vitamin A 4,798 IU*

South-of-France Baked Cod

FEATURED NUTRIENT: VITAMIN B$_6$

Makes 4 servings

1 large onion, chopped

1 green bell pepper, chopped

1 red bell pepper, chopped

$\frac{1}{4}$ cup apple juice

4 tomatoes, chopped

$\frac{1}{2}$ pound red potatoes, cubed

$\frac{1}{4}$ cup chopped fresh parsley

1 clove garlic, minced

1 tablespoon capers, rinsed and
 drained

1 tablespoon chopped black olives

4 cod fillets (4 ounces each)

Preheat the oven to 400°F. Coat a 13" × 9" baking dish with cooking spray.

Coat a large nonstick skillet with cooking spray. Set over medium-high heat. Add the onion, peppers, and juice. Cook, stirring, for 5 minutes, or until the peppers are soft. Add the tomatoes, potatoes, parsley, and garlic. Cook, stirring occasionally, for 10 minutes, or until the sauce thickens slightly. Add the capers and olives and stir well.

Spread half of the sauce in the bottom of the prepared dish. Place the fish on top. Cover with the remaining sauce. Cover and bake for 15 minutes, or until the fish flakes easily.

Per serving: *Calories 198; Protein 24 g; Carbohydrates 23 g; Fiber 5 g; Fat 1.6 g; Saturated Fat 0 g; Sodium 159 mg; Vitamin B$_6$ 0.69 mg*

Spaghetti with White Clam Sauce

FEATURED NUTRIENT: VITAMIN B$_{12}$

Makes 4 servings

1$\frac{1}{2}$ cups chicken broth, divided

3 dozen littleneck clams, scrubbed

1 tablespoon olive oil

2 cloves garlic, minced

2 bay leaves

Pinch of dried thyme

$\frac{1}{4}$ cup milk or milk substitute

1 tablespoon brown rice flour

1 tablespoon finely chopped
  fresh parsley

$\frac{1}{8}$ teaspoon salt

$\frac{1}{8}$ teaspoon ground black pepper

12 ounces gluten-free spaghetti,
  such as brown rice

Bring $\frac{1}{2}$ cup of the broth to a boil in a large pot. Add the clams. Cover and cook for 6 to 10 minutes, or until all the clams open. Remove to a platter. Drain the cooking liquid through a fine sieve lined with a coffee filter. Reserve the drained cooking liquid. Set the clams aside until cool enough to handle, then remove from the shells. Mince the clams and set aside.

In a large nonstick skillet over medium heat, combine the oil, garlic, bay leaves, and thyme. Cook for 1 to 2 minutes, or until the garlic is golden. Add the milk or milk substitute, flour, parsley, salt, pepper, the remaining 1 cup of broth, and the reserved cooking liquid. Cook, whisking constantly, for 4 to 5 minutes, or until the sauce thickens. Add the clams and keep warm over low heat. Remove and discard the bay leaves.

Meanwhile, cook the pasta according to package directions. Drain and return to the pot. Pour on the clam sauce, toss, and serve.

Per serving: *Calories 471; Protein 25 g; Carbohydrates 71 g; Fiber 2 g; Fat 6 g; Saturated Fat 1 g; Sodium 344 mg; Vitamin B$_{12}$ 64.6 mcg*

Spicy Bean Pancakes with Tomato-Pepper Sauce

FEATURED NUTRIENT: POTASSIUM

Makes 4 servings

Puree

1½ cups tomato puree

1 red bell pepper, chopped

2 tablespoons fresh lime juice

3 cloves garlic, minced

1 tablespoon chopped fresh cilantro
or parsley

1 teaspoon agave syrup or honey

½ teaspoon dried thyme

½ teaspoon ground black pepper

Pancakes

½ cup cooked navy or pinto beans,
rinsed and drained (page 372)

2 eggs, lightly beaten

⅓ cup brown rice flour

⅓ cup almond flour

1 teaspoon baking powder

½ cup low-fat buttermilk

½ cup shredded extrasharp
Cheddar cheese

½ small jalapeño chile pepper, seeded
and finely chopped (wear plastic
gloves when handling)

1 teaspoon olive oil

To make the puree: In a blender or food processor, combine the puree, bell pepper, juice, and garlic. Process for 1 to 2 minutes, or until smooth. Transfer to a medium saucepan. Stir in the cilantro or parsley, syrup or honey, thyme, and black pepper. Cook over medium heat, stirring occasionally, for 10 minutes for the flavors to blend.

To make the pancakes: Meanwhile, in a medium bowl, mash the beans well with a fork. Stir in the eggs until well blended. Stir in the flours and baking powder. Add the buttermilk, cheese, chile pepper, and oil. Stir until the mixture forms a thick sauce.

Place a large skillet over medium-high heat for 2 minutes, or until hot. Coat with cooking spray. For each pancake, dollop 2 tablespoonfuls of batter into the pan. Leave space between the pancakes. Cook for 1 to 2 minutes, or until bubbles appear on the surface. Turn and cook for 2 minutes, or until golden brown. Place on a plate. Cover to keep warm. Repeat with the remaining batter to make a total of 12 pancakes.

Serve the pancakes with the warm puree.

Per serving: *Calories 311; Protein 14 g; Carbohydrates 34 g; Fiber 7 g; Fat 14 g; Saturated Fat 5 g; Sodium 676 mg; Potassium 705 mg*

Squash and Greens Gratin

FEATURED NUTRIENT: POTASSIUM

Makes 8 servings

1 tablespoon olive oil

3 leeks (1½ pounds), white and light green parts only, halved lengthwise, sliced

1 red bell pepper, thinly sliced

½ teaspoon sea salt, divided

¼ tcaspoon ground black pepper, divided

3 large carrots, thinly sliced

1 pound kale (tough stems removed), chopped

¼ cup water

1 large butternut squash (3 pounds), peeled, seeded, and cut lengthwise into ½"-thick slices

1 cup shredded Gruyère or Swiss cheese

½ cup grated Parmesan cheese

1 cup vegetable broth

Preheat the oven to 375°F. Coat a shallow 3-quart baking dish with cooking spray.

Warm the oil in a large skillet over medium heat. Add the leeks and bell pepper. Add ¼ teaspoon of the salt and ⅛ teaspoon of the black pepper. Cook, stirring frequently, for about 5 minutes, or until softened. Stir in the carrots and cook for 5 minutes, or until tender-crisp. Remove the mixture to a plate and set aside.

Return the skillet to medium heat. Add the kale and water. Stir. Cover and increase the heat to high. Cook for 2 minutes, or until the kale wilts. Remove the lid and reduce the heat to medium-high. Cook, tossing, for 2 to 3 minutes, or until the kale is tender-crisp. Drain any liquid in the pan.

Place one-third of the squash in the prepared baking dish. Season with some of the remaining salt and black pepper. Top with half of the kale, ½ cup of the Gruyère or Swiss, half of the carrot mixture, and 3 tablespoons of the Parmesan. Repeat the layering. Top with the remaining squash. Add the broth. Sprinkle with the remaining salt and black pepper.

Cover the dish with foil and bake for 45 minutes.

Remove the foil and sprinkle the gratin with the remaining Parmesan. Bake for 15 minutes, or until the vegetables are tender. Let stand for 15 minutes before serving.

Per serving: *Calories 235; Protein 11 g; Carbohydrates 34 g; Fiber 6 g; Fat 8 g; Saturated Fat 4 g; Sodium 667 mg; Potassium 1,054.88 mg*

Stir-Fry Walnut Shrimp

FEATURED NUTRIENT: SELENIUM

Makes 4 servings

2 tablespoons medium-dry sherry (optional)

1 tablespoon wheat-free tamari

1 pound medium peeled and deveined shrimp

2 tablespoons grape seed oil

2 tablespoons chopped fresh ginger

1/2 cup chicken broth

3 scallions, whites thinly sliced diagonally, greens diagonally sliced 1" thick

1 tablespoon agave syrup or honey

1 teaspoon rice wine vinegar

1 1/2 teaspoons cornstarch, dissolved in 1 tablespoon water

1/2 cup walnut halves, coarsely chopped and toasted (see note)

In a medium bowl, combine the sherry (if using) and tamari. Add the shrimp and toss to coat. Let stand for 10 minutes. Drain the shrimp, reserving the marinade.

Set a large skillet on medium-high heat. Add the oil and ginger. Cook, stirring frequently, for 1 minute, or until the ginger is fragrant. Add the reserved shrimp and cook, tossing frequently, for 3 to 4 minutes, or until opaque. Add the broth, scallions, and reserved marinade. Bring to a boil for 1 minute.

Add the agave or honey and vinegar. Stir in the cornstarch mixture and cook, stirring constantly, for about 1 minute, or until thickened and bubbly. Remove from the heat and stir in the walnuts.

Note: *To toast nuts, place them in a dry skillet over medium heat. Toast, shaking the pan often, for 3 to 5 minutes, or until lightly browned.*

Per serving: *Calories 306; Protein 26 g; Carbohydrates 10 g; Fiber 1 g; Fat 18 g; Saturated Fat 2 g; Sodium 488 mg; Selenium 43.92 mcg*

Summer Squash alla Parmigiana

FEATURED NUTRIENT: FOLATE

Makes 4 servings

2 cups tomato sauce

2 teaspoons Italian seasoning

1 clove garlic, minced

$\frac{1}{4}$ teaspoon sea salt

$\frac{1}{4}$ teaspoon ground black pepper

3 small yellow squash or zucchini, unpeeled, sliced

2 tablespoons ground flaxseed

$\frac{1}{4}$ cup grated Parmesan cheese

$\frac{1}{2}$ cup shredded part-skim mozzarella cheese

Coat a 9" × 9" microwaveable shallow baking dish with cooking spray.

In a bowl, combine the tomato sauce, seasoning, garlic, salt, and pepper. Spread a few tablespoons of the sauce on the bottom of the prepared dish. Cover with a layer of the squash. Repeat with 2 more layers of sauce and squash, ending with the remaining sauce. Sprinkle with the flaxseed, Parmesan, and mozzarella.

Cook in the microwave oven on high power for about 18 minutes, or until the squash is tender and the cheese bubbles.

Per serving: *Calories 122; Protein 9 g; Carbohydrates 13 g; Fiber 4.2 g; Fat 5 g; Saturated Fat 2.4 g; Sodium 937 mg; Folate 41 mcg*

Swiss Chard on Toast with Goat Cheese Sauce

FEATURED NUTRIENT: MAGNESIUM

Makes 4 servings

2 tablespoons brown rice flour

1 cup cold low-sodium vegetable broth

1 cup cold milk or milk substitute

8 ounces goat cheese, crumbled

$\frac{1}{2}$ teaspoon chopped fresh rosemary

$\frac{1}{2}$ teaspoon dried basil

$\frac{1}{2}$ teaspoon sea salt

1 tablespoon olive oil

$\frac{1}{2}$ small onion, fincly chopped

$\frac{3}{4}$ pound Swiss chard, chopped

4 slices gluten-free whole grain bread

Paprika (optional)

Place the flour in a saucepan. While whisking constantly, gradually add about 2 tablespoons of the broth, until the mixture is smooth. Whisk in the milk or milk substitute and the remaining broth.

(continued)

Place the pan over medium-high heat. Cook, stirring constantly, for about 5 minutes, or until thickened. Reduce the heat to low. Add the cheese, rosemary, basil, and salt. Cook, whisking constantly, for about 2 minutes, or until the cheese melts. Remove from the heat. Cover and set aside to keep warm.

Warm the oil in a medium skillet over medium heat. Add the onion and cook, stirring occasionally, for about 3 minutes, or until translucent. Add the chard and stir. Cover and increase the heat to high. Cook for 2 minutes, or until the chard wilts. Remove the lid and reduce the heat to medium-high. Cook, tossing, for 2 minutes, or until the chard is tender-crisp.

Toast the bread. Place each slice on a plate. Top with the chard mixture and pour on the sauce. Sprinkle with paprika (if using).

Per serving: *Calories 465; Protein 24 g; Carbohydrates 34 g; Fiber 3 g; Fat 26 g; Saturated Fat 15.6 g; Sodium 806 mg ; Magnesium 114.95 mg*

Tomato and Spinach Crustless Quiche

FEATURED NUTRIENT: BIOTIN

Makes 4 servings

2 teaspoons olive oil

4 plum tomatoes, halved lengthwise

1 small onion, chopped

1 clove garlic, minced

1 bag (10 ounces) baby spinach, stems removed

³⁄₄ cup shredded Cheddar cheese

3 eggs

1 cup milk or milk substitute

2 tablespoons (¹⁄₂ ounce) grated Parmesan cheese

1¹⁄₂ teaspoons Dijon mustard

¹⁄₈ teaspoon ground black pepper

Preheat the oven to 350°F. Coat a 9" pie pan with cooking spray.

Heat the oil in a large nonstick skillet over medium-high heat. Place the tomatoes, cut side down, in the pan. Cook for 5 minutes, or until browned. Turn the tomatoes. Add the onion and garlic. Cook, stirring occasionally, for 2 minutes, or until the onion softens. Arrange the tomatoes, cut side up, in the pan. Spoon the onion and garlic around the tomatoes.

Add half of the spinach to the skillet and reduce the heat to medium. Cover and cook for 4 minutes, or until wilted. Transfer to a colander. Repeat with the remaining spinach. When cool enough to handle, squeeze the spinach until dry. Coarsely chop. Sprinkle over the tomato mixture. Top with the Cheddar.

In a medium bowl, whisk the eggs. Add the milk or milk substitute, Parmesan, mustard, and pepper. Whisk until well blended. Pour into the pan. Bake for 30 to 35 minutes, or until golden and puffed. Cool in the pan on a rack for about 30 minutes. Serve warm or at room temperature.

Per serving: *Calories 163; Protein 11 g; Carbohydrates 7 g; Fiber 2 g; Fat 11 g; Saturated Fat 5 g; Sodium 236 mg; Biotin 8.36 mcg*

Tomatoes Stuffed with Basil Salmon

FEATURED NUTRIENT: VITAMIN A

Makes 2 servings

1 egg, in the shell

1 salmon fillet (6 ounces)

2 large tomatoes

2 tablespoons sour cream

2 tablespoons mayonnaise

$\frac{1}{2}$ teaspoon prepared coarse mustard

$\frac{1}{4}$ cup chopped red onion

$\frac{1}{2}$ cup finely chopped fresh basil

Place the egg in a small saucepan with cold water to cover the top by 1". Cook over high heat until the water boils. Reduce the heat to low and simmer for 10 minutes. Carefully drain most of the water and set the pan under a faucet. Run cold water over the egg to stop the cooking. Let the egg sit in the cold water for 10 minutes to cool.

Place a steamer basket in a small saucepan with 1" of water. Bring to a boil over high heat. Place the fish in the basket. Cover and steam for 10 minutes, or until the fish is opaque. Remove the fish to cool slightly.

Meanwhile, cut the tops off the tomatoes. Carefully scoop out the pulp, leaving enough so that the tomatoes retain their shape. Squeeze the pulp to get rid of excess juice, then chop coarsely. Chop the egg coarsely.

In a medium bowl, whisk the sour cream, mayonnaise, and mustard. Add the fish, onion, basil, tomato pulp, and egg. Toss gently to mix. Spoon into the reserved tomato shells, letting extra stuffing fall to surround the tomato.

Per serving: *Calories 289; Protein 23 g; Carbohydrates 14 g; Fiber 3 g; Fat 16 g; Saturated Fat 4 g; Sodium 199 mg; Vitamin A 2,364 IU*

Turkey Sausage

FEATURED NUTRIENT: NIACIN

Makes 4 servings

2 tablespoons maple syrup

1½ teaspoons ground black pepper

1½ teaspoons ground sage

½ teaspoon salt

½ teaspoon onion powder

1¼ pounds lean ground turkey

2 teaspoons olive oil, divided

In a large bowl, combine the syrup, pepper, sage, salt, and onion powder. Mix with a fork until smooth.

Add the turkey and mix gently until the seasonings are evenly distributed. With clean hands, roll into 8 (3" diameter) patties.

Heat 1 teaspoon of the oil in a skillet over medium-high heat. Place half of the patties in the skillet. Cook for 2 to 3 minutes per side, or until no longer pink and the juices run clear. Transfer to a platter.

Add the remaining 1 teaspoon oil and repeat with the remaining patties.

Per serving: *Calories 262; Protein 25 g; Carbohydrates 8 g; Fiber 0 g; Fat 14 g; Saturated Fat 4 g; Sodium 331 mg; Niacin 4.97 mg*

Tuscan Tuna Cakes

FEATURED NUTRIENT: MAGNESIUM

Makes 4 servings

1 pound yellowfin tuna, coarsely chopped

2 eggs

¼ cup finely chopped fennel or celery

1 small onion, finely chopped

1 tablespoon capers, rinsed and drained

1 tablespoon fresh lemon juice

2 teaspoons grated lemon peel

½ teaspoon dried oregano

1½ cups almond flour, divided

½ teaspoon salt

½ teaspoon ground black pepper

2 tablespoons olive oil, divided

4 lemon wedges

In a large bowl, combine the fish, eggs, fennel or celery, onion, capers, juice, peel, and oregano. Mix well. Gently fold in 1 cup of the flour, the salt, and pepper until just combined.

Spread the remaining ½ cup flour on a plate. Divide the fish mixture into 8 equal portions (about ⅓ cup of mixture per cake). Roll each portion in the flour and shape into 3½" diameter patties.

Warm 1 tablespoon of the oil in a large nonstick skillet over medium heat. Add 4 fish cakes and cook for 3 to 4 minutes per side, or until golden and cooked through. Remove to a platter. Repeat with the remaining 1 tablespoon oil and the remaining 4 fish cakes. Serve with the lemon wedges.

Per serving: *Calories 472; Protein 39 g; Carbohydrates 13 g; Fiber 6 g; Fat 31 g; Saturated Fat 3 g; Sodium 337 mg; Magnesium 185 mg*

Walnut Chicken with Snow Peas

FEATURED NUTRIENT: SELENIUM

Makes 4 servings

1 pound boneless, skinless chicken breasts, cut into ½" pieces

2 tablespoons wheat-free tamari, divided

4 teaspoons cornstarch, divided

½ cup chicken broth

¼ cup orange juice

3 teaspoons grape seed oil, divided

3 cloves garlic, finely chopped

1 onion, chopped

1 red or orange bell pepper, sliced

¾ cup snow peas, cut crosswise into thirds

½ jicama, chopped

½ cup walnuts, coarsely chopped

1 teaspoon toasted sesame oil

In a bowl, combine the chicken, 1 tablespoon of the tamari, and 2 teaspoons of the cornstarch. In a separate bowl, combine the broth, juice, and the remaining 1 tablespoon tamari and 2 teaspoons cornstarch. Set aside.

Heat 2 teaspoons of the grape seed oil in a large nonstick skillet or wok over medium-high heat. Add the chicken and cook, stirring often, for 4 to 5 minutes, or until no longer pink and the juices run clear. Transfer to a plate and set aside.

Add the remaining 1 teaspoon grape seed oil to the skillet. Add the garlic and cook for 15 seconds. Stir in the onion and pepper and cook for 1 to 2 minutes, or until the vegetables just begin to soften. Stir in the snow peas and jicama and cook for 1 to 2 minutes, or until the snow peas are bright green. Add the walnuts and sesame oil and cook for 1 minute.

Stir in the reserved chicken and broth mixture. Cook for 1 to 2 minutes, or until thickened.

Per serving: *Calories 349; Protein 29 g; Carbohydrates 20 g; Fiber 7 g; Fat 17 g; Saturated Fat 2 g; Sodium 680 mg; Selenium 38.22 mcg*

Warm Grilled Beef with Quinoa Salad

FEATURED NUTRIENT: ZINC

Makes 4 servings

¼ cup red wine vinegar

1 tablespoon stone-ground mustard

3 bay leaves

¼ teaspoon ground black pepper

1 pound beef top round, about
    1" thick

1 cup quinoa

½ small red onion, chopped

1 tablespoon olive oil

1 large tomato, cut into wedges

In a large glass baking dish, combine the vinegar, mustard, bay leaves, and pepper. Whisk to mix. Place the meat in the dish. With a skewer or long-tined fork, poke some holes in the meat. Cover and refrigerate, turning occasionally, to marinate for several hours.

Cook the quinoa according to package directions. Drain and spread on a tray to cool to room temperature.

Preheat the boiler. Remove the meat from the marinade and place on the broiler pan. Reserve the marinade.

Cook the meat 5" from the heat source for about 8 minutes, turning once, or until a thermometer inserted in the center registers 145°F for medium-rare. Remove the meat from the broiler and let it sit for a few minutes before slicing.

Meanwhile, pour the reserved marinade in a small saucepan. Remove and discard the bay leaves. Set the pan over medium heat. Bring to a boil. Reduce the heat to medium-low. Cook for 2 minutes.

In a large bowl, combine the quinoa, onion, oil, and marinade. Toss well. Mound the mixture in the center of a serving dish. Thinly slice the meat. Place the meat and tomatoes over the quinoa salad.

Per serving: *Calories 406; Protein 32 g; Carbohydrates 30 g; Fiber 4 g; Fat 17 g; Saturated Fat 5 g; Sodium 113 mg; Zinc 4.57 mg*

Zucchini Strands in Creamy Basil Sauce

FEATURED NUTRIENT: GLUTATHIONE

Makes 4 servings

1 cup chicken or vegetable broth

2 cloves garlic, minced

Pinch of ground red pepper

1 small carrot, cut into matchsticks

4 zucchini, cut into 5" × $\frac{1}{8}$" strips

$\frac{1}{4}$ cup grated Parmesan cheese

$\frac{1}{4}$ cup mozzarella cheese, shredded

$\frac{1}{4}$ cup half-and-half

1 tablespoon finely chopped fresh basil

In a large skillet over high heat, combine the broth, garlic, and pepper. Bring to a boil. Reduce the heat to medium-high. Cook for about 3 minutes, or until slightly reduced. Add the carrots. Cover and reduce the heat to medium. Cook for 3 minutes. Add the zucchini. Cover and cook for 1 or 2 minutes, or until the carrots are tender. Drain off the liquid. Add the Parmesan and mozzarella, half-and-half, and basil. Toss gently until the cheese melts.

Per serving: *Calories 106; Protein 7 g; Carbohydrates 9 g; Fiber 2 g; Fat 5.5 g; Saturated Fat 3 g; Sodium 389 mg*

Desserts

Almond Mousse with Raspberry Sauce

FEATURED NUTRIENT: RIBOFLAVIN

6 servings

Mousse

¼ cup water

1 envelope (¼ ounce) unflavored
    gelatin

1¼ cups unsweetened almond milk

¼ cup agave syrup or honey

3 eggs, separated

1½ teaspoons almond extract

Sauce

½ cup red or black raspberry all-fruit
    spread

½ pint red or black raspberries

To make the mousse: Pour the water into a medium saucepan. Sprinkle the gelatin on in an even layer. Let stand to soften, about 5 minutes. Add the milk and syrup or honey. Set the pan over medium-low heat. Cook for about 3 minutes, or until warm.

In a bowl, beat the egg yolks with a fork. Slowly add some of the warm milk mixture, whisking constantly. Add the egg yolks, stirring constantly, to the pan. Cook, stirring, for about 2 minutes, or until slightly thickened. Remove from the heat. Add the almond extract. Whisk to combine. Cool to room temperature and then refrigerate for about 45 minutes, or until thickened but not set.

In a bowl or an electric mixer, beat the egg whites until stiff. Fold into the chilled mixture. Pour into a 1-quart mold and refrigerate for at least 6 hours, or until firm.

To make the sauce: Place the spread in a small saucepan. Cook, whisking, over low heat for 2 to 3 minutes, or until melted and smooth. Remove from the heat and add the raspberries. Stir gently. Cover and refrigerate for at least 1 hour, or until chilled.

To serve, unmold the mousse onto a flat serving dish. Spoon the sauce over the mousse.

Per serving: *Calories 155; Protein 5 g; Carbohydrates 27 g; Fiber 2 g; Fat 3.3 g; Saturated Fat 0.8 g; Sodium 75 mg; Riboflavin 0.13 mg*

Baked Coconut Custards

Makes 6 servings

3 eggs

2 cups milk or milk substitute

1 teaspoon coconut extract

$\frac{1}{4}$ cup agave syrup or honey, warmed

1 tablespoon unsweetened shredded coconut

Preheat the oven to 300°F. Coat 6 custard cups (6 ounces each) with cooking spray. Place in a 13" × 9" baking pan. Bring a kettle of water to the boil.

In a medium bowl, beat the eggs lightly with a fork. While beating, gradually add the milk or milk substitute, coconut extract, and syrup or honey. Pour into the prepared cups.

Place the pan on the oven rack and pour hot water into the pan to a depth of $\frac{1}{2}$".

Bake for about 25 minutes, or until a knife inserted halfway between the edge and center comes out clean. Remove from the oven. Transfer the custards from the pan to a rack to cool. Refrigerate for several hours, if desired, to chill. Or serve at room temperature.

Meanwhile, place the coconut in a small heavy skillet. Set over medium-high heat. Cook, stirring with a fork, for 3 to 4 minutes, or until golden. Remove and set aside.

To serve, unmold the custards onto serving dishes. Sprinkle with the reserved coconut.

Per serving: *Calories 132; Protein 6 g; Carbohydrates 15 g; Fiber 0.1 g; Fat 5.74 g; Saturated Fat 2.82 g; Sodium 70 mg; Vitamin D 54 IU*

Caramel Flan with Blueberries and Strawberries

FEATURED NUTRIENT: ZINC

Makes 6 servings

$^2/_3$ cup raw cane sugar or turbinado, divided

1 tablespoon water

3 eggs

$1^1/_2$ cups milk or milk substitute

$1^1/_2$ teaspoons vanilla extract

1 cup blueberries

1 cup sliced strawberries

$^1/_4$ teaspoon ground cinnamon

Preheat the oven to 325°F. Set 6 custard cups (6 ounces each) in a 13" × 9" baking pan. Bring a kettle of water to the boil.

In a medium skillet over medium-high heat, combine $^1/_3$ cup of the sugar and the water. Cook, stirring often, for about 5 minutes, or until the sugar is caramelized. Carefully pour the very hot caramel evenly into the cups. Swirl to coat the bottoms. Let stand for 10 minutes.

In a medium bowl, combine the eggs and the remaining $^1/_3$ cup sugar. Whisk until well blended. Whisk in the milk or milk substitute and vanilla. Transfer to a large glass measuring cup or pitcher for easier handling. Pour evenly into the cups. Place the pan on the oven rack and pour hot water into the pan to a depth of $^1/_2$".

Bake for 20 to 25 minutes, or until a knife inserted halfway between the edge and center comes out clean. Remove from the oven. Transfer the cups from the pan to a rack to cool. Serve warm or cool completely, cover, and refrigerate for up to 24 hours. Garnish with the blueberries and strawberries. Sprinkle with the cinnamon.

Per serving: *Calories 181; Protein 5 g; Carbohydrates 30 g; Fiber 1 g; Fat 5 g; Saturated Fat 2 g; Sodium 70 mg; Zinc 0.62 mg*

Cherry-Berry Almond Fruit Cake

FEATURED NUTRIENT: RIBOFLAVIN

Makes 16 servings

$1\frac{1}{2}$ cups blanched almonds, toasted (see note)

$1\frac{1}{2}$ cups raw cane sugar or turbinado, divided

1 cup almond flour

1 cup brown rice flour + some for dusting the pan

1 tablespoon baking powder

$\frac{1}{2}$ teaspoon baking soda

$\frac{1}{2}$ teaspoon sea salt

1 cup buttermilk

2 eggs

3 egg whites

$\frac{1}{3}$ cup grape seed oil

$\frac{1}{4}$ cup fresh lemon juice

1 teaspoon almond extract

$\frac{1}{2}$ cup blueberries

$\frac{1}{2}$ cup raspberries

1 cup cherries, halved

Preheat the oven to 350°F. Coat a 12-cup Bundt pan with cooking spray. Dust with flour.

In a food processor, combine the almonds and $\frac{1}{2}$ cup of the sugar. Process until the almonds are finely ground. Transfer to a large bowl. Add the flours, baking powder, baking soda, salt, and the remaining 1 cup sugar. Stir to mix. Add the buttermilk, eggs, egg whites, oil, juice, and almond extract. Whisk until well combined. Fold in the blueberries, raspberries, and cherries. Pour into the prepared pan.

Bake in the center of the oven for 65 to 70 minutes, or until a wooden pick inserted in the center comes out clean. Cool in the pan on a rack for 15 minutes. Remove to the rack and cool completely.

Note: *To toast nuts, place them in a dry skillet over medium heat. Toast, shaking the pan often, for 3 to 5 minutes, or until lightly browned.*

Per serving: *Calories 298; Protein 7 g; Carbohydrates 34 g; Fiber 3 g; Fat 16 g; Saturated Fat 1.7 g; Sodium 238 mg; Riboflavin 0.18 mg*

Cherry Pudding Cake

FEATURED NUTRIENT: PROBIOTICS

Makes 6 servings

2 cups frozen dark sweet cherries, thawed

1 cup plain yogurt

½ cup part-skim ricotta cheese

¼ cup brown rice flour

2 eggs

¼ teaspoon ground nutmeg

6 tablespoons raw cane sugar or turbinado, divided

¼ cup golden raisins

Preheat the oven to 400°F. Coat a 12" quiche dish with cooking spray. Place the cherries in the dish. In a blender or food processor, combine the yogurt, ricotta, flour, eggs, nutmeg, and 4 tablespoons of the sugar. Process for about 2 minutes, scraping the sides of the bowl, or until smooth. Pour over the cherries. Sprinkle with the raisins.

Bake for 12 minutes, or until the cake begins to set. Sprinkle with the remaining 2 tablespoons sugar. Bake for 8 minutes, or until the cake is firm and golden brown. Cool in the pan on a rack for at least 30 minutes. Serve warm or at room temperature.

Per serving: *Calories 198; Protein 7 g; Carbohydrates 33 g; Fiber 2 g; Fat 5 g; Saturated Fat 2.5 g; Sodium 74 mg*

Honeyed Summer Fruit Bowl

FEATURED NUTRIENT: VITAMIN C

Makes 8 servings

¼ cup honey

1 tablespoon fresh lemon juice or fresh lime juice

Pinch of ground cinnamon

1½ pints strawberries, quartered

½ large cantaloupe, cut into chunks or balls

2 nectarines, cut into thin wedges

2 peaches, cut into thin wedges

2 large or 3 small plums, cut into thin wedges

1 cup blueberries

In a large bowl, combine the honey, juice, and cinnamon. Whisk to mix. Add the strawberries, cantaloupe, nectarines, peaches, plums, and blueberries. Toss gently to coat the fruit with the honey mixture.

Let stand for 30 minutes to allow the flavors to blend.

Per serving: *Calories 120; Protein 2 g; Carbohydrates 30 g; Fiber 3 g; Fat 0.54 g; Saturated Fat 0 g; Sodium 9 mg; Vitamin C 60 mg*

Maple Rice Pudding with Pecans

FEATURED NUTRIENT: MELATONIN

6 servings

4 cups milk or milk substitute

1 cup short-grain brown rice

¼ cup maple syrup

2 teaspoons vanilla extract

1 tablespoon butter

¼ cup chopped pecans

¼ cup half-and-half (optional)

In a heavy-bottomed nonstick saucepan, combine the milk or milk substitute and rice. Cover and set over medium-high heat until the mixture simmers briskly. Reduce the heat to low. Cook for about 40 minutes, or until the milk is absorbed and the rice is very tender.

Add the maple syrup and vanilla. Stir to mix well.

Heat the butter over medium heat in a small skillet until the foam subsides. Add the pecans and cook, stirring, for about 3 minutes, or until toasted. Spoon the pudding into bowls. Top with the pecan mixture and drizzle with the half-and-half (if using).

Per serving: *Calories 301; Protein 8 g; Carbohydrates 44 g; Fiber 3 g; Fat 11.5 g; Saturated Fat 5 g; Sodium 75 mg*

Pear, Date, and Walnut Muffins

FEATURED NUTRIENT: MELATONIN

Makes 12 (1 muffin per serving)

1 cup stone-ground yellow cornmeal

1 cup brown rice flour

1/2 cup chopped pitted dates

4 teaspoons baking powder

Pinch of baking soda

1 cup milk or milk substitute

2 eggs

4 tablespoons butter, melted

3 tablespoons agave syrup or honey

1/2 teaspoon white or cider vinegar

1 large pear, grated

1/4 cup finely ground walnuts

1 tablespoon grated orange peel

Preheat the oven to 400°F. Coat a 12-cup muffin pan with cooking spray.

In a bowl, combine the cornmeal, flour, dates, baking powder, and baking soda. Stir with a fork to mix. Set aside.

In another bowl, combine the milk or milk substitute, eggs, butter, syrup or honey, and vinegar. Beat with a fork until smooth. Add the pear, walnuts, and peel. Stir to mix. Add the dry ingredients. Stir to combine just until no flour is visible. Spoon the batter into the prepared pan.

Bake for 20 to 25 minutes, or until golden. Cool in the pan on a rack for 10 minutes. Remove to the rack and cool completely.

Per serving: *Calories 204; Protein 4 g; Carbohydrates 32 g; Fiber 4 g; Fat 7 g; Saturated Fat 3 g; Sodium 222 mg*

Poached Pears in Vanilla Sauce

FEATURED NUTRIENT: CALCIUM

6 servings

1 cup apple cider

1 cup water

3 tablespoons agave syrup or honey

1 teaspoon vanilla extract

1 tablespoon lemon peel

6 ripe but firm pears, halved and
    cored (leave the stems on)

¼ cup fat-free plain yogurt

In a large saucepan, combine the cider, water, syrup or honey, vanilla, and peel. Add the pears and press gently to submerge in the liquid.

Over high heat, bring the mixture almost to a boil, or until the liquid is steaming vigorously. Reduce the heat to medium-low. Cover and cook, turning the pears occasionally for even cooking, for 15 to 20 minutes, or until the pears are just tender when pierced with a fork. Using a slotted spoon, carefully remove the pears and divide among 6 dessert dishes.

Return the pan to the stove. Increase the heat to high. Boil the liquid for about 5 minutes, or until reduced by half. Cool slightly. Add the yogurt and whisk to incorporate. Spoon the sauce over the pears.

Per serving: *Calories 162; Protein 1 g; Carbohydrates 41 g; Fiber 6 g; Fat 1 g; Saturated Fat 0 g; Sodium 8 mg; Calcium 31 mg*

Strawberries with Rhubarb Sauce

FEATURED NUTRIENT: VITAMIN C

8 servings

1¼ pounds rhubarb stalks, cut into
    1" pieces, or 1 package (20 ounces)
    frozen rhubarb, thawed

1 cup raw cane sugar or turbinado

½ cup water

¼ teaspoon ground cinnamon

2 pounds strawberries, quartered

In a medium saucepan, combine the rhubarb, sugar, water, and cinnamon. Bring to a boil over medium heat. Cook, stirring occasionally, for about 20 minutes, or until reduced to a sauce. Set aside to cool slightly.

Place the strawberries in dessert bowls. Spoon on the sauce.

Per serving: *Calories 143; Protein 1 g; Carbohydrates 36 g; Fiber 4 g; Fat 0.5 g; Saturated Fat 0 g; Sodium 14 mg; Vitamin C 72 mg*

Sam's Fruit and Nut Medley

FEATURED NUTRIENT: VITAMIN A

Makes 1½ cups (¼ cup per serving)

2 tablespoons agave syrup or honey

1 tablespoon grape seed oil

1 tablespoon water

½ teaspoon almond extract

½ teaspoon ground cinnamon

¼ teaspoon salt

½ cup coarsely chopped walnuts

¼ cup unsweetened flaked dried coconut

2 tablespoons hulled hemp seeds

1 tablespoon ground flaxseed

¼ cup dried currants

¼ cup dried cranberries

½ cup chopped dried apricots

Preheat the oven to 300°F. Coat a large baking pan with shallow sides with cooking spray.

In a microwaveable bowl, combine the syrup or honey, oil, water, almond extract, cinnamon, and salt. Cook in the microwave oven on high power for about 1 minute, or until hot. Whisk to combine.

In a large bowl, combine the walnuts, coconut, hemp seeds, and flaxseed. Drizzle with the syrup or honey mixture. Toss thoroughly to coat all the dry ingredients. Transfer the mixture to the prepared pan and spread it evenly in the pan.

Bake for about 20 minutes, or until golden brown. Remove to a rack. Stir in the currants, cranberries, and apricots. Cool completely. Store in an airtight container in a cool, dry place.

Per serving: *Calories 230; Protein 4 g; Carbohydrates 28 g; Fiber 4 g; Fat 12 g; Saturated Fat 3 g; Sodium 67 mg; Vitamin A 853 IU*

Watermelon-Cranberry Granita

FEATURED NUTRIENT: GLUTATHIONE

6 servings

2 tablespoons agave syrup or honey

1 tablespoon fresh lemon juice

1 tablespoon fresh lime juice

6 cups seedless watermelon chunks or balls (about 4 pounds with rind)

½ cup 100% cranberry juice

In a small bowl, combine the syrup or honey, lemon juice, and lime juice. Whisk until smooth.

Working in several batches, in a blender, combine the watermelon and syrup or honey mixture. Blend until smooth. Transfer to a bowl and repeat until all the watermelon is pureed. Add the cranberry juice and stir to blend completely.

Pour the mixture into a freezerproof 8" × 8" dish. Place in the freezer for 2½ hours, raking the mixture with a fork (be sure to scrape the sides of the pan) every 30 minutes, or until nearly frozen but not completely solid. Rake with a fork and serve.

Per serving: *Calories 76; Protein 1 g; Carbohydrates 20 g; Fiber 1 g; Fat 0 g; Saturated Fat 0 g; Sodium 2 mg*

Resources

Great Supplements: Companies That Put Their Best Foot Forward

You'll find only a handful of companies that are authentically great, that willingly share certification information, and that offer you truly good stuff. These companies offer a full line of nutraceuticals from A to Z. You can feel good about shopping for the nutrients you need from any one of the manufacturers I list here. You can search online at their Web sites or call the companies directly. Some are sold through doctors' offices only. Many are widely available at your local health food stores or pharmacies, and at grocery stores and natural health markets such as Whole Foods Market, Mother Earth's Storehouse, and the Vitamin Shoppe. For some, I have mentioned specialty formulas that I think are pure and helpful. Almost all of these companies offer their supplements in vegetarian capsules or offer products that are gluten free, dairy free, and yeast free. If any of these things concern you, please check each item.

Doctor's Data, Inc. or DDI
www.doctorsdata.com
800-323-2784

> They have numerous tests and a very good one for evaluating heavy metals spilled through the urine. When I do heavy metal testing, I use their 24-Hour Urine Test because it seems to be the most accurate for heavy metals. Their tests are utilized in the assessment, detection, prevention, and treatment of heavy metal burden, but they also (like the other labs) offer excellent tests for nutritional deficiencies, environmental toxic burdens, gastrointestinal function, detoxification, and metabolic testing.

Douglas Laboratories
www.douglaslabs.com
800-245-4440

> This company is an international leader in the dietary supplement industry. They have been in business for more than 50 years, and they manufacture their own line of supplements and hundreds of other proprietary blends. The supplements are manufactured with fine raw materials and under strict guidelines and ISO 9001-certified standards.

Dr. Ohhira's Probiotics

www.essentialformulas.com

This is one of those outstanding companies that produces various high-quality supplements that improve health at the cellular level. Their line of nourishing whole-health supplements is from Japan and is formulated by renowned microbiologist Dr. Iichiroh Ohhira. Their Essential Living oils are certified vegan alternatives to fish oil and help nourish the nervous, immune, and hormonal systems. They have an incredible blend of probiotics and prebiotics that are based on traditional Asian fermentation processes. These are the only supplements that I know of that do not spark an allergic or immunological response. I take this brand and give it to my children.

Dr. Ohhira's Probiotics is a truly unique blend that is safe for sensitive folks and gets through your stomach acid and down to your intestines, where you need it. This probiotic blend does not require refrigeration. It is sold at most health food stores.

EcoNugenics

www.econugenics.com
800-308-5518

If you go to this company's Web site, you'll find a number of products that are unique and pure. They are sticklers for detail and quality. One of their primary researchers is Isaac Eliaz, MD. He has created one product, PectaSol-C, out of the rinds of citrus fruits. Research done on this product has found it to be beneficial for prostate, breast, and colon cancers. It's an absorbable form of soluble fiber that can latch onto tumors and help break them down. EcoNugenics also makes MycoPhyto Complex, which contains six potent varieties of medicinal mushrooms that are grown on immune-system-boosting herbs and organic brown rice. This product calms your immune function if you have an autimmune disorder such as rheumatoid arthritis, lupus, multiple sclerosis, or Sjögren's syndrome. It can also rev up your immune system if you have constant infections, chronic fatigue syndrome, AIDS-related infections, and so forth. MycoPhyto Complex activates your body's natural killer cells and boosts energy reserves, too.

Another star product this company makes is Padma Basic. It's an impressive blend of Tibetan herbs. In the United States, this product is a dietary supplement; overseas, it's sold as a drug. There is research to support Padma Basic's use in people with multiple sclerosis. (It helps prevent demyelination.) It's also helpful for reducing inflammation; unclogging sticky, cholesterol-laden arteries; and possibly delaying the need for a root canal. The research behind Padma Basic is lengthy and impressive.

Enzymatic Therapy

www.enzymatictherapy.com
800-783-2286

This company is a leader in nutrition with more than 250 health products. They pay attention to detail, and you have to love them for allowing regular people to schedule visits to their facility. They are in the Green Bay, Wisconsin, area, and unlike many companies, Enzymatic Therapy will send you certification on bacteriological testing. Because they are so committed to quality and their products are so easy to find at health food stores, I have featured many of them. They make smart and sensible blends of herbs and vitamins so you get the best of both worlds.

Enzymedica

www.enzymedica.com
888-918-1118

This company pays attention to detail and brings us outstanding enzymes to help us digest our food. I've written about them several times in my syndicated column because I really like their plant-based line. A good all-around basic digestive enzyme that everyone could take is Digest. If you are gluten intolerant (celiac disease) and have concerns about a particular meal, you could take their GlutenEase, which grabs gluten out of the meal before you absorb it. Another star product is Natto-K (nattokinase), an enzyme that breaks up cysts and clots that could clog your arteries and contribute to a stroke. If you have allergies, try their MucoStop. It reduces the effects of histamine-induced misery. I met the president of Enzymedica, Tom Bohager, author of *Enzymes: What the Experts Know*, and he is as compassionate as he is brilliant. Every doctor should read his book to learn how to better serve his or her patients. It is also good for the educated consumer.

Genova Diagnostics

www.gdx.net
800-522-4762

One of the best tests they offer is called NutrEval, and it is very comprehensive. Pages and pages of results show you your levels of key micronutrients and amino acids. The lab also offers another test for bone strength. This urine and blood test examines compounds to help identify the current rate of bone loss; the presence of lytic bone disease; the efficacy of bone support medications or treatments; and your levels of vitamins, minerals, and essential fatty acids.

iNutritionals

www.inutritionals.com
800-647-6100

This company's product line was developed by a renegade neurologist, David Perlmutter, MD, author of *The Better Brain Book, Raise a Smarter Child by Kindergarten*, and *Power Up Your Brain*. He's created a natural supplement called BrainSustain to improve memory and brain function. This synergistic blend of nutrients contains many brain savers, including alpha-lipoic acid, ginkgo biloba, phosphatidylserine, calcium, some B vitamins, CoQ10, and NAC. The nutrients in this formula work together to help you maintain memory and mood. It protects you from the inside out because your brain cells will be less affected by toxic free radicals, which are basically molecular loose cannons that seek to destroy cells.

BrainSustain works by improving the energy production within each brain cell and increasing oxygen flow. You mix a scoop of powder in juice or water each day. I recommend this supplement for people who want to reduce the risks of free radicals, which have been associated with many neurodegenerative disorders such as Alzheimer's disease, Parkinson's disease, multiple sclerosis, ALS (Lou Gehrig's disease), and poor memory. Dr. Perlmutter makes a children's version of this product that may be helpful for kids with attention-deficit problems.

LivingFuel

www.livingfuel.com

866-580-3835

This product line of supplements and foods is impressive not only in quality, but also in taste. I met the brain behind the brilliant line of goodies at an expo and got to sample his delicious products. His name is K. C. Craichy, and he is the author of *The Super Health Diet*. When you meet him, it's clear that he practices what he preaches. He looks incredibly healthy and fit. It's challenging to create healthy all-in-one supplements that taste good. Many superfoods and healthy supplements taste awful and are loaded with artificial sweeteners, toxic chemicals, sugar, and colors. This is not the case with LivingFuel. You simply mix the powder products with water to get hundreds of essential nutrients, minerals, and antioxidants. It is an all-organic/non-GMO, nutrient-rich whole food. LivingFuel offers a delicious chocolate bar called CocoChia made with chia seeds (yes, just like the Chia Pet from the 1980s), which are high in omega-3 essential fatty acids and very healthy for you. I'm not kidding. I hide them from my husband whenever we get a case. Another product they make is coffee, a safe and pure kind called Super Coffee Rx. It comes in a dropper bottle and you mix it with hot water.

Metametrix Clinical Laboratory

www.metametrix.com

800-221-4640

They have a large selection of excellent tests, and I find their GI Effects Complete test to be the very best when it comes to convenient stool testing for digestive problems like celiac disease, irritable bowel syndrome, and liver or pancreatic problems. They also offer tests to measure PCBs, phthalates, and porphyrins (this is very hard to find).

Metabolic Maintenance

www.metabolicmaintenance.com

800-772-7873

This company makes a full line of vitamin and herbal products using vegetarian capsules. They use active forms of vitamins in many cases. One of their products, Brain Cell Support, is a combination of natural herbs and amino acids that improves memory, cognitive function, and mood. Another good product for diabetes is DIM Complex, which helps reduce estrogen load in the body. If you find that you are deficient in one or two B vitamins, their B complex is a great supplement.

Nature Made
www.naturemade.com
800-276-2878

This line of supplements is sold widely at pharmacies and health food stores. Nature Made pays attention to quality. Founded in 1971, this company has been making high-quality supplements for decades. They offer dozens of innovative blends to help you with diabetes, heart disease, insomnia, arthritis, osteoporosis, vision problems, and much more. Nutrients are USP-approved (USP is a verification program for dietary supplements to safeguard consumers from buying poor-quality formulas). The Nature Made Web site offers advice on how to choose vitamins and read vitamin labels, as well as a Vitamin Assessment Quiz to help you determine which nutrients you need based on your age, gender , and lifestyle.

Nordic Naturals
www.nordicnaturals.com
800-662-2544

This fresh and pure line of essential fatty acids (EFAs) was brought to the United States by a Norwegian man who was looking for high-quality fish oil and cod liver oil. He was accustomed to having these at his disposal in Norway, but when he moved here, it posed a challenge. So he formed his own company and is committed to quality and purity. He has dedicated his life to producing incredibly high-quality fish oils, which he sometimes combines with other wonderful ingredients like coenzyme Q10. Fish oils, however, are the foundation of the product line, which I have taken and enjoyed for many years. EFAs are not mugged by drugs, so there is no chapter on them. We don't make our own EFAs, but we still need them for good health. These fish-derived substances offer profound health benefits, including healthy cell membrane function and improved brain function and mood. They are also a powerful anti-inflammatory and can help with arthritis better than some medications can. There are many research studies on this topic available at the company's Web site. You can find this exceptional line at most health food stores and online.

Nutraceutical
www.nutraceutical.com
800-669-8877

Solaray products are sold at most health food stores. They make a number of products, including a full line of B vitamins, minerals, antioxidants, and specialty products. I recommend their vitamin B_1, folic acid 800 mcg, and calcium citrate supplements.

Nutrex Hawaii

www.nutrex-hawaii.com
800-453-1187

This Hawaii-based company makes natural astaxanthin. That's a big word for a powerful antioxidant that is much more effective than vitamins E and C put together, and it never goes "pro-oxidant" like other antioxidants. Many who subscribe to my free newsletter or read my syndicated column know that I like astaxanthin. It's so helpful to so many people. It can improve vision, reduce arthritis, help control blood sugar, and unclog arteries. It comes from marine algae and is red. It actually puts the pink in flamingos and the red in lobsters! I've partnered with the makers to get a 25 percent discount on all orders as preferred customers for reading my book. Use coupon code 24. Nutrex Hawaii makes a wonderful superfood that contains spirulina, a blue-green algae from the sea that's loaded with nutrients, especially important minerals. If you take a drug mugger that robs you of beta-carotene, iron, or calcium, consider the fact that spirulina contains 3,900 percent more beta-carotene than carrots, 2,300 percent more iron than spinach, and 300 percent more calcium than milk. Spirulina is superfood for humans, not just sea critters. I think everyone should take astaxanthin and spirulina for good health even if they are not being mugged by a drug.

Pure Encapsulations

www.purecaps.com
800-753-2277

Pure Encapsulations only sells their products to licensed health-care providers, so you won't find this line at your health food store. Your doctor or other health-care practitioner can fax in his or her license to obtain products for you. Chiropractors, nurses, pharmacists, acupuncturists, or any other licensed provider can also obtain them for you, not just MDs. They are also sold online. Pure Encapsulations has a very high standard, and their supplements are sold internationally.

Solgar

www.solgar.com
877-765-4274

Solgar products are sold at most health food stores in dark amber glass bottles. The product line is vast, with supplements from A to Z. This is an affordable, easy-to-find brand if you want to shop at your local health food store.

SpectraCell Laboratories

www.spectracell.com
800-227-5227

This laboratory sells blood test kits that you take to your local lab or physician's office. The tests measure specific nutrients through lymphocytes and show intracellular function for the past 4 to 6 months. Traditional blood tests measure an instant in time, and that snapshot is usually misleading. SpectraCell also measures levels of important fatty acids. SpectraCell tests are so comprehensive that they can tell you exactly what nutrient you are deficient in. I didn't believe it at first, so I tried it myself and now I'm a believer. I found that I had been suffering the drug mugging effects of those hazelnut lattes Sam whips up for me.

If you only do one blood test a year, do a SpectraCell analysis. There are various tests available. The FIA 5000 will check your levels of vitamin D, all of your B vitamins, calcium, magnesium, selenium, zinc, CoQ10, and glutathione.

You'll have to ask your doctor or practitioner to fax in his or her license to order their test kits for you.

Sunfood

www.sunfood.com
888-729-3663

One of this company's most interesting products is Ocean's Alive Marine Phytoplankton. This is concentrated raw food containing phytoplankton straight from the ocean. You get amazing nutritional benefits from superfoods like this. It's basically microalgae that contain 90 ionic and trace minerals without a lot of sodium. It's purified, so don't worry, and comes from a controlled ocean environment where it is carefully manufactured for human consumption. The intense chlorophyll content in this product detoxifies your body, chelates heavy metals, sends fuel to your muscles, and increases energy, heart health, and clarity. It gets right into your brain and improves functioning. While it does not contain a large amount of magnesium, the combination of all the minerals together in their live forms is perfect. I put a dropperful in water each day. It's completely tasteless.

Thorne Research

www.thorne.com
800-228-1966

Thorne offers a full range of vitamins, minerals, and herbal products using active and standardized ingredients without the lubricant magnesium stearate. They create medical foods for people with celiac disease or other digestive problems. Many of Thorne's products are available by phone or online. They are sometimes sold at holistic pharmacies, health food stores, and doctors' offices. One of their specialty products, Deproloft, is an herb and vitamin combination used to boost mood and ease depression. I also like a fiber product called Arabinex, which comes from the larch tree. It improves gastrointestinal function. Fibrovive is helpful for people with muscle pain, muscle atrophy, or fibromyalgia. The company also makes various vitamin B formulas that contain the active forms of B_6 (P5P) and folic acid (5-MTHF). Most of the products offer body-ready, usable, active ingredients like these, and I appreciate that they combine the nutrients in an intelligent way using high-quality salts or amino acid chelates.

Turtle Mountain

www.sodeliciousdairyfree.com

866-388-7853

The So Delicious line of foods is produced by Turtle Mountain. They make many delicious products, all free of many common allergens, especially dairy foods. It's a challenge to find healthy novelty items and desserts that taste really amazing. I'm impressed with their products. I recommend their cultured coconut milk yogurts because they're rich in probiotics and calcium and are dairy free, soy free, and just plain yummy. One arm of their frozen dessert line, Purely Decadent, is made with coconut milk and is dairy free, soy free, and sweetened with natural agave syrup, something people with diabetes can have. If you have children, look for their Kidz pops in fudge and fruit flavors. They are free of the eight most common food allergens.

Vitamin Code

www.thevitamincode.com

866-465-0051

Vitamin Code vitamins were created by Jordan Rubin using whole food extracts. When you consume raw foods like fruits, vegetables, nuts, and seeds, you are getting the vitamins, minerals, probiotics, enzymes, and phytonutrients in their most potent, unadulterated forms. Many experts believe that heating foods results in the loss of many nutrients and that whole food supplements give you nutrients most like what is present in nature. Your body can easily assimilate the nutrients into your bloodstream and maximize their potential. This product line caters to men and women, providing each with a comprehensive multivitamin.

Wakunaga of America

www.kyolic.com

800-421-2998

This company produces a fantastic brand of aged garlic, which is helpful for diabetes, heart disease, cholesterol, inflammation, and digestive problems. Aged garlic helps you fend off infections, improve circulation, lower cholesterol, and deal with cardiovascular problems. You name it, Wakunaga makes a garlic combination product for you. I appreciate their attention to detail and the fact that they use an active and standardized form of garlic. When you buy garlic, you want it to be active. They've also found a way to make it odorless. I like several of their products, including Kyo-Dophilus, a chewable probiotic that kids can take. Kyolic products are sold at most health food stores.

World Nutrition

www.worldnutrition.info

800-548-2710

Vitälzȳm is a unique blend of enzymes. It contains various digestive enzymes, which break down food, as well as serrapeptase, which eats clots, cysts, and other gunk in your body. It homes in on problem areas (for example, fibroids or arthritic joints) and reduces inflammation. In addition, Vitälzȳm contains bromelain and papain (to reduce inflammation) and Indian gooseberry, which is a source of vitamin C and is great for your hair. As if that isn't good enough, Vitälzȳm contains rutin, a flavonoid that strengthens capillaries and connective tissue. It may help protect blood vessels, reduce dark under-eye circles, and protect against viruses. It may also help with dozens of inflammatory and autoimmune conditions. The dosage varies based on your problems, but in general you should take Vitälzȳm on an empty stomach.

Xymogen
www.xymogen.com
800-647-6100

This is a high-quality nutraceutical company that uses active B vitamins in their formulas, as well as amino acid mineral chelates and easy-to-swallow capsules. Xymogen products are manufactured in an FDA-certified laboratory and are high quality. The products are sold through physicians' offices or to licensed health-care providers. You can buy their products online as well.

ZRT Laboratory
www.zrtlab.com
866-600-1636

The founder of ZRT Laboratory is David Zava, PhD, a leading authority on hormones and coauthor of several excellent books, including *What Your Doctor May Not Tell You about Breast Cancer.* I've met him, and he is very genuine about helping you get well.

ZRT can do saliva testing and/or blood spot testing to determine accurate levels of hormones such as estrogen, estrone, testosterone, DHEA, vitamin D, cortisol, PSA, SHBG, and many others. I really like this company because they sell directly to you and their tests are a cinch. You just collect saliva or do a little finger blood test, and you can see exactly what's going on in your body.

Just go to the Web site, look at the symptom checklist, and decide which kit is right for you. Their staff is sometimes available by phone. The test kits are sent to your home with very specific instructions. You mail back your samples in a prepaid envelope, and in a couple of weeks, ZRT sends you back boatloads of great health information that you can share with your practitioners.

References

Chapter 1

Adams, P. W., et al. "Effect of Pyridoxine Hydrochloride (Vitamin B_6) upon Depression Associated with Oral Contraception." *Lancet* 1973, 301: 897–904.

Blum, M., et al. "[Oral Contraceptive Lowers Serum Magnesium.]" *Harefuah* 1991, 121: 363–4 [in Hebrew].

Furlanetto, T. W., et al. "Estradiol Decreases Iodide Uptake by Rat Thyroid Follicular FRTL-5 Cells." *Brazilian Journal of Medical and Biological Research* 2001, 34: 259–63.

Furlanetto, T. W., et al. "Estradiol Increases Proliferation and Down-Regulates the Codium/Iodide Symporter Gene in FRTL-5 Cells." *Endocrinology* 140(12): 5705–11.

Olatunboaum, D. A., Adeniyi, F. A., Adadevoh, B. K. "Effect of Oral Contraceptives on Serum Magnesium Levels." *International Journal of Fertility* 1974, 19: 224–26.

Prinz-Langenohl, R., et al. "[6S]-5-Methyltetrahydrofolate Increases Plasma Folate More Effectively Than Folic Acid in Women with the Homozygous or Wild-Type 677C T Polymorphism of Methylenetetrahydrofolate Reductase." *British Journal of Pharmacology* 2009, December, 158(8): 2014–21.

Rimm, E. B., et al. "Folate and Vitamin B_6 from Diet and Supplements in Relation to Risk of Coronary Heart Disease among Women." *Journal of the American Medical Association* 1998, 279: 359–64.

Selhub, J., et al. "Vitamin Status and Intake as Primary Determinants of Homocysteinemia in an Elderly Population." *Journal of the American Medical Association* 1993, 270: 2693–98.

Wynn, V. "Vitamins and Oral Contraceptive Use." *Lancet* 1975, 305(7906): 561–64.

Zhang, S. M., et al. "Plasma Folate, Vitamin B_6, Vitamin B_{12}, Homocysteine, and Risk of Breast Cancer." *Journal of the National Cancer Institute* 2003, 95(5): 373–80.

Zhu, B. T. "Medical Hypothesis: Hyperhomocysteinemia Is a Risk Factor for Estrogen-Induced Hormonal Cancer." *International Journal of Oncology* 2003, March, 22(3): 499–508.

Chapter 2

Almeida, J. C. "Coma from the Health Food Store: Interaction Between Kava and Alprazolam." *Annals of Internal Medicine* 1996, 125: 940–41.

Aymard, J. P., et al. "Haematological Adverse Effects of Histamine H2-Receptor Antagonists." *Medical Toxicology and Adverse Drug Experience* 1988, November–December, 3(6): 430–48.

Bartle, W. "Grapefruit Juice Might Still Be Factor in Warfarin Response" [letter]. *American Journal of Health-System Pharmacy* 1999, April, 56(7): 676.

Brinker, F. *Herb Contraindications and Drug Interactions*, 2nd ed. Sandy, OR: Eclectic Medical Publications, 1998.

Burnham, B. E. "Garlic as a Possible Risk for Postoperative Bleeding." *Plastic and Reconstructive Surgery* 1995, 95: 213.

Caldwell, B., et al. "Risk of Cardiovascular Events and Celecoxib: A Systematic Review and Meta-analysis." *Journal of the Royal Society of Medicine*, 2006, March, 99: 132–40.

Campbell, N. R., Hasinoff, B. B. "Iron Supplements: A Common Cause of Drug Interactions." *British Journal of Clinical Pharmacology* 1991, 31: 251–55.

Celec, P., Behuliak, M. "Behavioural and Endocrine Effects of Chronic Cola Intake." *Journal of Psychopharmacology* 2009, May 7 [e-pub ahead of print].

Chen, M. F., et al. "Effect of Glycyrrhizin on the Pharmacokinetics of Prednisolone Following Low Dosage of Prednisolone Hemisuccinate." *Endocrinologia Japonica* 1990, 37: 331–41.

Cina, S. J., Russell, R. A., Conradi, S. "Sudden Death Due to Metronidazole/Ethanol Interaction." *American Journal of Forensic Medicine and Pathology* 1996, 17(4): 343–46.

Davis, R., Markham, A., Balfour, J. A. "Ciprofloxacin: An Updated Review of Its Pharmacology, Therapeutic Efficacy and Tolerability." *Drugs* 1996, 51: 1019–74.

Freeman, J. M., et al. "Does Carnitine Administration Improve the Symptoms Attributed to Anticonvulsant Medications? A Double-Blinded, Crossover Study." *Pediatrics* 1994, 93: 893–95.

Gadkari, J. V., Joshi, V. D. "Effect of Ingestion of Raw Garlic on Serum Cholesterol Level, Clotting Time and Fibrinolytic Activity in Normal Subjects." *Journal of Postgraduate Medicine* 1991, 37: 128–31.

Gannon, M. C., et al. "Effect of Added Fat on Plasma Glucose and Insulin Response to Ingested Potato in Individuals with NIDDM." *Diabetes Care* 1993, 16: 874–80.

Garg, S. K., et al. "Effect of Grapefruit Juice on Carbamazepine Bio-Availability in Patients with Epilepsy." *Clinical Pharmacology and Therapeutics* 1998, 64: 286–88.

Harris, J. E. "Interaction of Dietary Factors with Oral Anticoagulants: Review and Applications." *Journal of the American Dietetic Association* 1995, 95: 580–84.

Holt, G. A. *Food and Drug Interactions*. Chicago: Precept Press, 1998. pp. 197–98.

Houston, J. B., Levy, G. "Drug Biotransformation Interactions in Man: Acetaminophen and Ascorbic Acid." *Journal of Pharmaceutical Sciences* 1976, 65: 1218–21.

Huang, S. M., Lesko, L. J. "Drug-Drug, Drug-Dietary Supplement, and Drug-Citrus Fruit and Other Food Interactions: What Have We Learned?" *Journal of Clinical Pharmacology* 2004, 44: 559–69.

Jabbar, M. A., Larrea, J., Shaw, R. A. "Abnormal Thyroid Function Tests in Infants with Congenital Hypothyroidism: The Influence of Soy-Based Formulas." *Journal of the American College of Nutrition* 1997, 16: 280–82.

Juurlink, D. N., et al. "Adverse Cardiovascular Events during Treatment with Pioglitazone and Rosiglitazone: Population Based Cohort Study." *British Medical Journal* 2009, 339: b2942.

Kleijnen, J., Knipschild, P. "*Ginkgo biloba*." *Lancet* 1992, 340: 1136–39.

Landbo, C., Almdal, T. P. "[Interaction between Warfarin and Coenzyme Q10.]" *Ugeskrift for Laeger* 1998, 160(22): 3226–27 [in Danish].

Leibovich, E. R., Deamer, R. L., Sanserson, L. A. "Food-Drug Interactions: Careful Drug Selection and Patient Counseling Can Reduce the Risk in Older Patients." *Geriatrics* 2004, 59: 19–33.

Leistner, E., and Drewke, C. "Ginkgo biloba and Ginkgotoxin." *Journal of Natural Products*. 2010, 73 (3): 500–16.

Liedholm, H., Wahlin-Boll, E., Melander, A. "Mechanisms and Variations in the Food Effect on Propranolol Bioavailability." *European Journal of Clinical Pharmacology* 1990, 38: 469–75.

Lilja, J. J., Juntti-Patinen, L., Neuvonen, P. J. "Orange Juice Substantially Reduces the Bioavailability of the Beta-Adrenergic-Blocking Agent Celiprolol." *Clinical Pharmacology and Therapeutics* 2004, March, 75(3): 184–90.

Lilja, J. J., Raaska, K., Neuvonen, P. J. "Effects of Orange Juice on the Pharmacokinetics of Atenolol." *European Journal of Clinical Pharmacology* 2005, July, 61(5–6): 337–40.

Mahmood, H., et al. "Health Effects of Soda Drinking in Adolescent Girls in the United Arab Emirates." *Journal of Critical Care* 2008, September, 23(3): 434–40.

Marchbanks, C. R. "Drug-Drug Interactions with Fluoroquinolones." *Pharmacotherapy* 1993, 13(Pt 2): 23S–28S.

Menon, I. S., et al. "Effect of Onions on Blood Fibrinolytic Activity." *British Medical Journal* 1968, 3: 351.

Konrad, L., Muller, H. H , Lenz, C., et al. "Antiproliferative Effect on Human Prostate Cancer Cells by a Stinging Nettle Root (Urtica dioica) Extract." *Planta Medica* 2000, 66: 44–47.

Newall, C. A., Anderson, L. A., Phillipson, J. D. *Herbal Medicines: A Guide for Health-Care Professionals.* London: Pharmaceutical Press, 1996.

Partin, J. F., Pushkin, Y. R. "Tachyarrhythmia and Hypomania with Horny Goat Weed." *Psychosomatics* 2004, November–December, 45(6): 536–37.

Pronsky, Z. *Powers and Moore's Food Medication Interactions,* 11th edition Pottstown, PA: Food-Medication Interactions, 1999.

Refsum, H., et al. "Homocysteine and Cardiovascular Disease." *Annual Review of Medicine* 1998, 49: 31–62.

Roe, D. A. "Drug and Nutrient Interactions in the Elderly Diabetic." *Drug-Nutrient Interactions* 1988, 5(4): 195–203.

Schulze, M. B., et al. "Processed Meat Intake and Incidence of Type 2 Diabetes in Younger and Middle-Aged Women." *Diabetologia* 2003, 46: 1465–73.

Sedghizadeh, P. P., Stanley, K., Caligiuri, M., et al. "Oral Bisphosphonate Use and the Prevalence of Osteonecrosis of the Jaw." *Journal of the American Dental Association,* 140 (1): 61–66.

Siegel, I. J. "Israel Bans Import of Sildenafil Citrate after Six Deaths in the US." *British Medical Journal* 1998, May, 316(7145): 1625.

Speroni, E., et al. "Sedative Effects of Crude Extract of *Passiflora incarnata* after Oral Administration." *Phytotherapy Research* 1996, 10: S92–S94.

Sullivan, D., et al. "Grapefruit Juice and the Response to Warfarin." *American Journal of Health-System Pharmacy* 1998, 55: 1581–83.

Upritchard, J. E., Sutherland, W. H., Mann, J. I. "Effect of Supplementation with Tomato Juice, Vitamin E, and Vitamin C on LDL Oxidation and Products of Inflammatory Activity in Type 2 Diabetes." *Diabetes Care* 2000, 23: 733–38.

Welihinda, J., et al. "Effect of *Momordica charantia* on the Glucose Tolerance in Maturity Onset Diabetes." *Journal of Ethnopharmacology* 1986, 17: 277–82.

Wells, P. S., et al. "Interactions of Warfarin with Drugs and Food." *Annals of Internal Medicine* 1994, 121: 676–83.

Whitcomb, D. C., Block, G. D. "Association of Acetaminophen Hepatotoxicity with Fasting and Ethanol Use." *Journal of the American Medical Society* 1994, December 21, 272(23): 1845–50.

Chapter 5

Albanes, D., et al. "Alpha-Tocopherol and Beta-Carotene Supplements and Lung Cancer Incidence in the Alpha-Tocopherol, Beta-Carotene Cancer Prevention Study: Effects of Base-Line Characteristics and Study Compliance." *Journal of the National Cancer Institute* 1996, 88: 1560–70.

Bailey, D. G., Spence, J. D., Munoz, C., et al. "Interaction of Citrus Juices with Felopidine and Nifedipine." *Lancet* 1991, 337: 268–9.

Lee, I. M., et al. "Beta-Carotene Supplementation and Incidence of Cancer and Cardiovascular Disease: The Women's Health Study." *Journal of the National Cancer Institute* 1999, 91: 2102–6.

Nau, G., et al. "Antiepileptic Drugs Alter Endogenous Retinoid Concentrations: A Possible Mechanism of Teratogenesis of Anticonvulsant Therapy." *Life Sciences* 1995, May, 57(1): 53–60.

Omenn, G. S., et al. "Effects of a Combination of Beta Carotene and Vitamin A on Lung Cancer and Cardiovascular Disease." *New England Journal of Medicine* 1996, 334: 1150–55.

Seitz, H. K. "Alcohol and Retinoid Metabolism." *Gut* 2000, 47: 748–50.

Sundström, A., et al. "Association of Suicide Attempts with Acne and Treatment with Isotretinoin: Retrospective Swedish Cohort Study." *British Medical Journal* 2010, 341: c5812.

Chapter 6

Báez-Saldaña, A., et al. "Biotin Deficiency in Mice Is Associated with Decreased Serum Availability of Insulin-Like Growth Factor-I." *European Journal of Nutrition* 2009, April, 48(3): 137–44.

Fenton, P. F., et al. "The Nutrition of the Mouse VIII. Studies on Pantothenic Acid, Biotin, Inositol and P-Aminobenzoic Acid." *American Journal of Clinical Nutrition* 1950, June, 42(2): 257–69.

Mock, D. M., Dyken, M. E. "Biotin Catabolism Is Accelerated in Adults Receiving Long-Term Therapy with Anticonvulsants." *Neurology* 1997, 49: 1444–47.

Mock, D. M., et al. "Disturbances in Biotin Metabolism in Children Undergoing Long-Term Anticonvulsant Therapy." *Journal of Pediatric Gastroenterology and Nutrition* 1998, 26: 245–50.

Spigset, O. "Reduced Effect of Warfarin Caused by Ubidecarenone." *Lancet* 1994, 344: 1372–73.

Chapter 7

Beall, D. P., Scofield, R. H. "Milk-Alkali Syndrome Associated with Calcium Carbonate Consumption. Report of 7 Patients with Parathyroid Hormone Levels and an Estimate of Prevalence among Patients Hospitalized with Hypercalcemia." *Medicine* (Baltimore) 1995, March, 74(2): 89–96.

Bhakta, M., et al. "Oral Calcium Supplements Do Not Affect the Progression of Aortic Valve Calcification or Coronary Artery Calcification." *Journal of the American Board of Family Medicine* 2009, 22(6): 610–16.

Elisaf, M., Milionis, H., Siamopoulos, K. "Hypomagnesemic Hypokalemia and Hypocalcemia: Clinical and Laboratory Characteristics." *Mineral and Electrolyte Metabolism* 1997, 23: 105–12.

Gennari, C. "Differential Effect of Glucocorticoids on Calcium Absorption and Bone Mass." *British Journal of Rheumatology* 1993, 32(Suppl 2): 11–14.

Gonnelli, S., Caffarelli, C., Maggi, S., et al. "Effect of Inhaled Glucocorticoids and Beta(2) Agonists on Vertebral Fracture Risk in COPD Patients: The EOLO Study." *Calcified Tissue International* August 2010, 87(2): 137–43.

Lems, W. F., et al. "[Pharmacological Prevention of Osteoporosis in Patients on Corticosteroid Mediciation.]" *Nederlands Tijdschrift voor Geneeskunde* 1998, 142(34): 1905–8 [in Dutch].

Manson, J. E., et al. For the Women's Health Initiative and Women's Health Initiative-Coronary Artery Calcium Study Investigators. "Calcium/Vitamin D Supplementation and Coronary Artery Calcification in the Women's Health Initiative." *Menopause* 2010, July, 17(4): 683–91.

Reasner, C. A., et al. "Acute Changes in Calcium Homeostasis During Treatment of Primary Hyperparathyroidism with Risedronate." *Journal of Clinical Endocrinology and Metabolism* 1993, 77: 1067–71.

Schneyer, C. R. "Calcium Carbonate and Reduction of Levothyroxine Efficacy." *Journal of the American Medical Association* 1998, 279: 750.

Singh, N., Singh, P. N., Hershman, J. M. "Effect of Calcium Carbonate on the Absorption of Levothyroxine." *Journal of the American Medical Association* 2000, 283: 2822–25.

Tucker, K. L., et al. "Intake of Cola, but Not of Other Carbonated Soft Drinks, Is Associated with Low BMD in Women." *American Journal of Clinical Nutrition* 2006, October, 84(4): 936–42.

Umesawa, M., et al. "Dietary Intake of Calcium in Relation to Mortality from Cardiovascular Disease." *Stroke* 2006, 37: 20–26.

Weaver, C. M., et al. "Human Calcium Absorption from Whole-Wheat Products." *Journal of Nutrition* 1991, November, 121(11): 1769–75.

Chapter 8

Caso, G., et al. "Effect of Coenzyme Q10 on Myopathic Symptoms in Patients Treated with Statins." *American Journal of Cardiology* 2007 May 15, 99(10): 1409–12. [E-pub 2007 Apr 3.]

Farmer, J. A. "Simvastatin with or without Ezetimibe in Familial Hypercholesterolemia." *Current Atherosclerosis Reports* 2009, March, 11(2): 81–82.

Folkers, K., et al. "Activities of Vitamin Q10 in Animal Models and a Serious Deficiency in Patients with Cancer." *Biochemical and Biophysical Research Communications* 1997, May 19, 234(2): 296–99.

Folkers, K., Simonsen, R. "Two Successful Double-Blind Trials with Coenzyme Q10 (Vitamin Q10) on Muscular Dystrophies and Neurogenic Atrophies." *Biochimica et Biophysica Acta* 1995, May 24, 1271(1): 281–86.

Folkers, K., Yamamura, Y. "Italian Multi-Center Study on the Efficacy and Safety of Coenzyme Q10 as Adjuvant Therapy in Heart Failure." *Journal of Molecular Medicine* 1992, 4: 291–330.

Hamilton-Craig, I., et al. "At Sea with SEAS: The First Clinical Endpoint Trial for Ezetimibe, Treatment of Patients with Mild to Moderate Aortic Stenosis, Ends with Mixed Results and More Controversy." *Heart, Lung and Circulation* 2009, 18(5): 343–46.

Hamilton-Craig, I., et al. "Simvastatin with or without Ezetimibe in Familial Hypercholesterolemia." *New England Journal of Medicine* 2008, July 31, 359(5): 531.

Judy, W. V., et al. "Double Blind-Double Crossover Study of Coenzyme Q10 in Heart Failure." In: Folkers K., Yamamura Y., eds. *Biomedical and Clinical Aspects of Coenzyme Q.* Amsterdam: Elsevier, 1986. pp. 315–23.

Kamikawa, T., et al. "Effects of Coenzyme Q10 on Exercise Tolerance in Chronic Stable Angina Pectoris." *American Journal of Cardiology* 1985, 56: 247–51.

Langsjoen, P., Vadhanavikit, S., Folkers, K. "Response of Patients in Classes III and IV of Cardiomyopathy to Therapy in a Blind and Crossover Trial with Coenzyme Q10." *Proceedings of the National Academy of Sciences* 1985, 82: 4240–44.

Morisco, C., Trimarco, B., Condorelli, M. "Effect of Coenzyme Q10 Therapy in Patients with Congestive Heart Failure: A Long-Term Multicenter Randomized Study." *Clinical Investigator* 1993, 71(8 Suppl): S134–S36.

Rossi, E., et al. "Coenzyme Q10 in Ischaemic Cardiopathy." In: Folkers, K., et al., eds. *Biomedical and Clinical Aspects of Coenzyme Q,* Volume 6. Amsterdam: Elsevier, 1991. pp. 321–26.

Schardt, F., et al. "Effect of Coenzyme Q10 on Ischaemia-Induced ST-Segment Depression: A Double Blind, Placebo-Controlled Crossover Study." In: Folkers, K., et al., eds. *Biomedical and Clinical Aspects of Coenzyme Q,* Volume 6. Amsterdam: Elsevier, 1991. pp. 385–403.

Schneeberger, W., et al. "Clinical Double Blind and Crossover Trial with Coenzyme Q10 on Patients with Cardiac Disease." In: Folkers, K., et al., eds. *Biomedical and Clinical Aspects of Coenzyme Q,* Volume 5. Amsterdam: Elsevier, 1991. pp. 325–33.

Spigset, O. "Reduced Effect of Warfarin Caused by Ubidecarenone." *Lancet* 1994, 344: 1372–73.

Swedberg, K., et al. "Coenzyme Q10 as an Adjunctive in Treatment of Congestive Heart Failure." In: *64th Scientific Sessions, American Heart Association,* 1991. Abstract 774–76.

Tavintharan, S., Ong, C. N., Jeyaseelan, K., et al. "Reduced Mitochondrial Coenzyme Q10 Levels in Hep G2 Cells Treated with High–Dose Simvastatin; A Possible Role in Statin Induced Hepatotoxicity?" *Toxicology and Applied Pharmacology* September 1, 2007, 223(2):173-9.

Watts, G. F., Castelluccio, C., Rice-Evans, C., et al. "Plasma Coenzyme Q (Ubiquinone) Concentrations in Patients Treated with Simvastatin." *Journal of Clinical Pathology* November 1993, 46(11): 1055–7.

Witte, K. K., Clark, A. L., Cleland, J. G. "Chronic Heart Failure and Micronutrients." *Journal of the American College of Cardiology* 2001, 37: 1765–74.

Chapter 9

Baggott, J. E., et al. "Inhibition of Folate-Dependent Enzymes by Non-Steroidal Anti-Inflammatory Drugs." *Biochemical Journal* 1992, 282: 197–202.

Bethke, L. "Functional Polymorphisms in Folate Metabolism Genes Influence the Risk of Meningioma and Glioma." *Cancer Epidemiology, Biomarkers and Prevention* 2008, 17(5): 1195–202.

Brinker, F. *Herb Contraindications and Drug Interactions,* Eclectic Medical Publications, 1998.

Dormuth, C. R., Carney, G., Carleton, B., et al. "Thiazolidinediones and Fractures in Men and Women." *Archives of Internal Medicine* August 10, 2009, 169(15): 1395–402.

Flatley, J. E., et al. "Folate Status and Aberrant DNA Methylation Are Associated with HPV Infection and Cervical Pathogenesis." *Cancer Epidemiology, Biomarkers and Prevention* 2009, October, 18(10): 2782–89.

Flynn, M. A., et al. "Atherogenesis and the Homocysteine-Folate-Cobalamin Triad: Do We Need Standardized Analyses?" *Journal of the American College of Nutrition* 1997, 16: 258–67.

Fohr, I. P., et al. "5,10-Methylenetetrahydrofolate Reductase Genotype Determines the Plasma Homocysteine-Lowering Effect of Supplementation with 5-Methyltetrahydrofolate or Folic Acid in Healthy Young Women." *American Journal of Clinical Nutrition* 2002, 75: 275–82.

Folstein, et al. "The Homocysteine Hypothesis of Depression." *American Journal of Psychiatry* June 2007, 164: 861–7.

Hodges, R. *Nutrition in Medical Practice.* Philadelphia: W. B. Saunders, 1980, 323–31 [review].

Kohaar, I., et al. "Homocysteine Levels Are Associated with Cervical Cancer Independent of Methylene Tetrahydrofolate Reductase Gene (MTHFR) Polymorphisms in Indian Population." *Biomarkers* 2010, February, 15(1): 61–68.

Lawrence, V. A., Loewenstein, J. E., Eichner, E. R. "Aspirin and Folate Binding: In Vivo and In Vitro Studies of Serum Binding and Urinary Excretion of Endogenous Folate." *Journal of Laboratory and Clinical Medicine* 1984, 103: 944–48.

Prinz-Langenohl, R., et al. "[6S]-5-Methyltetrahydrofolate Increases Plasma Folate More Effectively Than Folic Acid in Women with the Homozygous or Wild-Type 677C T Polymorphism of Methylenetetrahydrofolate Reductase." *British Journal of Pharmacology* 2009, December, 158(8): 2014–21.

Rimm, E. B., et al. "Folate and Vitamin B_6 from Diet and Supplements in Relation to Risk of Coronary Heart Disease among Women." *JAMA* 1998, 279: 359–64.

Rivey, M. P., Schottelius, D. D., Berg, M. J. "Phenytoin-Folic Acid: A Review." *Drug Intelligence and Clinical Pharmacy* 1984, 18(4): 292–301.

Roe, D. A. 1985. *Drug-Induced Nutritional Deficiencies.* 2nd ed. Westport, Conn.: AVI Publishing Co.

Shils M., et al. (eds.). 1999. *Modern Nutrition in Health and Disease,* 9th ed. Baltimore: Williams and Wilkins, p. 1634.

Siri, P. W., Verhoef, P., Kok, F. J. "Vitamins B₆, B₁₂, and Folate: Association with Plasma Total Homocysteine and Risk of Coronary Atherosclerosis." *Journal of the American College of Nutrition* 1998, 17: 435–41.

Wang, M., et al. "Polymorphisms of Methylenetetrahydrofolate Reductase and Methionine Synthase Genes and Bladder Cancer Risk: A Case-Control Study with Meta-Analysis." *Clinical and Experimental Medicine* 2009, 9: 9–19.

Willems, F. F., et al. "Pharmacokinetic Study on the Utilisation of 5-Methyltetrahydrofolate and Folic Acid in Patients with Coronary Artery Disease." *British Journal of Pharmacology* 2004, March, 145 (5): 825–30.

Chapter 10

Dickinson, D. A., et al. "Curcumin Alters EpRE and AP-1 Binding Complexes and Elevates Glutamate-Cysteine Ligase Gene Expression." *FASEB Journal* 2003, 17(3): 473–75.

El-Dermerdash, E., Mohamadin, A. M. "Does Oxidative Stress Contribute in Tricyclic Antidepressants-Induced Cardiotoxicity?" *Toxicology Letters* 2004, September 10, 152(2): 159–66.

Ferenci, P., et al. "Randomized Controlled Trial of Silymarin Treatment in Patients with Cirrhosis of the Liver." *Journal of Hepatology* 1989, July, 9(1): 105–13.

Jiang, R., et al. "Consumption of Cured Meats, Lung Function and Chronic Obstructive Pulmonary Disease among US Adults." *American Journal of Respiratory and Critical Care Medicine* 2007, 175: 798–804.

Michaud, D. S., et al. "Meat Intake and Bladder Cancer Risk in 2 Prospective Cohort Studies." *American Journal of Clinical Nutrition* 2006, 84: 1177–83.

Walters, M. T., et al. "A Double-Blind, Cross-Over, Study of Oral N-Acetylcysteine in Sjogren's Syndrome." *Scandinavian Journal of Rheumatology Supplement* 1986, 61: 253–58.

Valenzuela, A., Aspillaga, M., Vial, S., et al. "Selectivity of Silymarin on the Increase of the Glutathione Content in Different Tissues of the Rat." *Planta Medica* October 1989, 55(5): 420–2.

Zheng, S., Yumei, F., Chen, A. "De Novo Synthesis of Glutathione Is a Prerequisite for Curcumin to Inhibit Hepatic Stellate Cell (HSC) Activation." *Free Radical Biology and Medicine* 2007, 43(3): 444–53.

Chapter 11

Beard, J., Borel, M., Derr, J. "Impaired Thermoregulation and Thyroid Function in Iron Deficiency Anemia." *American Journal of Clinical Nutrition* 1990, 52: 813–19.

Beard, J., Borel, M., Peterson, F. J. "Changes in Iron Status During Weight Loss with Very-Low-Energy Diets." *American Journal of Clinical Nutrition* 1997, 66: 104–10.

Bovell-Benjamin, A. C., et al. "Iron Absorption from Ferrous Bisglycinate and Ferric Trisglycinate in Whole Maize Is Regulated by Iron Status." *American Journal of Clinical Nutrition* 2000, June, 71(6): 1563–69.

Campbell, N. R., Hasinoff, B. B. "Iron Supplements: A Common Cause of Drug Interactions." *British Journal of Clinical Pharmacology* 1991, 31: 251–55.

Olivares, M., Pizarro, F. "Bioavailability of Iron Bis-Glycinate Chelate in Water." *Archivos Latinoamericanos de Nutrición* 2001, March, 51(1 Suppl 1): 22–25.

Szarfarc, S. C., et al. "Relative Effectiveness of Iron Bis-Glycinate Chelate (Ferrochel) and Ferrous Sulfate in the Control of Iron Deficiency in Pregnant Women." *Archivos Latinoamericanos de Nutrición* 2001, March, 51(1 Suppl 1): 42–47.

Chapter 12

Elisaf, M., Milionis, H., Siamopoulos, K. "Hypomagnesemic Hypokalemia and Hypocalcemia: Clinical and Laboratory Characteristics." *Mineral and Electrolyte Metabolism* 1997, 23:105–12.

Hoorn, E. J., et al. "A Case Series of Proton Pump Inhibitor-Induced Hypomagnesemia." *American Journal of Kidney Diseases* 2010, July, 56(1): 112–16.

Kozielec, T., Starobrat-Hermelin, B. "Assessment of Magnesium Levels in Children with Attention Deficit Hyperactivity Disorder (ADHD)." *Magnesium Research* 1997, June, 10(2): 143–48.

Linderman, R. D. "Hypokalemia—Causes, Consequences, and Correction." *American Journal of Medical Sciences,* 1976, 272(1): 5–17.

Lucker, P. W., Witzmann, H. K. "Influence of Magnesium and Potassium Deficiency on Renal Elimination and Cardiovascular Function Demonstrated by Impedance Cardiography," *American Society for Magnesium Research,* 1984, 3(4–6): 265–73.

Martin, B., Milligan, K. "Diuretic-Associated Hypomagnesiumia in the Elderly." *Archives of Internal Medicine* 1987, 147: 1768–71.

Quamme, G. A.: "Renal Magnesium Handling: New Insights in Understanding Old Problems," *Kidney International* 1997, 52(5): 1180–95.

Rude, R. K. "Magnesium Deficiency: A Cause of Heterogeneous Disease in Humans." *Journal of Bone and Mineral Research* 1998, 13: 749–58.

Saris, N. E., et al. "Magnesium: An Update on Physiological, Clinical, and Analytical Aspects." *Clinica Chimica Acta* 2000, 294: 1–26.

Schwinger, R. H., Erdmann, E. "Heart Failure and Electrolyte Disturbances." *Methods and Findings of Experimental and Clinical Pharmacology,* 1992, 14(4): 315–25.

Shils, M. E. "Magnesium." In Shils, M.E., et al., eds. *Modern Nutrition in Health and Disease,* 9th edition. Baltimore: Williams and Wilkins, 1999. pp. 169–92.

Stratobrat-Hermelin, B. "The Effects of Magnesium Physiological Supplementation on Hyperactivity in Children with Attention Deficit Hyperactivity Disorder (ADHD). Positive Reponse to Magnesium Oral Loading Test." *Magnesium Research* 1997, 10(2): 149–56.

Wester, P. "Magnesium." *American Journal of Clinical Nutrition* 1987, 45: 1305–10.

Whang, R., Whang, D. D., Ryan, M. P. "Refractory Potassium Repletion—A Consequence of Magnesium Deficiency." *Archives of Internal Medicine* 1992;152: 40–5.

Chapter 13

Bartsch, C., et al. "Prostate Cancer and Tumor Stage-Dependent Circadian Neuroendocrine Disturbances." *Aging Male* 1998, 1(3): 188–99.

Ebadi, M., et al. "Peroxynitrite in the Pathogenesis of Parkinson's Disease and the Neuroprotective Role of Metallothioneins." *Methods in Enzymology* 2005, 396: 276–98.

Fava, M., et al. "Folate, B12, and Homocysteine in Major Depression." *American Journal of Psychiatry* March 1997, 154(3): 426–8.

Garfinkel, D., et al. "Facilitation of Benzodiazepine Discontinuation by Melatonin: A New Clinical Approach." *Archives of Internal Medicine* 1999, 159: 2456–60.

Kabuto, M., Namura, I., Saitoh, Y. "Nocturnal Enhancement of Plasma Melatonin Could Be Suppressed by Benzodiazepines in Humans." *Endocrinologia Japonica* 1986, June, 33(3): 405–14.

Lusardi, P., Piazza, E., Fogari, R. "Cardiovascular Effects of Melatonin in Hypertensive Patients Well Controlled by Nifedipine: A 24-Hour Study." *British Journal of Clinical Pharmacology* 2000, 49(5): 423–27.

Martín, V., et al. "Melatonin Sensitizes Human Malignant Glioma Cells against TRAIL-Induced Cell Death." *Cancer Letters* 2010, 287: 216–23.

McIntyre, I. M., et al. "Alterations to Plasma Melatonin and Cortisol After Evening Alprazolam Administration in Humans." *Chronobiology International* 1993, June, 10(3): 205–13.

McIntyre, I. M., Norman, T. R., Burrows, G. D, et al. "Alterations to Plasma Melatonin and Cortisol After Evening Alprazolam Administration in Humans." *Chronobiology International* June 1993, 10(3): 205–13.

Mills, E., et al. "Melatonin in the Treatment of Cancer: A Systematic Review of Randomized Controlled Trials and Meta-Analysis." *Journal of Pineal Research* 2005, November, 39(4): 360–66.

Olatunbosum, D. A., Adeniyi, F. A., Adadevoh, B. K. "Effect of Oral Contraceptives on Serum Magnesium Levels." *International Journal of Fertility* 1974, 19: 224–26.

Rojdmark, S., et al. "Inhibition of Melatonin Secretion by Ethanol in Man." *Metabolism* 1993, 42: 1047–51.

Shamir, E., et al. "Melatonin Treatment for Tardive Dyskinesia: A Double-Blind, Placebo-Controlled, Crossover Study." *Archives of General Psychiatry* 2001, 58(11): 1049–52.

Stevens, R. G., et al. "Alcohol Consumption and Urinary Concentration of 6-Sulfatoxymelatonin in Healthy Women." *Epidemiology* 2000, 11: 660–65.

Ursing, C., et al. "Influence of Cigarette Smoking on Melatonin Levels in Man." *European Journal of Clinical Pharmacology* 2005, May, 61(3): 197–201.

Yin, J., et al. "Melatonin Arrests Peroxynitrite-Induced Tau Hyperphosphorylation and the Overactivation of Protein Kinases in Rat Brain." *Journal of Pineal Research* 2006, September, 41(2): 124–29.

Chapter 14

Bellou, A., et al. "Cobalamin Deficiency with Megaloblastic Anaemia in One Patient Under Long-Term Omeprazole Therapy." *Journal of Internal Medicine* September 1996, 240(3): 161–4.

Mikhailov, V. V., Mikhailov, V. V., Avakumov, V. M. "[Mechanism of the Effect of Methylcobalamin on the Recovery of Neuromuscular Functions in Mechanical and Toxic Denervation.]" *Farmakologia i Toksikologiia* 1983 November, 46(6): 9–12 [in Russian].

Hernández-Lahoz, C., et al. "[Sustained Clinical Remission in a Patient with Remittent-Recurrent Multiple Sclerosis and Celiac Disease Gluten-Free Diet for 6 Years.]" *Neurologia* 2009, April, 24(3): 213–15 [in Spanish].

Hokin, B. D., Butler, T. "Cyanocobalamin (Vitamin B$_{12}$) Status in Seventh-Day Adventist Ministers in Australia." *American Journal of Clinical Nutrition* 1999, September, 70: 576S–78S.

Kaptan, K., et al. "*Helicobacter pylori*: Is It a Novel Causative Agent in Vitamin B$_{12}$ Deficiency?" *Archives of Internal Medicine* 2000, May 8, 160: 1349–53.

Koyama, K., et al. "Efficacy of Methylcobalamin on Lowering Total Homocysteine Plasma Concentrations in Haemodialysis Patients Receiving High-Dose Folic Acid Supplementation." *Nephrology Dialysis Transplantation* 2002, 17(5): 916–22.

Kuwabara, S., et al. "Intravenous Methylcobalamin Treatment for Uremic and Diabetic Neuropathy in Chronic Hemodialysis Patients." *Internal Medicine* 1999, 38(6): 472–75.

Li, G. "Effect of Mecobalamin on Diabetic Neuropathies. Beijing Methycobal Clinical Trial Collaborative Group." *Zhonghua Nei Ke Za Zhi* 1999, 38(1): 14–17 [in Chinese].

Saltzman J. R., et al. "Effect of Hypochlorhydria Due to Omeprazole Treatment or Atrophic Gastritis on Protein-Bound Vitamin B12

Absorption." *Journal of the American College of Nutrition* 1994, 13: 584–91.

Scalabrino, G. "Cobalamin (Vitamin B$_{12}$) in Subacute Combined Degeneration and Beyond: Traditional Interpretations and Novel Theories." *Experimental Neurology* 2005, April, 192(2): 463–79.

Scalabrino, G. "The Multi-Faceted Basis of Vitamin B$_{12}$ (Cobalamin) Neurotrophism in Adult Central Nervous System: Lessons Learned from Its Deficiency." *Progress in Neurobiology* 2009, July, 88(3): 203–20.

Scalabrino, G., Veber, D., Mutti, E. "New Pathogenesis of the Cobalamin-Deficient Neuropathy." *Medicina nei Secoli* 2007, 19(1): 9–18.

Siri, P. W., Verhoef, P., Kok, F. J. "Vitamins B$_6$, B$_{12}$, and Folate: Association with Plasma Total Homocysteine and Risk of Coronary Atherosclerosis." *Journal of the American College of Nutrition* 1998, 17: 435–41.

Stopeck, A. "Links between *Helicobacter pylori* Infection, Cobalamin Deficiency, and Pernicious Anemia." *Archives of Internal Medicine* 2000, May 8, 160: 1229–30.

Vogiatzoglou, A., et al. "Vitamin B12 Status and Rate of Brain Volume Loss in Community-Dwelling Elderly." *Neurology* 2008 September 9, 71(11): 826–32.

Yamatsu, K., et al. "Pharmacological Studies on Degeneration and Regeneration of Peripheral Nerves. (1) Effects of Methylcobalamin and Cobamide on EMG Patterns and Loss of Muscle Weight in Rats with Crushed Sciatic Nerve." *Nippon Yakurigaku Zasshi* 1976, 72(2): 259–68.

Yamatsu, K., et al. "Pharmacological Studies on Degeneration and Regeneration of the Peripheral Nerves. (2)" *Nippon Yakurigaku Zasshi* 1976, 72(2): 269–78.

www.ncbi.nlm.nih.gov/pubmed/15896807

www.ncbi.nlm.nih.gov/pubmed/8021696

Chapter 15

Carlson, L. A., Hamsten, A., Asplund, A. "Pronounced Lowering of Serum Levels of Lipoprotein Lp(a) in Hyperlipidaemic Subjects Treated with Nicotinic Acid." *Journal of Internal Medicine* 1989, 226: 271–76.

Crouse, J. R., 3rd. "New Developments in the Use of Niacin for Treatment of Hyperlipidemia: New Considerations in the Use of an Old Drug." *Coronary Artery Disease* 1996, April, 7(4): 321–26.

Elam, M. B., et al. "Effect of Niacin on Lipid and Lipoprotein Levels and Glycemic Control in Patients with Diabetes and Peripheral Arterial Disease. The ADMIT Study: A Randomized Trial." *JAMA* 2000, 284(10): 1263–70.

Grundy, S. M., et al. "Efficacy, Safety, and Tolerability of Once-Daily Niacin for the Treatment of Dyslipidemia Associated with Type 2 Diabetes: Results of the Assessment of Diabetes Control and Evaluation of the Efficacy of Niaspan Trial." *Archives of Internal Medicine* 2002, 162: 1568–76.

Holti, G. "An Experimentally Controlled Evaluation of the Effect of Inositol Nicotinate Upon the Digital Blood Flow in Patients with Raynaud's Phenomenon." *Journal of International Medical Research* 1979: 473–83.

Illingworth, D. R., et al. "Comparative Effects of Lovastatin and Niacin in Primary Hypercholesterolemia." *Archives of Internal Medicine* 1994, 154: 1586–95.

Kiff, R. S., Wuick, C. R. G. "Does Inositol Nicotinate Influence Intermittent Claudication?" *British Journal of Clinical Practice* 1988, 42: 141–45.

Pan, J., et al. "Niacin Treatment of the Atherogenic Lipid Profile and Lp(a) in Diabetes." *Diabetes, Obesity and Metabolism* 2002, 4: 255–61.

Schwartz, M. L. "Severe Reversible Hyperglycemia as a Consequence of Niacin Therapy."

Archives of Internal Medicine 1993, September 13, 153(17): 2050–52.

Sunderland, G. T., et al. "A Double-Blind Randomised Placebo Controlled Trial of Hexopal in Primary Raynaud's Disease." *Clinical Rheumatology* 1988, 7: 46–49.

Chapter 16

Elisaf, M., Milionis, H., Siamopoulos, K. "Hypomagnesemic Hypokalemia and Hypocalcemia: Clinical and Laboratory Characteristics." *Mineral and Electrolyte Metabolism* 1997, 23:105–12.

Shenfield, G. M., Knowles, G. K., Thomas, N., et al. "Potassium Supplements in Patients Treated with Corticosteroids." *British Journal of Diseases of the Chest.* July 1975, 69: 171–6.

Widmer, P., et al. "Diuretic-Related Hypokalaemia—The Role of Diuretics, Potassium Supplements, Glucocorticoids, and Beta-2-Adrenoceptor Agonists. Results from the Comprehensive Hospital Drug Monitoring Program, Berne (CHDM)." *European Journal of Clinical Pharmacology* 1995, 49(1–2): 31–36.

Chapter 17

Aiba, Y., et al. "Lactic Acid-Mediated Suppression of *Helicobacter pylori* by the Oral Administration of *Lactobacillus salivarius* as a Probiotic in a Gnotobiotic Murine Model." *American Journal of Gastroenterology* 1998, 93(11): 2097–101.

De Vrese, M., et al. "Effect of *Lactobacillus gasseri* PA 16/8, *Bifidobacterium longum* SP 07/3, *B. bifidum* MF 20/5 on Common Cold Episodes: A Double Blind, Randomized, Controlled Trial." *Clinical Nutrition* 2005 August, 24(4): 481–91.

Forsythe, P., Inman, M. D., and Bienenstock, J. "Oral Treatment with Live *Lactobacillus reuteri* Inhibits the Allergic Airway Response in Mice." *American Journal of Respiratory and Critical Care Medicine* 2007, 175: 561–69.

Kabir, A. M., et al. "Prevention of *Helicobacter pylori* Infection by Lactobacilli in a Gnotobiotic Murine Model." *Gut* 1997, 41(1): 49–55.

Karmini, K., et al. "*Lactobacillus reuteri*–Induced Regulatory T Cells Protect Against an Allergic Airway Response in Mice." *American Journal of Respiratory and Critical Care Medicine* 2009, 179: 186–93.

McFarland, L. V. "Systematic Review and Meta-Analysis of *Saccharomyces boulardii* in Adult Patients." *World Journal of Gastroenterology* 2010, May 14, 16(18): 2202–22.

Smith, H. F., et al. "Comparative Anatomy and Phylogenetic Distribution of the Mammalian Cecal Appendix." *Journal of Evolutionary Biology* 2009, October, 22(10): 1984–99.

Sreeramulu, G., Zhu, Y., Knol, W. "Kombucha Fermentation and Its Antimicrobial Activity." *Journal of Agricultural and Food Chemistry* 2000, 48(6): 2589–94.

Chapter 18

Bernstein, A. L. "Vitamin B_6 in Clinical Neurology." *Annals of the New York Academy of Sciences* 1990, 585: 250–60.

Boers, G. H. "Hyperhomocysteinaemia: A Newly Recognized Risk Factor for Vascular Disease." *Netherlands Journal of Medicine* 1994, 45: 34–41.

Adams, P. W., et al. "Effect of Pyridoxine Hydrochloride (Vitamin B_6) upon Depression Associated with Oral Contraception." *Lancet* 1973, 301: 897–904.

De Lau, L. M., et al. "Dietary Folate, Vitamin B12 and Vitamin B6 and the Risk of Parkinson's Disease." *Neurology* 2006, 67(2): 315–18.

Fortin, L. J., Genest, J. "Measurement of Homocysteine in the Prediction of Arteriosclerosis." *Journal of Cellular Biochemistry* 1995, 28: 155–62.

Frye, P. E., Arnold, L. E. "Persistent Amphetamine-Induced Compulsive Rituals: Response to Pyridoxine (B_6)." *Biological Psychiatry* 1981, 16: 583–87.

Kohaar, I., et al. "Homocysteine Levels Are Associated with Cervical Cancer Independent of Methylene Tetrahydrofolate Reductase Gene (MTHFR) Polymorphisms in Indian Population." *Biomarkers* 2010, February, 15(1): 61–68.

Leklem, J. E. "Vitamin B_6." In: Shils, M. E., et al., eds. *Modern Nutrition in Health and Disease*, 9th ed. Baltimore: Williams and Wilkins, 1999. pp. 413–21.

Malinow, M. R. "Plasma Homocysteine and Arterial Occlusive Diseases: A Mini-Review." *Clinical Chemistry* 1995, 41: 173–76.

Reinken, L. "The Influence of Antiepileptic Drugs on Vitamin B_6 Metabolism." *Acta Vitaminologica et Enzymologica* 1975, 291: 252–54.

Rimm, E. B., et al. "Folate and Vitamin B_6 from Diet and Supplements in Relation to Risk of Coronary Heart Disease among Women." *JAMA* 1998, 279: 359–64.

Shimizu, T., et al. "Theophylline Attenuates Circulating Vitamin B_6 Levels in Children with Asthma." *Pharmacology* 1994, December, 49(6): 392–97.

Siri, P. W., Verhoef, P., Kok, F. J. "Vitamins B_6, B_{12}, and Folate: Association with Plasma Total Homocysteine and Risk of Coronary Atherosclerosis." *Journal of the American College of Nutrition* 1998, 17: 435–41.

Slade, B. A., et al. "Postlicensure Safety Surveillance for Quadrivalent Human Papillomavirus Recombinant Vaccine." *JAMA* 2009, August 19, 302(7): 795–96.

Ubbink, J. B., et al. "The Effect of a Subnormal Vitamin B-6 Status on Homocysteine Metabolism." *Journal of Clinical Investigation* 1996, 98: 177–84.

Chapter 19

Boehnke, C., et al. "High-Dose Riboflavin Treatment Is Efficacious in Migraine Prophylaxis: An Open Study in a Tertiary Care Centre." *European Journal of Neurology* 2004, July, 11(7): 475–77.

Newman, L. C., Lipton, R. B. "Migraine MLT-Down: An Unusual Presentation of Migraine in Patients with Aspartame-Triggered Headaches." *Headache* 2001, October, 41(9): 899–901.

Schoenen, J., Jacquy, J., Lenaerts, M. "Effectiveness of High-Dose Riboflavin in Migraine Prophylaxis. A Randomized Controlled Trial." *Neurology* 1998, 50(2): 466–70.

Sun-Edelstein, C., Mauskop, A. "Foods and Supplements in the Management of Migraine Headaches." *Clinical Journal of Pain* 2009, 25(5): 446–52.

Chapter 20

Baum, M. K., et al. "Selenium and Interleukins in Persons Infected with Human Immunodeficiency Virus Type 1." *Journal of Infectious Diseases* 2000, September, 182 (Suppl 1): S69–S73.

Bec, M. A., Levander, O. A., and Handy, J. "Selenium Deficiency and Viral Infection." *Journal of Nutrition* 2003, May (5 Suppl 1): 1463–67.

Broome, C. S., et al. "An Increase in Selenium Intake Improves Immune Function and Poliovirus Handling in Adults with Marginal Selenium Status." *American Journal of Clinical Nutrition* 2004, July, 80(1): 154–62.

Gärtner, R., et al. "Selenium Supplementation in Patients with Autoimmune Thyroiditis Decreases Thyroid Peroxidase Antibodies Concentrations." *Journal of Clinical Endocrinology and Metabolism* 2002, April, 87(4): 1687–91.

Mazokopakis, E. E., et al. "Effects of 12 Months Treatment with L-Selenomethionine on Serum Anti-TPO Levels in Patients with Hashimoto's Thyroiditis." *Thyroid* 2007, July, 17(7): 609–12.

Office of Dietary Supplements, National Institutes of Health. "Dietary Supplement Fact Sheet: Selenium."

Peretz, A., Neve, J., Vertongen, F., et al. "Selenium Status in Relation to Clinical Variables and Corticosteroid Treatment in Rheumatoid Arthritis." *Journal of Rheumatology* December 1987, 14(6): 1104–7.

www.jama.ama-assn.org/cgi/content/full/301/1/39

Chapter 21

Babaei-Jadidi, R., et al. "Prevention of Incipient Diabetic Neuropathy by High-Dose Thiamine and Benfotiamine." *Diabetes* 2003, 52: 2110–20.

Brady, J. A., Rock, C. L., Horneffer, M. R. "Thiamine Status, Diuretic Medications and the Management of Congestive Heart Failure." *Journal of the American Dietetic Association* 1995, 95: 541–44.

Greb, A., Bitsch, R. "Comparative Bioavailability of Various Thiamine Derivatives after Oral Administration." *International Journal of Clinical Pharmacology and Therapeutics* 1998, 36: 216–21.

Seligmann, H., et al. "Thiamine Deficiency in Patients with Congestive Heart Failure Receiving Long-Term Furosemide Therapy: A Pilot Study." *American Journal of Medicine* 1991, 91: 151–55.

Sprince, H., et al. "Protection against Acetaldehyde Toxicity in the Rat by L-Cysteine, Thiamin and L-2-Methylthiazolidine-4-Carboxylic Acid." *Agents and Actions* 1974, April, 4(2): 125–30.

Sprince, H., et al. "Protective Action of Ascorbic Acid and Sulfur Compounds Against Acetaldehyde Toxicity: Implications in Alcoholism and Smoking." *Inflammation Research* 5(2): 164–73.

Stracke, H., et al. "Efficacy of Benfotiamine Versus Thiamine on Function and Glycation Products of Peripheral Nerves in Diabetic Rats." *Experimental and Clinical Endocrinology and Diabetes* 2001, 109: 330–36.

Zenuk, C., et al. "Thiamine Deficiency in Congestive Heart Failure Patients Receiving Long Term Furosemide Therapy." *Canadian Journal of Clinical Pharmacology* 2003, 10: 184–88.

Chapter 22

Buist, R. A. "Drug-Nutrient Interactions: An Overview." *International Clinical Nutrition Review* 1984, 4(3): 114.

Coffey, G., Wilson, C. W. M. "Ascorbic Acid Deficiency and Aspirin Induced Haematemesis." *British Medical Journal* 1975, I: 208.

McRae, M. P. "Vitamin C Supplementation Lowers Serum Low-Density Lipoprotein Cholesterol and Triglycerides: A Meta-Analysis of 13 Randomized Controlled Trials." *Journal of Chiropractic Medicine* 2008, 7(2): 48–58.

Simon, J. A., Hudes, E. S. "Relationship of Ascorbic Acid to Blood Lead Levels." *Journal of the American Medical Association* 1999, June 23–30, 281(24): 2289–93.

www.ncbi.nlm.nih.gov/pmc/articles/PMC2631578

Chapter 23

Cannell, J. J. "The Truth about Vitamin D Toxicity." Vitamin D Council, 2009.

Heaney, R. P., et al. "Vitamin D_3 Is More Potent Than Vitamin D_2 in Humans." *Journal of Clinical Endocrinology & Metabolism* doi: 10.1210/jc.2010–2230.

Helmholtz Association of German Research Centers. "High Blood Levels of Vitamin D Protect Women from Breast Cancer, Study Suggests." *Science Daily* 2008, April 22.

Lin, R., White, J. H. "The Pleiotropic Actions of Vitamin D." *BioEssays* 2004, 26: 21–8.

Mitka, M. "Vitamin D Deficits May Affect Heart Health." *Journal of the American Medical Association* 2008, 299: 753–4.

Vantieghem, K., et al. "UVB-Induced 1,25(OH)2D3 Production and Vitamin D Activity in Intestinal CaCo-2 Cells and in THP-1 Macrophages Pretreated with a Sterol-Reductase Inhibitor." *Journal of Cellular Biochemistry* 2006, 99(1): 229–40.

Chapter 24

Golik, A., Zaidenstein, R., Dishi, V., et al. "Effects of Captopril and Enalapril on Zinc Metabolism in Hypertensive Patients." *Journal of the American College of Nutrition* 1998, 17(1):75–8.

Haase, H., Rink, L. "The Immune System and the Impact of Zinc During Aging." *Immunity and Ageing* 2009, June 12, 6: 9.

Office of Dietary Supplements, National Institutes of Health. "Dietary Supplement Fact Sheet: Zinc."

Parham, M., et al. "Effect of Zinc Supplementation on Microalbuminuria in Patients with Type 2 Diabetes: A Double Blind, Randomized, Placebo-Controlled, Cross-Over Trial." *Review of Diabetic Studies* 2008, 5(2): 102–09.

Prasad, A. S. "Zinc in Human Health: Effect of Zinc on Immune Cells." *Molecular Medicine* 2008, May–June, 14(5–6): 353–57.

Rink, L., Gabriel, P. "Zinc and the Immune System." *Proceedings of the Nutrition Society* 2000, November, 59(4): 541–52.

Sturniolo, G. C., et al. "Inhibition of Gastric Acid Secretion Reduces Zinc Absorption in Man." *Journal of the American College of Nutrition* 1991, August, 10(4): 372–75.

Chapter 25

Holt, G. A. *Food and Drug Interactions*. Chicago: Precept Press, 1998. pp. 197–98.

Jacob, S. E., Stechschulte, S. "Formaldehyde, Aspartame, and Migraines: A Possible Connection." *Dermatitis* 2008, 19(3): E10–E11.

Lockey, S. D., Sr. "Hypersensitivity to Tartrazine (FD&C Yellow 5) and Other Dyes and Additives Present in Foods and Pharmaceutical Products." *Annals of Allergy, Asthma and Immunology* 1977, March, 38(3): 206–10.

McDonald's Web site. "Nutrition." http://mcdonalds.com/us/en/food/food_quality/nutrition_choices.html.

Neuman, I., et al. "The Danger Of 'Yellow Dyes' (Tartrazine) to Allergic Subjects." *Clinical Allergy*. 1978, January, 8(1): 65–68.

Prinz-Langenohl, R., et al. "[6S]-5-Methyltetrahydrofolate Increases Plasma Folate More Effectively Than Folic Acid in Women with the Homozygous or Wild-Type 677C T Polymorphism of Methylenetetrahydrofolate Reductase." *British Journal of Pharmacology* 2009, December, 158(8): 2014–21.

Tebbey, P. W., Buttke, T. M. "Molecular Basis for the Immunosuppressive Action of Stearic Acid on T Cells." *Immunology* 1990, July, 70(3): 379–84. Erratum in *Immunology* 1990, October, 71(2): 306.

Chapter 26

Danovaro, R., et al. "Sunscreens Cause Coral Bleaching by Promoting Viral Infections." *Environmental Health Perspectives* 2008, 116: 441–47.

Drown, D. J. "Vitamin D Deficiency in the United States: A Growing Epidemic with Serious Health Consequences." *Progress in Cardiovascular Nursing* 2009 September, 24(3): 117–18.

"Facts and Comparisons." *Review of Natural Products*, CliniSphere 2.0. New York: Wolters Kluwer Company, 2000.

Institute of Medicine, Food and Nutrition Board. *Dietary Reference Intakes: Calcium, Phosphorus, Magnesium, Vitamin D and Fluoride*. Washington, DC: National Academy Press, 1999.

———. *Dietary Reference Intakes: Thiamin, Riboflavin, Niacin, Vitamin B6, Folate, Vitamin B12, Pantothenic Acid, Biotin, and Choline*. Washington, DC: National Academy Press, 1998.

————. *Dietary Reference Intakes for Vitamin A, Vitamin K, Arsenic, Boron, Chromium, Copper, Iodine, Iron, Manganese, Molybdenum, Nickel, Silicon, Vanadium, and Zinc.* Washington, DC: National Academy Press, 2001.

Kohaar, I., et al. "Homocysteine Levels Are Associated with Cervical Cancer Independent of Methylene Tetrahydrofolate Reductase Gene (MTHFR) Polymorphisms in Indian Population." *Biomarkers* 2010, February, 15(1): 61–68.

Koutkia, P., Chen, T. C., Hollick, M. F. "Vitamin D Intoxication Associated with an Over-the-Counter Supplement." *New England Journal of Medicine* 2001, July 5, 345(1): 66–67.

Chapter 27

Shih, C. M., Cheng, S. N., Wong, C. S., et al. "Antiinflammatory and Antihyperalgesic Activity of C-Phycocyanin." *Anesthesia & Analgesia* April 2009, 108(4): 1303–10.

Chapter 29

Natural Resources Defense Council Web site. www.nrdc.org

General Background

Consumerlab.com/results/index.asp.

"Facts and Comparisons." *Review of Natural Products,* CliniSphere 2.0. New York: Wolters Kluwer Company, 2000.

Institute of Medicine, Food and Nutrition Board. *Dietary Reference Intakes: Calcium, Phosphorus, Magnesium, Vitamin D and Fluoride.* Washington, DC: National Academy Press, 1999.

Institute of Medicine, Food and Nutrition Board. *Dietary Reference Intakes: Thiamin, Riboflavin, Niacin, Vitamin B6, Folate, Vitamin B12, Pantothenic Acid, Biotin, and Choline.* Washington, DC: National Academy Press, 1998.

Institute of Medicine, Food and Nutrition Board. *Dietary Reference Intakes for Vitamin A, Vitamin K, Arsenic, Boron, Chromium, Copper, Iodine, Iron, Manganese, Molybdenum, Nickel, Silicon, Vanadium, and Zinc.* Washington, DC: National Academy Press, 2001.

Lacy, C. F., et al. *Lexi-Drugs.* Hudson, OH: Lexi-Comp, 2006.

PDR for Herbal Medicines, 2nd edition. Oradell, NJ: Medical Economics Company, 2000.

Pelton, R., et al. *Drug-Induced Nutrient Depletion Handbook.* Hudson, OH: Lexi-Comp, 2001.

Sifton, D. W., ed. *Physicians Desk Reference.* Montvale, NJ: Medical Economics Company, 2000. pp. 2504–06; 2953–54.

Sullivan, D., et al. "Grapefruit Juice and the Response to Warfarin." *American Journal of Health-System Pharmacy* 1998, 55: 1581–83.

Werbach, M. R. *Foundations of Nutritional Medicine.* Tarzana, CA: Third Line Press, 1997. pp. 210–11.

Wynn, V. "Vitamins and Oral Contraceptive Use." *Lancet* 1975, 305(7906): 561–64.

Chapter 27

Jabbar, M. A., Larrea, J., Shaw, R. A. "Abnormal Thyroid Function Tests in Infants with Congenital Hypothyroidism: The Influence of Soy-Based Formulas." *Journal of the American College of Nutrition* 1997, 16: 280–82.

About the Author

Suzy Cohen, RPh, is a bestselling author, syndicated columnist, and speaker. She has been a licensed pharmacist for more than 22 years and has experience in hospital, retail, and consultant pharmacy practice. She understands the value of medication, but she prides herself on thinking "outside the pill." Suzy has been a guest on *The 700 Club, The View, The Dr. Oz Show,* and *Good Morning America Health.* Suzy can also be seen regularly doing medical minutes on the syndicated *Know the Cause* show offering sensible advice about improving health. She is a member of the American College for Advancement in Medicine, the Institute for Functional Medicine, the American Academy of Anti-Aging Medicine, and the American Pharmacists Association.

Her groundbreaking book on diabetes, *Diabetes without Drugs,* was selected for reading by the American Academy of Anti-Aging Medicine for doctors seeking board certification in Anti-Aging and Regenerative Medicine.

You can follow Suzy on Twitter and Facebook. You can also sign up to receive Suzy's free health newsletter, submit your own health questions, or read hundreds of her archived articles at her Web site, www. dearpharmacist.com.

Also by the Author

The 24-Hour Pharmacist (Rodale, 2008)
Diabetes without Drugs (Rodale, 2010)

Index